Molecular Biomarkers of Tumors: Advancing Genetic Studies

Molecular Biomarkers of Tumors: Advancing Genetic Studies

Guest Editors

Sainan Wei
Jing Di

MDPI

Basel • Beijing • Wuhan • Barcelona • Belgrade • Novi Sad • Cluj • Manchester

Guest Editors

Sainan Wei
Department of Pathology and Laboratory Medicine
University of Kentucky
Lexington
USA

Jing Di
Department of Pathology and Laboratory Medicine
University of Kentucky
Lexington
USA

Editorial Office
MDPI AG
Grosspeteranlage 5
4052 Basel, Switzerland

This is a reprint of the Special Issue, published open access by the journal *Biomedicines* (ISSN 2227-9059), freely accessible at: https://www.mdpi.com/journal/biomedicines/special_issues/8U21IK9156.

For citation purposes, cite each article independently as indicated on the article page online and as indicated below:

Lastname, A.A.; Lastname, B.B. Article Title. *Journal Name* **Year**, *Volume Number*, Page Range.

ISBN 978-3-7258-5265-9 (Hbk)
ISBN 978-3-7258-5266-6 (PDF)
https://doi.org/10.3390/books978-3-7258-5266-6

Contents

About the Editors

Sainan Wei

Sainan Wei is a full professor and Laboratory Director in the department of Pathology and Laboratory Medicine, School of Medicine at the University of Kentucky. She has been dedicated to clinical genetic laboratory services and clinical genetic research. Her interest in genetic research strive her for keeping up cutting age technologies used in clinical laboratory services, translating bench discovery into clinical patient care. she has expertise in genetics from congenital genetic disorders and somatic conditions.

Jing Di

Jing Di is a surgical pathology fellow at the University of California San Diego with a focus on breast and gynecologic pathology. She completed her pathology residency at the University of Kentucky and has conducted research on digital pathology and artificial intelligence, including projects on prognostic prediction in tongue squamous cell carcinoma, soft tissue tumor classification, and melanoma metastasis detection. An active member of the College of American Pathologists Council on Informatics and Pathology Innovation, she has published more than 70 peer-reviewed articles and presented her work at national and international meetings.

biomedicines

MDPI

Article

GSTM5 as a Potential Biomarker for Treatment Resistance in Prostate Cancer

Patricia Porras-Quesada [1,2,†], Lucía Chica-Redecillas [1,2,†], Beatriz Álvarez-González [2,3,*], Francisco Gutiérrez-Tejero [4], Miguel Arrabal-Martín [4,5], Rosa Rios-Pelegrina [5,6], Luis Javier Martínez-González [1,2,5], María Jesús Álvarez-Cubero [1,2,5] and Fernando Vázquez-Alonso [7]

1 Biochemistry and Molecular Biology III and Immunology Department, Faculty of Medicine, University of Granada, PTS, 18016 Granada, Spain; pmporras@ugr.es (P.P.-Q.); luciachica@ugr.es (L.C.-R.); luisjavier.martinez@genyo.es (L.J.M.-G.); mjesusac@ugr.es (M.J.Á.-C.)
2 GENYO, Centre for Genomics and Oncological Research-Pfizer, University of Granada, Andalusian Regional Government, PTS, 18016 Granada, Spain
3 Legal Medicine and Toxicology Department, Faculty of Medicine, University of Granada, PTS, 18016 Granada, Spain
4 Department of Urology, San Cecilio University Hospital, 18007 Granada, Spain; franciscogutej@gmail.com (F.G.-T.); arrabalm@ugr.es (M.A.-M.)
5 Biosanitary Research Institute (ibs. GRANADA), University of Granada, PTS, 18012 Granada, Spain; rosa.rios.pelegrina@gmail.com
6 Department of Pathology, University Hospital Virgen de las Nieves, 18014 Granada, Spain
7 Urology Department, University Hospital Virgen de las Nieves, 18014 Granada, Spain; fvazquezalonso@gmail.com
* Correspondence: bealvarez@ugr.es; Tel.: +34-958-248-945
† These authors contributed equally to this work.

Abstract: Background/Objectives: Androgen deprivation therapy (ADT) is widely used to manage prostate cancer (PC), but the emergence of treatment resistance remains a major clinical challenge. Although the GST family has been implicated in drug resistance, the specific role of *GSTM5* remains poorly understood. This study investigates whether *GSTM5*, alone or in combination with clinical variables, can improve patient stratification based on the risk of early treatment resistance. **Methods**: In silico analyses were performed to examine *GSTM5*'s role in protein interactions, molecular pathways, and gene expression. The rs3768490 polymorphism was genotyped in 354 patients with PC, classified by ADT response. Descriptive analysis and logistic regression models were applied to evaluate associations between genotype, clinical variables, and ADT response. *GSTM5* expression related to the rs3768490 genotype and ADT response was also analyzed in 129 prostate tissue samples. **Results**: The T/T genotype of rs3768490 was significantly associated with a lower likelihood of early ADT resistance in both individual (p = 0.0359, Odd Ratios (OR) = 0.18) and recessive models (p = 0.0491, OR = 0.21). High-risk classification according to D'Amico was strongly associated with early progression (p < 0.0004; OR > 5.4). Combining genotype and clinical risk improved predictive performance, highlighting their complementary value in stratifying patients by treatment response. Additionally, *GSTM5* expression was slightly higher in T/T carriers, suggesting a potential protective role against ADT resistance. **Conclusions**: The T/T genotype of rs3768490 may protect against ADT resistance by modulating *GSTM5* expression in PC. These preliminary findings highlight the potential of integrating genetic biomarkers into clinical models for personalized treatment strategies, although further studies are needed to validate these observations.

Keywords: castration-resistant prostate cancer; *GSTM5*; biomarker

1. Introduction

Prostate cancer (PC) treatment resistance represents a significant clinical challenge, affecting not only therapeutic efficacy but also patient survival. Androgen deprivation therapy (ADT) is one of the mainstays of treatment for PC, particularly for cases where the tumor is not localized [1]. ADT effectively reduces testosterone levels, an androgenic hormone essential for the growth of prostate cells. By lowering testosterone, AR (androgen receptor) stimulation is diminished, which in turn reduces PSA (prostate-specific antigen) levels and halts tumor growth [2]. However, despite its initial effectiveness, more than half of the patients eventually progress to castration-resistant prostate cancer (CRPC), in which tumor growth persists and PSA levels increase despite reduced testosterone levels [1,3,4]. It is important to note that there is still some controversy regarding the exact proportion of patients who develop resistance, as this largely depends on the timing and criteria used to assess it. Nevertheless, some studies suggest that, over time, nearly all patients undergoing long-term ADT ultimately develop resistance [5]. This resistance is associated with limited long-term survival, as the median overall survival for patients with metastatic CRPC is generally less than two to three years [4,6]. The emergence of CRPC underscores the need to characterize patient subgroups who may benefit from alternative or complementary therapeutic approaches [7]. In this context, and considering the clinical impact of treatment resistance in PC, risk stratification plays a crucial role in therapeutic decision-making [8,9]. Currently, the D'Amico risk classification is widely used to categorize patients with PC based on baseline PSA levels, Gleason Score, and clinical stage. However, its predictive power could be significantly enhanced by integrating genetic biomarkers and advanced imaging [10]. In particular, identifying genetic variants associated with ADT resistance could provide novel opportunities for more personalized and effective therapies [11]. For instance, alterations in genes such as *RB1*, *TP53*, and *PTEN*, as well as increased *MYCN* amplification, have been identified as key drivers in the development of neuroendocrine PC (NEPC), a molecular PC subtype that emerges after ADT failure [12].

In line with these advancements, several studies have demonstrated that the AR can be activated independently of androgens, allowing tumor progression to continue despite hormonal deprivation. This phenomenon suggests that resistance to ADT is not solely dependent on androgen levels but is instead mediated by a range of alternative mechanisms that enable the AR to maintain its function in driving tumor progression [2,13,14], including those driven by oxidative stress [15,16]. In PC, oxidative stress has been linked to tumor initiation and progression, as well as to the development of CRPC, in part through activation of AR signaling pathways. However, the precise molecular interplay between oxidative stress and AR signaling remains poorly understood [15].

It has been shown that redox balance in advanced tumor cells may be mediated by the glutathione (GSH) system, enabling tumor cells to evade oxidative stress-induced cell death [17]. In this context, members of the glutathione S-transferase (GST) family, including *GSTM5*, are thought to play a key role in the detoxification of free radicals and the regulation of redox status in PC [18]. Interestingly, *GSTM2* has been shown to contribute to resistance against second-generation androgen receptor inhibitors (SG-ARIs), such as enzalutamide, apalutamide, and darolutamide [19]. Specifically, it has been shown that *GSTM2* overexpression in enzalutamide-resistant cells contributes to oxidative stress damage evasion and activates the p38 MAPK pathway. Furthermore, glutathione reductase activity has been described as a key factor in oxidative stress adaptation in metastatic PC cells, providing resistance to peroxide-induced cytotoxicity and facilitating tumor survival under adverse therapeutic conditions [17]. Similarly, Zhang et al. observed a significant correlation between AR expression and *GSTM1* copy number, suggesting a functional interaction between AR regulation and GSH-dependent detoxification pathways in PC [20].

Regarding *GSTM5*, its expression has been shown to be significantly downregulated in various cancer types, including bladder, ovarian, and lung cancer [21,22]. For instance, in bladder cancer, *GSTM5* overexpression has been linked to reduced cell proliferation, migration, and colony formation [21], while in lung adenocarcinoma, aberrant *GSTM5* expression correlates with poor overall survival [22]. These findings suggest that *GSTM5* may also represent a potential therapeutic target in certain cancer contexts, particularly through redox-modulating or epigenetic-based strategies such as demethylating agents, although its role in PC remains largely unexplored.

Despite the established relevance of *GSTM5* in cancer, its specific function in PC and treatment response remains poorly understood. This study, therefore, focuses on exploring the impact of *GSTM5* on ADT resistance in patients with PC. By examining both *GSTM5* expression levels and genetic variants, we aim to gain valuable insights into its role in modulating tumor response to ADT, potentially offering new therapeutic strategies for treatment resistance and improving the clinical management of advanced PC [19]. This effort not only has the potential to improve risk stratification but also to guide the use of novel targeted therapies, which are essential for managing this type of cancer more effectively and improving patient quality of life and survival.

2. Methods

2.1. In Silico Analysis of GSTM5 Role in PC

In order to investigate the functional role of *GSTM5* in PC, a protein–protein interaction (PPI) network was constructed using STRING (v12.0) with a high-confidence interaction threshold (0.7), selecting the top 15 interactors. To identify significantly enriched pathways, functional enrichment analysis was performed using GeneCodis (v4.0) [23], integrating KEGG, Gene Ontology, and InterPro. The results were filtered using a false discovery rate (FDR) threshold of 0.05. Additionally, DisGeNET (v24.1) was used to assess the association of *GSTM5* and its top 15 interactors with prostate neoplasm and malignant prostate neoplasm. To further explore the role of *GSTM5* in PC, its expression levels were analyzed using The Cancer Genome Atlas (TCGA, n = 549), comparing tumor vs. normal prostate tissue and across different tumor aggressiveness stages. Furthermore, promoter methylation of *GSTM5* was investigated in TCGA data to examine potential epigenetic regulation. The methylation levels in the *GSTM5* promoter region were compared between tumor and normal prostate tissue, and the results were analyzed to identify potential correlations between *GSTM5* silencing through hypermethylation and advanced PC progression. The *GTSM5* expression analysis was expanded using the Prostate Cancer Atlas (PCA, n = 1365), incorporating multiple independent cohorts (GSE21034, MSKCC, SU2C/PCF, and E-MTAB-6128) for validation.

2.2. In Silico Characterization of the rs3768490 Variant (GSTM5)

The rs3768490 (G > T) polymorphism in *GSTM5* was analyzed in silico to assess its potential functional impact. MutationTaster (v2.0, [24]) was used to predict effects on transcriptional regulation, mRNA processing, and potential splicing site alterations. Additionally, population databases (1000 Genomes, ExAC) were consulted to determine SNP frequency and evolutionary conservation scores (phyloP, phastCons). Splicing site alterations were also evaluated using MutationTaster, which provided scores indicative of potential changes in the splicing donor and acceptor sites.

2.3. Study Design

The present study included a cohort of 354 Caucasian patients diagnosed with PC. The diagnosis was established based on serum PSA levels > 4 ng/dL and histologically confirmed prostatic adenocarcinoma. A biological sample was obtained from each patient, consisting of peripheral blood and/or buccal swab, which were used for genetic analysis. Blood samples were processed by centrifugation at 1400 rpm for 10 min at 4 °C, separating the cellular fraction and plasma, which were stored independently at −80 °C until further use. Buccal swabs were stored at −20 °C. Additionally, prostate tissue samples were obtained from 129 patients with PC, consisting of fresh prostate tissue, which was immediately frozen and stored at −80 °C. These samples were later used for gene expression studies.

For all patients, key clinical variables were collected, including age, diagnostic PSA, Gleason score, ISUP grade, D'Amico risk classification, TNM staging, and treatment received. Additionally, the presence of metastases and mortality were recorded when applicable. Further details are shown in Table 1.

Table 1. Descriptive summary of clinical variables in the PC cohort.

Clinical Variable	N (%)
PSA serum levels:	
PSA < 10 ng/dL	135 (40.79%)
PSA ≥ 10 ng/dL	196 (59.21%)
Gleason score:	
Gleason < 7	107 (31.66%)
Gleason ≥ 7	231 (68.34%)
T Stage (TNM)	
T1–T2	209 (83.60%)
T3–T4	41 (16.40%)
D'Amico Risk	
Low-Mid	157 (45.77%)
High	186 (54.23%)
Metastasis	
Yes	133 (51.55%)
No	125 (48.45%)

Some clinical variables were unavailable for certain samples, leading to a varying total n across categories.

Within this cohort, a total of 222 patients underwent ADT and met the criteria for the analysis of treatment response. Patients were classified into three groups based on their clinical evolution: *Early-onset CRPC* (patients who develop resistance to ADT within the first three years of treatment), *Long-Term responders* (patients who have been on ADT for at least three years and have not developed resistance up to the current date), and *Non-progression responders* (a subgroup of *Long-term responders* who remained responsive to ADT beyond five years of treatment). The criterion used to define treatment resistance was three consecutive increases in PSA serum levels or the development of metastases during ADT.

All study participants provided written informed consent before being enrolled, and the study was previously approved by the Research Ethics Committee of Granada Center (CEI-Granada internal code 1638-N-18) in accordance with the Declaration of Helsinki.

2.4. DNA Extraction from Blood Samples and Buccal Swabs

Genomic DNA was extracted from peripheral blood samples using the Real Blood DNA kit (Real Laboratory, Valencia, ES), following the manufacturer's instructions. For buccal swabs, DNA extraction was performed as described by Freeman et al. [25] with additional optimizations developed by Gómez-Martín et al. [26]. The quality and quantity of extracted DNA were assessed using a NanoDrop 2000c (ThermoFisher Scientific, Waltham, MA, USA) to ensure its suitability for downstream applications. The extracted DNA was stored at −20 °C until genotyping studies.

2.5. Genotyping Analysis by qPCR

DNA genotyping of rs3768490 was performed using a specific TaqMan probe (C___3184500_20; ThermoFisher Scientific, Waltham, MA, USA) in combination with TaqMan Genotyping Master Mix (ThermoFisher Scientific, Waltham, MA, USA). Allelic discrimination assays were conducted in 384-well plates using the QuantStudio 6 Flex Real-Time PCR System (Applied Biosystems, Waltham, MA, USA). The qPCR reaction was performed as follows: 60 °C for 30 s and 95 °C for 10 min; followed by 40 cycles of 15 s at 95 °C and 1 min at 60 °C. A negative template control (NTC) was included in each plate.

2.6. RNA Extraction and Reverse Transcription from Fresh Prostatic Tissue

Total mRNA was extracted from fresh prostate tissue samples using the Trizol®/chloroform method following standard protocols. RNA quality and purity were assessed by measuring the A260/A280 ratio using a NanoDrop 2000c spectrophotometer (ThermoFisher Scientific, Waltham, MA, USA). The extracted RNA was stored at −80 °C to ensure stability until further processing. All samples were normalized to 100 ng/µL. Reverse transcription was performed using the PrimeScript RT Reagent Kit (Takara Bio, Kusatsu, Japan), following the manufacturer's instructions. The cDNA obtained was stored at −20 °C until gene expression analysis.

2.7. Gene Expression Analysis by qPCR

Gene expression analysis was conducted using SYBR Green designed probes (Life Technologies, Carlsbad, CA, USA), on a 96-well plate with the QuantStudio 6 Flex Real-Time PCR System (Applied Biosystems, Waltham, MA, USA). The qPCR reaction was performed as follows: 95 °C for 10 min for enzyme activation; followed by 40 cycles of 15 s at 95 °C and 1 min at 60 °C for denaturation and annealing/extension. Primers for *GSTM5* and *HPRT1*, the latter used as housekeeping control, were designed using Primer-Blast (NIH) software v2.5.0 [27] and supplied by Sigma Aldrich (San Luis, MO, USA) with the following sequences: *GSTM5* (forward): CTCTCAAAGTCTGAGCCCCG; *GSTM5* (reverse): GTCATAGTCAGGAGCGTCCC; *HPRT1* (forward): TTATGGACAGGACTGAACGTCTT; *HPRT1* (reverse): CTTGAGCACACAGAGGGCTA.

All samples were analyzed in triplicate, and each plate included an NTC. A common threshold was set for each gene, and threshold cycle (Ct) values were obtained for each sample. A Ct $\geq$ 35 was considered undetermined. The expression level of *GSTM5* was quantified using the relative quantification (RQ) method, normalized to the housekeeping gene *HPRT1*.

2.8. Statistical Analysis

A comprehensive statistical analysis was conducted, integrating both descriptive and inferential approaches. All statistical procedures were executed in R (v4.4.1) using the stats (v4.4.1) and MASS (v7.3-61).

The association of treatment response in patients with PC with the rs3768490 genotype and disease classification was analyzed by chi-square tests (χ^2) or Fisher's exact test for small sample sizes. To strengthen the analysis, simple logistic regression was performed to quantify the strength and direction of these associations beyond mere statistical significance. Results were expressed as Odds Ratios (OR) with 95% confidence intervals (95% CI), and statistical significance was set at $p < 0.05$. This combined approach facilitated the selection of relevant variants for subsequent analyses.

To enhance the predictive accuracy of the models, the D'Amico risk classification—an established prognostic tool that integrates PSA levels, clinical stage, and Gleason score into a single risk measure—was incorporated alongside genotyping data for multiple logistic regression analysis. Stepwise selection based on the Akaike Information Criterion (AIC) was employed to confirm that both the genotypic and clinical classifications contributed meaningfully to patient stratification. Models were accepted at $p < 0.05$.

For the *GSTM5* expression analysis, data normality was assessed using the Shapiro–Wilk test. The median and 95% confidence intervals were calculated for each group, and the Kruskal–Wallis test and Mann–Whitney U test were used to identify significant differences. These analyses were performed using GraphPad Prism (v8.0.1).

3. Results

3.1. Expression and Functional Role of GSTM5 in PC

To explore the functional role of *GSTM5* in PC, a PPI network was constructed using STRING with a high-confidence threshold of 0.7 to identify the top 15 interactors. Among the identified proteins, three major pathways were highlighted, involving carcinogenesis, drug metabolism via cytochrome P450, and other enzymatic detoxification systems, all of which included *GSTM5*. A visual representation of the PPI network, highlighting the functional classification of genes, is shown in Figure 1A. Furthermore, functional enrichment analysis of these interacting genes revealed significant KEGG pathways closely related to cancer progression and treatment response, including chemical carcinogenesis, drug metabolism, and pathways in cancer, among others (Figure 1B, Table S1).

To further evaluate the clinical relevance of these interactors, disease association analysis was performed using DisGeNET. The results showed that the identified genes were significantly associated with prostatic neoplasm (FDR = 2.1×10^{-2}) and malignant prostate neoplasm (FDR = 2.1×10^{-2}). These findings suggest that *GSTM5* and its interacting partners may play a crucial role in tumorigenesis and drug metabolism in PC, potentially affecting treatment response and resistance mechanisms.

To investigate the expression levels of *GSTM5* in PC, data from TCGA were analyzed. The results revealed that *GSTM5* was significantly downregulated in tumor tissue compared to normal prostate tissue ($p < 0.0001$), suggesting a potential tumor suppressor role (Figure 1C). Furthermore, when patients were stratified based on tumor aggressiveness, *GSTM5* expression remained consistently downregulated, with a progressive decrease as tumor aggressiveness increased (Figure 1D). These findings indicate that *GSTM5* downregulation may be associated with PC progression, reinforcing its potential involvement in tumor suppression and disease severity. TCGA data were also used to analyze methylation changes in the *GSTM5* promoter sequence in PC. Our results revealed that the *GSTM5* promoter is significantly hypermethylated in tumor samples compared to normal prostate tissue ($p = 1.9 \times 10^{-12}$, Figure 1E). This suggests that epigenetic regulation through hypermethylation may contribute to *GSTM5* silencing in PC, potentially promoting tumor progression and treatment resistance.

To further validate these findings, we repeated the analysis using data from the PCA, which integrates TCGA with additional cohorts, including GSE21034, MSKCC, SU2C/PCF, and E-MTAB-6128. This expanded dataset allowed us to examine a broader spectrum of molecular subtypes in PC. The results confirmed that all molecular subtypes of PC showed lower *GSTM5* expression compared to normal prostate tissue, supporting the notion that *GSTM5* downregulation is a common feature across different forms of PC (Figure 1F).

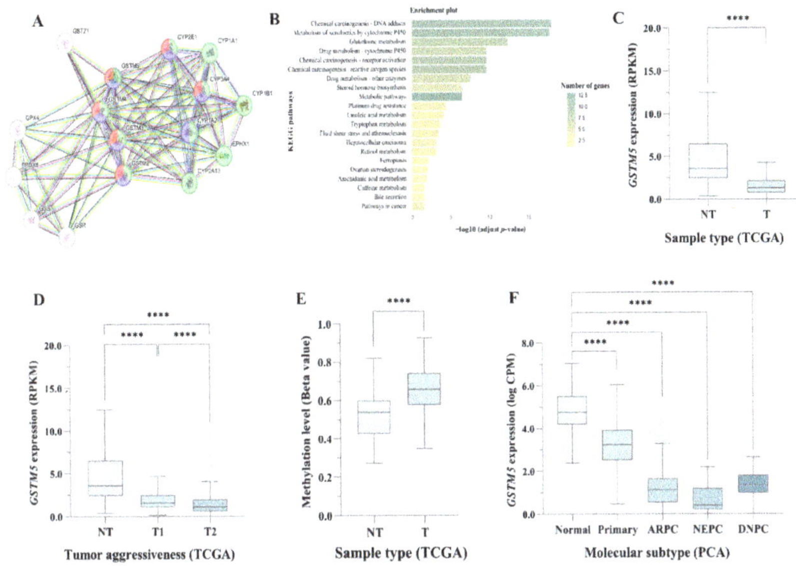

Figure 1. Functional and Expression Analysis of *GSTM5* in PC. (**A**) PPI network of *GSTM5* and its top 15 interactors, highlighting key genes involved in chemical carcinogenesis (green) and drug metabolism via cytochrome P450 (blue) or other enzymes (red). (**B**) Functional enrichment analysis of the top 15 *GSTM5* interactors. (**C**,**D**) TCGA expression data analysis across different sample types (**C**) and tumor aggressiveness stages (**D**). (**E**) TCGA promoter methylation analysis of *GSTM5* in tumoral versus normal prostate tissue. (**F**) PCA expression data analysis across different PC molecular subtypes. NT = Non-tumoral prostate sample, T = tumoral prostate sample, T1 = low-aggressive tumoral prostate sample, T2 = high-aggressive tumoral prostate sample, ARPC = androgen receptor-positive PC, NEPC = neuroendocrine PC, DNPC = double-negative PC. **** $p \leq 0.0001$.

3.2. Functional Impact of rs3768490 (GSTM5)

The in silico analysis using MutationTaster indicated that rs3768490 is located in the 3′UTR of *GSTM5*. Although it does not alter the protein sequence, it may affect post-transcriptional regulation. The SNP was associated with H3K27me3 epigenetic modification, suggesting a possible role in gene repression. Moreover, the variant increased the strength of an existing splicing donor site (wild-type score: 0.45; mutant score: 0.76) and led to the gain of a novel donor site (score: 0.34), which could influence mRNA stability and alternative splicing. Its low evolutionary conservation (phyloP = −0.339, phastCons = 0) suggests that it is not highly preserved across species, although it may have a regulatory role in PC.

3.3. Association of rs3768490 Genotype with ADT Response

To evaluate the association between clinical variables and ADT response in patients with PC, two grouping strategies were applied: (i) *Early-onset CRPC* (n = 54) vs. *Long-term responders* (n = 67), and (ii) *Early-onset CRPC* vs. *Non-progression responders* (n = 64). The same grouping was used to analyze genotype distribution according to treatment response.

Descriptive analysis revealed a strong association between clinical variables, except PSA, and treatment response in *Long-term responders* (Table S2) and *Non-progression responders* (Table S3) compared to *Early-onset CRPC* patients. In particular, patients with Gleason scores ≥ 7, tumor stage T3–T4, and high-risk classification according to D'Amico showed a greater likelihood of developing early resistance to ADT (Figure 2A,B). These findings indicate that patients with more adverse clinical features at diagnosis have a significantly higher probability of developing treatment resistance within the first three years of treatment.

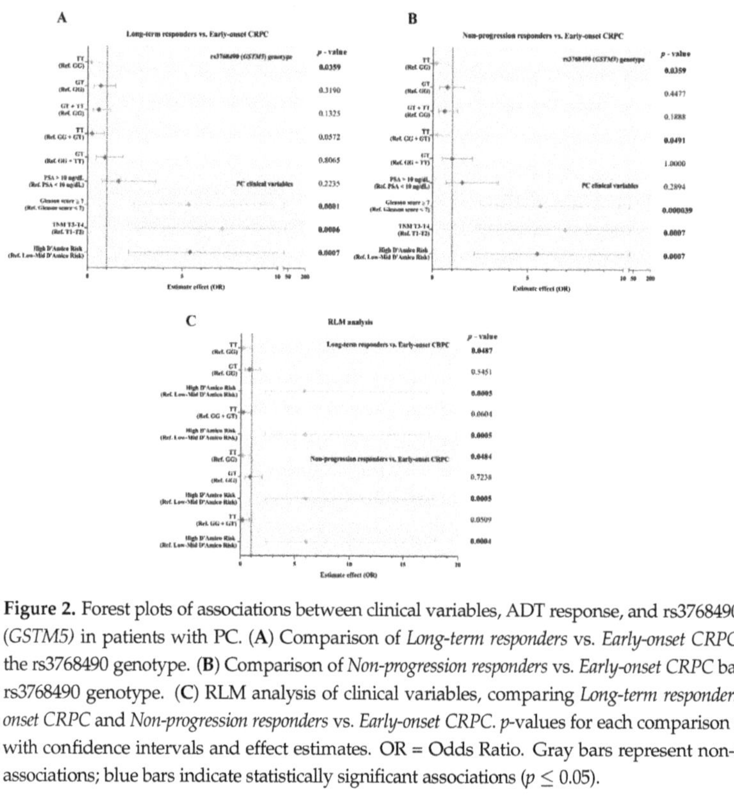

Figure 2. Forest plots of associations between clinical variables, ADT response, and rs3768490 genotype (*GSTM5*) in patients with PC. (**A**) Comparison of *Long-term responders* vs. *Early-onset CRPC* based on the rs3768490 genotype. (**B**) Comparison of *Non-progression responders* vs. *Early-onset CRPC* based on the rs3768490 genotype. (**C**) RLM analysis of clinical variables, comparing *Long-term responders* vs. *Early-onset CRPC* and *Non-progression responders* vs. *Early-onset CRPC*. *p*-values for each comparison are shown, with confidence intervals and effect estimates. OR = Odds Ratio. Gray bars represent non-significant associations; blue bars indicate statistically significant associations ($p \leq 0.05$).

Regarding genotype analysis, the T/T genotype showed a significant association with a lower probability of belonging to the *Early-onset CRPC* group compared to the *Long-term responders* group ($p = 0.0359$ in simple logistic regression; OR = 0.18, 95% CI: 0.02–0.76). The recessive model (TT vs. GG + GT) also showed a trend toward significance ($p = 0.0636$ in Fisher's test), with a reduced risk of early progression in T/T genotype carriers ($p = 0.0572$ in simple logistic regression; OR = 0.22, 95% CI: 0.03–0.88) compared to those with GG + GT genotypes. Multiple logistic regression analysis confirmed this association, with an OR of 0.18 (95% CI: 0.02–0.86; $p = 0.0487$) for the T/T genotype and an OR of 0.21 (95% CI: 0.03–0.96; $p = 0.0604$) in the recessive model (Figure 2C and Table S4).

A similar trend was observed when comparing the *Early-onset CRPC* and *Non-progression responders* groups (Figure 2B). Patient with the T/T genotype showed a significantly lower probability of developing treatment resistance within five years ($p = 0.0359$;

OR = 0.18, 95% CI: 0.02–0.76). The recessive model also showed a significant association ($p = 0.0491$; OR = 0.21, 95% CI: 0.03–0.83), supporting the lower risk of early resistance for the T/T carriers. Multiple logistic regression confirmed these findings, with an OR of 0.18 (95% CI: 0.02–0.86, $p = 0.0484$) for the T/T genotype and an OR of 0.19 (95% CI: 0.03–0.86; $p = 0.0509$) in the recessive model (Figure 2C and Table S4).

In both analysis models, high-risk classification according to D'Amico was a significant predictor of early progression to CRPC, with OR values greater than 5 in all cases ($p < 0.001$) (Figure 2C and Table S4).

These results suggest that the T/T genotype of the rs3768490 SNP in *GSTM5* may be associated not only with a lower risk of early resistance to ADT, but also with sustained sensitivity to ADT, potentially preventing the development of CRPC in patients with PC. Further studies are needed to confirm its role as a prognostic biomarker.

3.4. Impact of rs3768490 on GSTM5 Expression and ADT Outcome

GSTM5 expression levels were analyzed in relation to rs3768490 genotype, D'Amico risk classification, and response to ADT (Table S5). *GSTM5* expression was higher in T/T carriers, both when considering the three genotypes separately and under the recessive model (Figure 3A,B). However, this difference did not reach statistical significance, possibly due to the low frequency of the T/T genotype. Additionally, *GSTM5* expression was lower in high-risk patients according to the D'Amico classification (Figure 3C). Although this decrease was not statistically significant, it is consistent with the genotyping results, where the T/T genotype was associated with a better prognosis, potentially due to higher *GSTM5* expression levels.

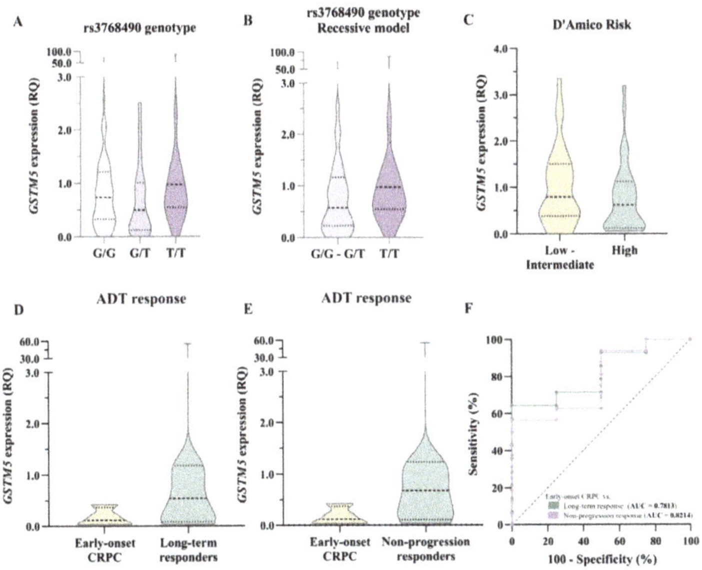

Figure 3. Statistical analysis of *GSTM5* expression. (**A**,**B**) *GSTM5* expression analysis across three rs3768490 genotypes (**A**) and in the recessive model (**B**). (**C**) *GSTM5* expression concerning D'Amico risk classification. (**D**,**E**) *GSTM5* expression in patients with *Early-onset CRPC* vs. *Long-term* (**D**) and *Non-progression responders*. (**F**) ROC curve comparing *Early-onset CRPC* vs. *Long-term* and *Non-progression responders*. RQ = Relative quantification, AUC = Area under the curve.

Regarding ADT response, *Early-onset CRPC* patients exhibited lower *GSTM5* expression levels than *Long-term responders* (Figure 3D). This difference was even more pronounced when comparing *Early-onset CRPC* patients with *Non-progression responders* (Figure 3E). These findings suggest a potential trend toward increased *GSTM5* expression in patients with a prolonged response to ADT.

ROC curve analysis was performed to evaluate the predictive ability of *GSTM5* expression in distinguishing *Early-onset CRPC* from ADT responders (Figure 3F). The model showed a moderate discriminative ability when *Early-onset CRPC* was compared with *Long-term responders* (AUC = 0.7813), and improved discriminative ability when compared with *Non-progression responders* (AUC = 0.8214).

4. Discussion

GSH metabolism plays a fundamental role in the cellular response to therapy, particularly in xenobiotic detoxification, oxidative stress protection, and drug resistance promotion [28,29]. In this context, *GSTM5* may contribute to modulating treatment response in PC through several mechanisms. First, *GSTM5* regulates cellular redox balance by influencing intracellular GSH availability, a critical metabolite that protects cells against oxidative stress and chemotherapy-induced damage [21]. Second, its involvement in resistance to platinum-based drugs suggests that *GSTM5* expression levels could affect the efficacy of these treatments in advanced PC [30]. Additionally, *GSTM5*'s interaction with DNA repair mechanisms may influence activation of the NRF2 pathway, thereby impacting the tumor cell's ability to respond to treatment-induced damage [31].

Despite the well-established role of *GSTM5* in oxidative stress modulation and drug resistance mechanisms, the impact of its genetic variants in the context of PC remains poorly understood. Other genetic variants in GST family members have been associated with increased PC risk. For example, the rs1138272 polymorphism in *GSTP1* is linked to a nearly five-fold increase in risk among carriers of the variant allele [32], and the *GSTM1* null genotype has been shown to significantly increase PC risk in Asian populations [33]. Interestingly, genetic variants within the GSTM gene cluster—particularly in *GSTM3*—have been associated with cancer susceptibility in breast cancer, where certain *GSTM3* SNPs conferred increased risk only in individuals lacking *GSTM1* expression [34]. However, to date, no studies have evaluated the role of *GSTM5* genetic variants in PC. Our study is the first to assess the influence of rs3768490 polymorphism in the *GSTM5* on ADT response. The results suggest that the T/T genotype may play a protective effect against ADT resistance, as carriers of this genotype exhibited a significantly lower likelihood of early treatment failure ($p < 0.05$; OR < 0.2). Conversely, D'Amico's high-risk classification was consistently associated with early progression ($p < 0.0004$; OR > 5.4), reinforcing its clinical value as a predictor of poor outcomes. The combination of genotype and clinical risk improved predictive capacity, emphasizing the potential utility of integrating genetic and clinical factors in ADT response stratification.

Beyond genetic associations, *GSTM5* expression levels were also evaluated. Previous studies have shown that *GSTM5* expression can be epigenetically regulated through promoter hypermethylation, leading to gene silencing and increased tumor aggressiveness. In breast cancer, *GSTM5* downregulation via promoter methylation has been linked to increased cell proliferation and migration [35]. Similarly, in bladder cancer, *GSTM5* acts as a tumor suppressor, and its promoter hypermethylation results in decreased expression, reduced glutathione levels, and enhanced tumor progression [21]. In lung adenocarcinoma, *GSTM5* promoter hypermethylation has also been identified as a key gene-silencing mechanism, correlating with poor prognosis and reduced survival. Notably, treatment with demethylating agents such as 5-Aza-CdR has been shown to restore GSTM5 expression and inhibit tumor cell proliferation and migration, reinforcing the potential therapeutic value of targeting DNA methylation in cancer.

This effect is not only epigenetic but also functional, as restoration of GSTM5 expression has been associated with reduced proliferation, migration, and improved oxidative balance through GSH metabolism [25]. Demethylating agents like 5-Aza-CdR could offer a potential strategy for reactivating GSTM5 expression in PC, improving the therapeutic response and overcoming resistance. While these findings suggest that *GSTM5* expression may be epigenetically regulated by methylation, our results indicate that it may also be influenced by specific genetic variants, such as rs3768490. This is consistent with the fact that rs3768490 lies within a distal enhancer-like signature region (EH38E1375040), a regulatory element previously validated as capable of modulating gene expression [36]. These preliminary findings provide new insight into how regulatory genetic variants may modulate *GSTM5* expression and, consequently, influence treatment response in PC.

From a clinical perspective, incorporating the *GSTM5* rs3768490 genotype into predictive resistance models of ADT resistance could improve patient stratification and support a more personalized therapeutic approach. Specifically, individuals carrying the G allele (G/G or G/T genotypes) may represent a subgroup with increased vulnerability to early progression and could benefit from closer monitoring or the consideration of additional therapeutic strategies. Although platinum-based agents and redox-targeted therapies are not standard in PC management, their potential role in genetically defined subgroups with altered *GSTM5* function, as well as the combination with demethylating agents, merits further investigation in preclinical and translational studies [21,30]. Of particular interest, redox modulation strategies may offer therapeutic opportunities in tumors with altered *GSTM5* function. For example, depleting intracellular glutathione using buthionine sulfoximine (BSO) has been shown to enhance the efficacy of histone deacetylase inhibitors in resistant breast cancer cells, suggesting that glutathione buffering contributes to drug resistance [37]. In ovarian cancer, *GSTM5* expression has been associated with stemness features and therapeutic response. Notably, treatment with investigational anticancer agents such as AICAR, an AMPK activator, and PI-103, a dual PI3K/mTOR inhibitor, was shown to restore *GSTM5* expression and increase treatment sensitivity in resistant ovarian cancer cells [38]. Although direct evidence in PC is still limited, the genetic and molecular similarities between prostate, breast, and ovarian cancers support further exploration of redox and epigenetic therapies in PC, particularly in molecularly defined subgroups with *GSTM5* dysregulation [39,40].

Despite the promising findings of this study, certain limitations must be considered. The small sample size limits the statistical robustness of some analyses; therefore, future studies with larger cohorts and external validation are needed to confirm the clinical relevance of *GSTM5* as a predictive biomarker of ADT resistance. Additionally, although our data suggests its involvement in treatment resistance, functional studies in cellular and preclinical models will be required to elucidate the underlying molecular mechanisms [21]. Specifically, future in vivo studies should focus on investigating how *GSTM5* interacts with key resistance pathways, such as oxidative stress regulation and AR signaling [2,13–16]. Moreover, treatment resistance in PC is a multifactorial process involving diverse molecular pathways; thus, it will be crucial to investigate how *GSTM5* interacts with other resistance pathways, such as alterations in *BRCA2*, *TP53*, and *PTEN*, which have been shown to influence therapeutic response [30]. Additionally, further functional studies are necessary to determine how GSTM5 modulates oxidative stress and its crosstalk with other signaling pathways, such as *NRF2* or DNA repair mechanisms, in the context of PC and ADT resistance [31]. Although our study focuses on *GSTM5*, it is part of the larger GST family, which includes *GSTM1* and *GSTM2*, both of which have been implicated in tumor progression and treatment response [19,20]. This underscores the importance of considering other members of the GST family in future studies that adopt more integrative approaches.

In clinical practice, genotyping this variant before initiating ADT could help physicians identify patients more likely to benefit from standard hormonal therapy versus those who may require early intensification strategies, including the addition of second-line agents. These preliminary findings lay the groundwork for future clinical trials that incorporate *GSTM5* status as a stratification variable or therapeutic target.

From a translational perspective, these preliminary findings open new avenues for personalizing the management of advanced PC. In clinical practice, genotyping the rs3768490 polymorphism prior to initiating ADT could assist physicians in identifying patients more likely to benefit from standard hormonal treatment versus those who may require early intensification strategies, such as the addition of second-line agents. Prospective studies are warranted to evaluate whether *GSTM5* genotyping can be effectively integrated into clinical workflows, enabling earlier identification of patients at higher risk of developing resistance to ADT.

5. Conclusions

This study highlights the potential role of the *GSTM5* rs3768490 T/T genotype as a protective factor against resistance to ADT in PC. Integrating this genetic marker with clinical risk factors, such as the D'Amico classification, significantly improved the ability to identify patients at higher risk of treatment failure. In parallel, the reduced expression of *GSTM5* in tumor tissue, along with its established involvement in oxidative stress regulation and drug metabolism, support its biological relevance in therapeutic response. Together, these findings suggest that *GSTM5* may serve as a promising biomarker for refining risk stratification and guiding personalized treatment strategies. Specifically, integrating the rs3768490 genotype with established clinical classifiers could support more tailored decision-making for patients with PC undergoing ADT. In addition, the biological role of *GSTM5* in oxidative stress regulation and its potential for pharmacological modulation open the door to future therapeutic avenues involving redox-targeted therapies. Further functional and clinical validation is warranted to confirm its utility and explore potential therapeutic interventions targeting redox balance and epigenetic regulation in PC.

Supplementary Materials: The following supporting information can be downloaded at https://www.mdpi.com/article/10.3390/biomedicines13081872/s1, Table S1. KEGG Pathway Enrichment Analysis of *GSTM5* and its 15 Top Interactors. Table S2. Association of *GSTM5* rs3768490 Genotype and Clinical Variables: *Long-term responders* vs. *Early-onset CRPC*. Table S3. Association of *GSTM5* rs3768490 Genotype and Clinical Variables: *Non-progression responders* vs. *Early-onset CRPC*. Table S4. Multiple logistic regression analysis for ADT response in PC. Table S5. Statistical report of *GSTM5* expression analysis.

Author Contributions: Conceptualization, F.V.-A., M.J.Á.-C. and L.J.M.-G.; methodology, P.P.-Q. and L.C.-R.; validation, P.P.-Q.; formal Analysis, P.P.-Q. and L.C.-R.; investigation, P.P.-Q., F.G.-T., M.A.-M. and R.R.-P.; data Curation, F.V.-A., M.A.-M., R.R.-P., P.P.-Q., L.C.-R. and B.Á.-G.; writing—original draft preparation, P.P.-Q., L.C.-R. and B.Á.-G.; writing—review and editing, P.P.-Q., L.C.-R., B.Á.-G., M.J.Á.-C. and L.J.M.-G.; visualization, P.P.-Q. and F.G.-T.; supervision, F.V.-A., M.J.Á.-C. and L.J.M.-G.; project administration, M.J.Á.-C. and L.J.M.-G.; funding acquisition, M.J.Á.-C. and L.J.M.-G. All authors have read and agreed to the published version of the manuscript.

Funding: This research was funded by the Ministry of Education, grant number FPU21/05808 (PPQ), the Ministry of Science and Innovation, grant number PRED2020-094013 (LCR), and the Ministry of Education, grant number FPU20/06611 (BAG). This research received contributions from PIP-0043-2022 funded by Proyectos en Salud FIBAO—Junta de Andalucia.

Institutional Review Board Statement: The study was conducted according to the guidelines of the Declaration of Helsinki and approved by the Ethics Committee of the Biomedical Research Ethics Committee of Andalusia (protocol code 0166-N-19, date of approval: 13 May 2019).

Informed Consent Statement: Informed consent was obtained from all subjects involved in the study.

Data Availability Statement: The original contributions presented in this study are included in the article/Supplementary Material. Further inquiries can be directed to the corresponding author(s).

Acknowledgments: We would like to acknowledge the support of nursery of Urology Service of Virgen de las Nieves for making this study possible. We are also very grateful to all familiars and donors for their support and unconditional collaboration with the project.

Conflicts of Interest: The authors declare no conflict of interest.

References

1. Vellky, J.E.; Ricke, W.A. Development and Prevalence of Castration-Resistant Prostate Cancer Subtypes. *Neoplasia* **2020**, *22*, 566–575. [CrossRef]
2. Wadosky, K.M.; Koochekpour, S. Molecular mechanisms underlying resistance to androgen deprivation therapy in prostate cancer. *Oncotarget* **2016**, *7*, 64447–64470. [CrossRef] [PubMed]
3. Congregado Ruiz, B.; Rivero Belenchón, I.; Lendínez Cano, G.; Medina López, R.A. Strategies to Re-Sensitize Castration-Resistant Prostate Cancer to Antiandrogen Therapy. *Biomedicines* **2023**, *11*, 1105. [CrossRef]
4. Chandrasekar, T.; Yang, J.C.; Gao, A.C.; Evans, C.P. Mechanisms of resistance in castration-resistant prostate cancer (CRPC). *Transl. Androl. Urol.* **2015**, *4*, 365–380. [CrossRef] [PubMed]
5. Dawson, N.A. Castration-resistant prostate cancer: Treatments targeting the androgen pathway. In *UpToDate*; UpToDate Inc.: Waltham, MA, USA, 2025.
6. Le, T.K.; Duong, Q.H.; Baylot, V.; Fargette, C.; Baboudjian, M.; Colleaux, L.; Taïeb, D.; Rocchi, P. Castration-Resistant Prostate Cancer: From Uncovered Resistance Mechanisms to Current Treatments. *Cancers* **2023**, *15*, 5047. [CrossRef]
7. Rodrigo-Aliaga, M.; Alvarez-Ossorio, J.L.; Rodríguez-Alonso, A.; García-Porrero, Á.; Quesada-García, A.; del Toro, J.M.; Rodríguez-Antolín, A. Prevalence and Management of Castration-Resistant Prostate Cancer of Unknown Metastatic Status in the Real-World Setting: The AfroDiTA Study. *Urol. Oncol. Semin. Orig. Investig.* **2025**, *43*, 64.e11–64.e18. [CrossRef] [PubMed]
8. Zumsteg, Z.S.; Spratt, D.E.; Pei, I.; Zhang, Z.; Yamada, Y.; Kollmeier, M.; Zelefsky, M.J. A New Risk Classification System for Therapeutic Decision Making with Intermediate-Risk Prostate Cancer Patients Undergoing Dose-Escalated External-Beam Radiation Therapy. *Eur. Urol.* **2013**, *64*, 895–902. [CrossRef]
9. Rodrigues, G.; Warde, P.; Pickles, T.; Crook, J.; Brundage, M.; Souhami, L.; Lukka, H. Pre-Treatment Risk Stratification of Prostate Cancer Patients: A Critical Review. *Can. Urol. Assoc. J.* **2012**, *6*, 121–127. [CrossRef]
10. Schaeffer, E.M.; Srinivas, S.; Adra, N.; An, Y.; Barocas, D.; Bitting, R.; Bryce, A.; Chapin, B.; Cheng, H.H.; D'Amico, A.V.; et al. Prostate Cancer, Version 4.2023, NCCN Clinical Practice Guidelines in Oncology. *J. Natl. Compr. Cancer Netw.* **2023**, *21*, 1067–1096. [CrossRef]
11. Urabe, F.; Sumiyoshi, T.; Tashiro, K.; Goto, T.; Kimura, T.; Kobayashi, T. Prostate Cancer and Liquid Biopsies: Clinical Applications and Challenges. *Int. J. Urol.* **2024**, *31*, 617–626. [CrossRef]
12. Imamura, J.; Ganguly, S.; Muskara, A.; Liao, R.S.; Nguyen, J.K.; Weight, C.; Wee, C.E.; Gupta, S.; Mian, O.Y. Lineage Plasticity and Treatment Resistance in Prostate Cancer: The Intersection of Genetics, Epigenetics, and Evolution. *Front. Endocrinol.* **2023**, *14*, 1191311. [CrossRef]
13. Maitland, N.J. Resistance to Antiandrogens in Prostate Cancer: Is It Inevitable, Intrinsic or Induced? *Cancers* **2021**, *13*, 327. [CrossRef]
14. Shore, N.D.; Morgans, A.K.; Ryan, C.J. Resetting the Bar of Castration Resistance—Understanding Androgen Dynamics in Therapy Resistance and Treatment Choice in Prostate Cancer. *Clin. Genitourin. Cancer* **2021**, *19*, 199–207. [CrossRef]
15. Shiota, M.; Yokomizo, A.; Naito, S. Oxidative stress and androgen receptor signaling in the development and progression of castration-resistant prostate cancer. *Free Radic. Biol. Med.* **2011**, *51*, 1320–1328. [CrossRef]
16. Khurana, N.; Sikka, S.C. Targeting Crosstalk between Nrf-2, NF-κB and Androgen Receptor Signaling in Prostate Cancer. *Cancers* **2018**, *10*, 352. [CrossRef] [PubMed]
17. Freitas, M.; Baldeiras, I.; Proença, T.; Alves, V.; Mota-Pinto, A.; Sarmento-Ribeiro, A. Oxidative Stress Adaptation in Aggressive Prostate Cancer May Be Counteracted by the Reduction of Glutathione Reductase. *FEBS Open Bio* **2012**, *2*, 119–128. [CrossRef] [PubMed]
18. Townsend, D.M.; Tew, K.D. The Role of Glutathione-S-Transferase in Anti-Cancer Drug Resistance. *Oncogene* **2003**, *22*, 7369–7375. [CrossRef]
19. Li, C.; Liu, J.; He, D.; Mao, F.; Rao, X.; Zhao, Y.; Lanman, N.A.; Kazemian, M.; Farah, E.; Liu, J.; et al. GSTM2 Is a Key Molecular Determinant of Resistance to SG-ARIs. *Oncogene* **2022**, *41*, 4498–4511. [CrossRef] [PubMed]

20. Zhang, Y.; Meng, X.; Ma, Z.; Sun, Z.; Wang, Z. Association of Androgen-Receptor Gene Mutations with the Copy Number of Androgen-Receptor Silk Protein A Complex and Glutathione-S-Transferases T1 and M1 in Prostate Cancer Patients. *Genet. Res.* **2023**, *2023*, 5956951. [CrossRef]
21. Jou, Y.C.; Wang, S.C.; Dia, Y.C.; Wang, S.T.; Yu, M.H.; Yang, H.Y.; Chen, L.C.; Shen, C.H.; Liu, Y.W. Anti-cancer Effects and Tumor Marker Role of Glutathione S-transferase Mu 5 in Human Bladder Cancer. *Int. J. Mol. Sci.* **2021**, *22*, 3056. [CrossRef]
22. Hao, X.; Zhang, J.; Chen, G.; Cao, W.; Chen, H.; Chen, S. Aberrant Expression of GSTM5 in Lung Adenocarcinoma Is Associated with DNA Hypermethylation and Poor Prognosis. *BMC Cancer* **2022**, *22*, 685. [CrossRef]
23. Garcia-Moreno, A.; López-Domínguez, R.; Villatoro-García, J.A.; Ramirez-Mena, A.; Aparicio-Puerta, E.; Hackenberg, M.; Pascual-Montano, A.; Carmona-Saez, P. Functional Enrichment Analysis of Regulatory Elements. *Biomedicines* **2022**, *10*, 590. [CrossRef]
24. Schwarz, J.M.; Cooper, D.N.; Schuelke, M.; Seelow, D. Mutationtaster2: Mutation Prediction for the Deep-Sequencing Age. *Nat. Methods* **2014**, *11*, 361–362. [CrossRef]
25. Freeman, B.; Smith, N.; Curtis, C.; Huckett, L.; Mill, J.; Craig, I.W. DNA from Buccal Swabs Recruited by Mail: Evaluation of Storage Effects on Long-Term Stability and Suitability for Multiplex Polymerase Chain Reaction Genotyping. *Behav. Genet.* **2003**, *33*, 67–72. [CrossRef]
26. Gómez-Martín, A.; Hernández, A.F.; Martínez-González, L.J.; González-Alzaga, B.; Rodríguez-Barranco, M.; López-Flores, I.; Aguilar-Garduno, C.; Lacasana, M. Polymorphisms of Pesticide-Metabolizing Genes in Children Living in Intensive Farming Communities. *Chemosphere* **2015**, *139*, 534–540. [CrossRef] [PubMed]
27. National Center for Biotechnology Information (NCBI). Primer-BLAST. Available online: https://www.ncbi.nlm.nih.gov/tools/primer-blast/ (accessed on 10 October 2024).
28. Kennedy, L.; Sandhu, J.K.; Harper, M.E.; Cuperlovic-culf, M. Role of Glutathione in Cancer: From Mechanisms to Therapies. *Biomolecules* **2020**, *10*, 1429. [CrossRef] [PubMed]
29. Allocati, N.; Masulli, M.; Di Ilio, C.; Federici, L. Glutathione Transferases: Substrates, Inihibitors and pro-Drugs in Cancer and Neurodegenerative Diseases. *Oncogenesis* **2018**, *7*, 8. [CrossRef]
30. Akkus, E.; Arslan, Ç.; Ürün, Y. Advancements in Platinum Chemotherapy for Metastatic Castration-Resistant Prostate Cancer: Insights and Perspectives. *Cancer Treat. Rev.* **2024**, *130*, 102818. [CrossRef] [PubMed]
31. Bansal, A.; Celeste Simon, M. Glutathione Metabolism in Cancer Progression and Treatment Resistance. *J. Cell Biol.* **2018**, *217*, 2291–2298. [CrossRef]
32. Santric, V.; Djokic, M.; Suvakov, S.; Pljesa-Ercegovac, M.; Nikitovic, M.; Radic, T.; Acimovic, M.; Stankovic, V.; Bumbasirevic, U.; Milojevic, B.; et al. GSTP1 RS1138272 Polymorphism Affects Prostate Cancer Risk. *Medicina* **2020**, *56*, 128. [CrossRef]
33. Cao, D.L.; Ye, D.W.; Dai, B.; Zhang, H.L.; Shen, Y.J.; Zhu, Y.; Zhu, Y.P.; Shi, G.H.; Ma, C.G.; Xiao, W.J.; et al. Association of Glutathione S-Transferase T1 and M1 Polymorphisms with Prostate Cancer Susceptibility in Populations of Asian Descent: A Meta-Analysis. *Oncotarget* **2015**, *6*, 35843–35850. [CrossRef]
34. Yu, K.D.; Fan, L.; Di, G.H.; Yuan, W.T.; Zheng, Y.; Huang, W.; Chen, A.X.; Yang, C.; Wu, J.; Shen, Z.Z.; et al. Genetic Variants in GSTM3 Gene within GSTM4-GSTM2-GSTM1-GSTM5-GSTM3 Cluster Influence Breast Cancer Susceptibility Depending on GSTM1. *Breast Cancer Res. Treat.* **2010**, *121*, 485–496. [CrossRef]
35. Gohari, N.; Abbasi, E.; Akrami, H. Comprehensive Analysis of the Prognostic Value of Glutathione S-transferases Mu Family Members in Breast Cancer. *Cell Biol. Int.* **2024**, *48*, 1313–1325. [CrossRef]
36. Bulger, M.; Groudine, M. Functional and Mechanistic Diversity of Distal Transcription Enhancers. *Cell* **2011**, *144*, 327–339. [CrossRef]
37. Chiaradonna, F.; Barozzi, I.; Miccolo, C.; Bucci, G.; Palorini, R.; Fornasari, L.; Botrugno, O.A.; Pruneri, G.; Masullo, M.; Passafaro, A.; et al. Redox-Mediated Suberoylanilide Hydroxamic Acid Sensitivity in Breast Cancer. *Antioxid. Redox Signal.* **2015**, *23*, 15–29. [CrossRef] [PubMed]
38. Zhang, J.; Li, Y.; Zou, J.; Lai, C.-T.; Zeng, T.; Peng, J.; Zou, W.-D.; Cao, B.; Liu, D.; Zhu, L.-Y.; et al. Comprehensive analysis of the glutathione S-transferase Mu (GSTM) gene family in ovarian cancer identifies prognostic and expression significance. *Front. Oncol.* **2022**, *12*, 968547. [CrossRef] [PubMed]
39. Barber, L.; Gerke, T.; Markt, S.C.; Peisch, S.F.; Wilson, K.M.; Ahearn, T.U.; Giovannucci, E.L.; Parmigiani, G.; Mucci, L.A. Family history of breast or prostate cancer and prostate cancer risk. *Clin. Cancer Res.* **2018**, *24*, 5910–5917. [CrossRef] [PubMed]
40. Frank, C.; Sundquist, J.; Hemminki, A.; Hemminki, K. Familial Associations Between Prostate Cancer and Other Cancers. *Eur. Urol.* **2017**, *71*, 162–165. [CrossRef]

biomedicines

MDPI

Article

Unveiling *DENND2D* as a Novel Prognostic Biomarker for Prostate Cancer Recurrence: From Gene to Prognosis

Chi-Fen Chang [1], Lih-Chyang Chen [2], Yei-Tsung Chen [3], Chao-Yuan Huang [4], Chia-Cheng Yu [5,6,7], Victor C. Lin [8,9], Te-Ling Lu [10], Shu-Pin Huang [11,12,13,*] and Bo-Ying Bao [10,*]

1 Department of Anatomy, School of Medicine, China Medical University, Taichung 406, Taiwan; cfchang@mail.cmu.edu.tw
2 Department of Medicine, Mackay Medical College, New Taipei City 252, Taiwan; lihchyang@mmc.edu.tw
3 Department of Life Sciences and Institute of Genome Sciences, National Yang Ming Chiao Tung University, Taipei 112, Taiwan; yeitsungchen@ym.edu.tw
4 Department of Urology, National Taiwan University Hospital, College of Medicine, National Taiwan University, Taipei 100, Taiwan; cyh0909@ntu.edu.tw
5 Division of Urology, Department of Surgery, Kaohsiung Veterans General Hospital, Kaohsiung 813, Taiwan; ccyu@vghks.gov.tw
6 Department of Urology, School of Medicine, National Yang Ming Chiao Tung University, Taipei 112, Taiwan
7 Department of Pharmacy, College of Pharmacy and Health Care, Tajen University, Pingtung 907, Taiwan
8 Department of Urology, E-Da Hospital, Kaohsiung 824, Taiwan; ed102161@edah.org.tw
9 School of Medicine for International Students, I-Shou University, Kaohsiung 840, Taiwan
10 Department of Pharmacy, China Medical University, Taichung 404, Taiwan; lutl@mail.cmu.edu.tw
11 Graduate Institute of Clinical Medicine, College of Medicine, Kaohsiung Medical University, Kaohsiung 807, Taiwan
12 Department of Urology, Kaohsiung Medical University Hospital, Kaohsiung 807, Taiwan
13 Institute of Medical Science and Technology, College of Medicine, National Sun Yat-Sen University, Kaohsiung 804, Taiwan
* Correspondence: shpihu@kmu.edu.tw (S.-P.H.); bao@mail.cmu.edu.tw (B.-Y.B.)

Abstract: Background: Prostate cancer is a major global health burden, with biochemical recurrence (BCR) following radical prostatectomy affecting 20–40% of patients and posing significant challenges to prognosis and treatment. Emerging evidence suggests a critical role for differentially expressed in normal and neoplastic cell (*DENN*) domain-containing genes in oncogenesis; however, their implications in prostate cancer and BCR risk remain underexplored. **Methods:** This study systematically evaluated 151 single-nucleotide polymorphisms in *DENN* domain-containing genes in 458 patients with prostate cancer and BCR, followed by validation in an independent cohort of 185 patients. **Results:** Multivariate Cox regression analyses identified *DENND2D* rs610261 G>A as significantly associated with improved BCR-free survival in both cohorts (adjusted hazard ratio = 0.39, 95% confidence interval = 0.23–0.66, $p = 0.001$). Functional analysis revealed rs610261's regulatory potential, with the protective A allele correlating with increased *DENND2D* expression in various human tissues. Compared to normal prostate tissues, *DENND2D* expression was reduced in prostate cancer, with higher expression being linked to favorable patient prognosis ($p = 0.03$). Gene set enrichment analysis revealed an association between *DENND2D* expression and the negative regulation of *MYC* target genes, including *MAD2L1*, *ERH*, and *CLNS1A*, which are overexpressed in prostate cancer and associated with poor survival. Furthermore, the elevated *DENND2D* expression promotes immune infiltration in prostate cancer, supporting its role in immune modulation. **Conclusions:** *DENND2D* is a prognostic biomarker for BCR in prostate cancer and offers new avenues for personalized treatment strategies.

Keywords: prostate cancer; recurrence; *DENN* domain-containing genes; gene set enrichment analysis; biomarker

1. Introduction

Prostate cancer is the second most common cancer among men worldwide, with significant morbidity and mortality rates [1]. Radical prostatectomy (RP) is the primary treatment for localized prostate cancer. However, a substantial number of patients, ranging from 20% to 40%, experienced biochemical recurrence (BCR) characterized by an increase in serum prostate-specific antigen (PSA) levels and signaling potential disease progression [2]. Despite advancements in imaging and clinical staging, predicting which patients are at risk for BCR remains challenging. Current prognostic tools depend on preoperative and pathological factors, such as the Gleason score, tumor stage, and surgical margins. However, these metrics often fail to account for molecular heterogeneity, which limits their predictive accuracy [3]. Various molecular biomarkers, such as gene expression profiles and epigenetic markers, have shown potential to supplement clinical parameters and improve prediction accuracy [4–6]. Conversely, their applicability is limited owing to the variability in outcomes and lack of validation across diverse populations. Identifying novel biomarkers associated with BCR transformed the clinical decision-making process and offered a pathway for personalized therapy in patients with prostate cancer.

Differentially expressed in normal and neoplastic cells (*DENN*) domain-containing genes serve as guanine nucleotide exchange factors for Rab GTPases. Genes containing the *DENN* domain facilitate the activation of Rab by replacing GDP with GTP, as activated Rabs are instrumental in various cellular processes, including vesicle trafficking, autophagy, and cellular signaling—which are crucial for maintaining cellular homeostasis and regulating immune responses [7]. Recent studies have suggested that the dysregulation of *DENN* domain-containing genes may be implicated in oncogenesis, including cancer proliferation, invasion, and metastasis. Alterations in *DENN* domain-containing genes, such as loss-of-function mutations, may contribute to cancer pathogenesis through the dysregulation of cellular signaling pathways, apoptosis, and autophagy [8]. *DENN* splice variants modulate tumor necrosis factor-mediated apoptosis, and are associated with resistance to chemotherapeutic agents [9]. *DENND2D* is a potential tumor suppressor in gastric cancer, and its downregulation correlates with poor prognosis and early recurrence [10]. Recently, *DENN* domain-containing gene variants were determined to be involved in multiple cancers, including breast and pancreatic cancer, suggesting their involvement in tumorigenesis and disease prognosis [11,12]. However, *DENN* domain-containing gene variants' involvement in prostate cancer, specifically in BCR prediction, is largely unexplored.

Considering the emerging significance of *DENN* domain-containing genes in cancer treatment, we hypothesized that the genetic variants of these genes may be associated with the risk of BCR post-RP in patients with prostate cancer. We systematically evaluated 151 single-nucleotide polymorphisms (SNPs) across various *DENN* domain-containing genes in a discovery cohort comprising 458 patients with prostate cancer who underwent BCR. We then validated our data using an independent cohort of 185 patients and performed functional assays to elucidate the involvement of *DENND2D* in prostate cancer progression.

2. Materials and Methods

2.1. Study Population and Data Collection

Overall, 644 patients with histopathologically confirmed prostate cancer who underwent RP were recruited from three medical centers in Taiwan: National Taiwan University Hospital, E-Da Hospital, and Kaohsiung Medical University Hospital [5,13]. All participants were Han Taiwanese, had no genetic relationships, and did not receive adjuvant hormone or radiation therapy following RP. Clinical and demographic data, such as age at diagnosis, PSA levels, pathologic Gleason scores, cancer staging, surgical margin status, lymph node involvement, and BCR status, were collected from patient records. BCR was defined as two consecutive PSA levels of ≥0.2 ng/mL post-RP [14,15]. BCR-free survival time was calculated from the date of RP until BCR onset or last recorded follow-up. A two-phase study design was used to examine the effects of the genetic variants of the *DENN* family genes on patient outcomes. The discovery cohort, comprising 457 patients, was recruited from the National Taiwan University Hospital and E-Da Hospital, whereas the replication cohort, comprising 187 patients, was recruited from the Kaohsiung Medical University Hospital. Table S1 summarizes the baseline clinical and pathological characteristics of both cohorts, showing no significant differences in variables, such as age at diagnosis, PSA levels, pathological Gleason score, and lymph node metastasis between the cohorts. The PSA level at diagnosis, pathological Gleason score, and stage were significantly associated with BCR-free survival in both cohorts. The median follow-up times were 38 and 74 months with 137 (30.0%) and 92 (49.2%) BCR cases, for the discovery and replication cohorts, respectively. The study protocol was approved by the Institutional Review Board of Kaohsiung Medical University Hospital (KMUHIRB-2013132), and all participants provided written informed consent.

2.2. SNP Selection and Genotyping

Haplotype-tagging SNPs were selected from 17 genes within the *DENN* family (*DENND1A*, *DENND1B*, *DENND1C*, *DENND2A*, *DENND2B*, *DENND2C*, *DENND2D*, *DENND3*, *DENND4A*, *DENND4B*, *DENND4C*, *DENND5A*, *DENND5B*, *DENND6A*, *DENND6B*, *DENND10*, and *DENND11*) using Haploview v4.2. The criteria included a minor allele frequency (MAF) > 0.05 and pairwise linkage disequilibrium correlation coefficient (r^2) exceeding 0.8, based on data from the 1000 Genomes Project for Han Chinese in Beijing and Southern Han Chinese populations [16,17].

Genomic DNA was extracted from 5 mL of whole blood collected in EDTA tubes using the QIAamp DNA Blood Maxi Kit (Qiagen, Valencia, CA, USA) according to the manufacturer's instructions. Standardized protocols were applied across all centers, ensuring processing within 24 h of collection and storage at −80 °C prior to genotyping. Genotyping was conducted at Taiwan's National Center for Genome Medicine using the Affymetrix Axiom Genotyping Array system (Thermo Fisher Scientific, Waltham, MA, USA) according to established methods [18]. SNPs with a genotyping call rate < 95%, MAF < 0.05, or deviation from the Hardy–Weinberg equilibrium ($p < 0.001$) were excluded; thus, 151 SNPs remain for further analysis.

2.3. Bioinformatic Analyses

To functionally annotate rs610261, we integrated data from HaploReg v4.2 and FIVEx databases. HaploReg leverages ENCODE and Roadmap Epigenomics data to predict potential regulatory roles of the variant on regulatory elements (e.g., enhancers, promoters), assess changes in transcription factor binding affinity, and evaluate evolutionary conservation [19]. Expression quantitative trait loci (eQTL) and splicing quantitative trait loci (sQTL) analyses were performed using FIVEx, which incorporates comprehensive genomic and transcriptomic datasets [20]. eQTL analysis employed linear regression models to associate the rs610261 genotype with *DENND2D* expression levels. Similarly, sQTL analysis used linear regression to assess the association between rs610261 and *DENND2D* transcript isoform abundance.

To assess the impact of *DENND2D* expression on prostate cancer outcomes, 40 public datasets from PCaDB [21], Gene Expression Database of Normal and Tumor Tissues 2 [22], and The Cancer Genome Atlas (TCGA) were examined. The TCGA Prostate Adenocarcinoma (PRAD) data were also used to explore *DENND2D*-related molecular mechanisms via gene ontology and hallmark pathway enrichment analyses using LinkedOmics [23]. Gene set enrichment analysis (GSEA) was conducted using LinkedOmics to identify gene sets correlated with *DENND2D* expression. Genes were ranked based on Pearson correlation coefficients between their expression levels and *DENND2D* expression. GSEA employs a weighted Kolmogorov–Smirnov-like running sum statistic [24] to calculate the Enrichment Score (ES), which quantifies the overrepresentation of gene set members at the extremes of the ranked gene list. This weighting scheme prioritizes genes at the top and bottom of the ranked list by incorporating gene rank into the running sum calculation. The ES represents the maximum deviation from zero encountered during this process. Statistical significance was determined by 1000 gene set label permutations, and multiple testing correction was performed using the Benjamini–Hochberg method to control the false discovery rate (FDR). Prognostic assessments of *DENND2D* and *MYC* target genes, such as mitotic arrest deficient 2 like 1 (*MAD2L1*), enhancer of rudimentary homolog mRNA splicing and mitosis factor (*ERH*), and chloride nucleotide-sensitive channel 1A (*CLNS1A*), were conducted using the TCGA-PRAD dataset.

DENND2D copy number variations were analyzed using Genomic Identification of Significant Targets In Cancer (GISTIC) 2.0 [25] applied to TCGA PRAD segmented copy number data. GISTIC values were used to define copy number categories: -2 (deep deletion), -1 (arm-level deletion), 0 (diploid), 1 (arm-level gain), and $\geq$2 (high amplification). Tumor-infiltrating immune cell levels were assessed in relation to *DENND2D* alterations and expression using the Tumor Immune Estimation Resource (TIMER) [26]. TIMER employs a statistical deconvolution method to estimate immune cell infiltration based on gene expression data from TCGA. This method uses pre-defined gene sets specific to various immune cell types (B cells, $CD4^+$ T cells, $CD8^+$ T cells, macrophages, neutrophils, and dendritic cells) and infers their relative abundance within the tumor microenvironment.

2.4. Statistical Analyses

Kaplan–Meier and log-rank tests were used to evaluate survival differences across genotypes or gene expression groups. Cox regression analyses, both univariate and multivariate, were used to calculate hazard ratios (HRs) and 95% confidence intervals (CIs) to analyze the associations between clinical characteristics and patient prognosis. The relationships between *DENND2D* expression and tumor characteristics were determined using Pearson's and Spearman's correlations. Statistical analyses were conducted using SPSS v19.0.0 (IBM, Armonk, NY, USA), with a two-sided p-value < 0.05 being considered statistically significant. Additionally, *DENND2D* expression in prostate cancer and normal tissues was compared using standardized mean differences (SMD) and 95% CIs. Associations between *DENND2D* mRNA levels and survival outcomes were evaluated by pooling the HRs and CIs in a random-effects model using Review Manager v5.4.1 (Cochrane, London, UK).

3. Results

We conducted a Cox regression analysis to investigate the association between genetic variants in the *DENN* family and the risk of BCR (Table S2). Among the 151 SNPs analyzed in the discovery cohort, three SNPs within *DENND1A*, one in *DENND1C*, two in *DENND2A*, two in *DENND2D*, two in *DENND3*, one in *DENND6B*, and one in *DENND11* were found to be associated with BCR-free survival ($p < 0.05$). Notably, *DENND2D* rs610261 was the only SNP that was identified as consistently significant in the replication cohort ($p = 0.032$; Table 1 and Figure 1B). In a combined analysis, the *DENND2D* rs610261 G>A variant was associated with the significantly improved BCR-free survival. This finding was supported by the results of the multivariable Cox regression analyses adjusted for clinical factors such as age, PSA levels at diagnosis, pathological stage, Gleason score, surgical margin status, and lymph node metastasis (adjusted HR = 0.39, 95% CI = 0.23–0.66, $p = 0.001$; Table 1 and Figure 1C).

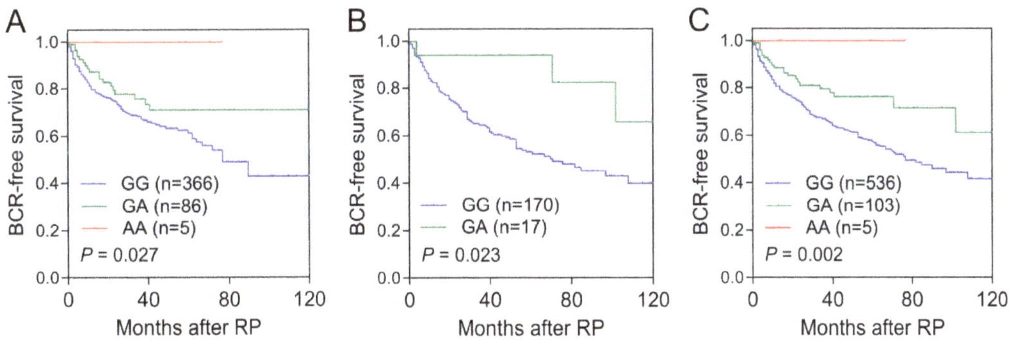

Figure 1. Kaplan–Meier curves show a significant association between *DENND2D* rs610261 and biochemical recurrence (BCR)-free survival in the (**A**) discovery, (**B**) replication, and (**C**) combined cohorts. RP, radical prostatectomy.

To investigate the functional significance of rs610261, we utilized the HaploReg database, which indicated that this SNP resides within regions enriched for promoter/enhancer histone marks and DNase I hypersensitivity sites across various tissues, highlighting its potential regulatory role (Table S3). Findings from the FIVEx database further supported this hypothesis by showing that the protective A allele of rs610261 was linked to the elevated expression of the *DENND2D* transcript ENST00000357640 in prostate ($p = 0.030$, Figure 2A) and in other human tissues, with the strongest association observed for the *DENND2D* transcript ENST00000473682 in the liver ($p = 0.0005$). In eQTL analysis, the A allele only showed a suggestive increase in *DENND2D* expression in the prostate ($p = 0.061$), though significant associations were observed in multiple tissues, including the brain, immune cells, kidneys, reproductive organs, and skin (Figure 2B). These findings suggest that splicing in *DENND2D* may play an important role in the tissue-specific regulation mediated by rs610261.

To evaluate the clinical relevance of *DENND2D* expression in prostate cancer, we analyzed the data from 2509 prostate cancer samples and 989 normal prostate tissue samples from 36 public datasets. *DENND2D* expression was significantly lower in prostate cancer tissues than in normal tissues (SMD = −0.17, 95% CI = −0.28 to −0.06, $p = 0.003$; Figure 3A). Furthermore, a pooled analysis of nine studies indicated that higher *DENND2D* expression correlated with improved prognosis (HR = 0.78, 95% CI = 0.63–0.97, $p = 0.03$; Figure 3B), suggesting a potential tumor-suppressive role for *DENND2D* in prostate cancer progression.

To investigate the biological role of *DENND2D* in prostate cancer, we identified genes that show correlated expression with *DENND2D* in the TCGA-PRAD dataset. In total, 4610 genes were positively correlated and 2353 genes were negatively correlated with *DENND2D*, with an FDR of <0.01 (Pearson's correlation). GSEA was performed using the complete ranked list of genes based on correlation coefficients and p-values. Gene Ontology analysis revealed that the negatively correlated genes were enriched in cellular components, such as the acetyltransferase complex, condensed chromosomes, and nuclear chromosomes (Figure 4A). Additionally, they were involved in biological processes, such as heterochromatin organization, protein localization to the cytoskeleton, and cytoplasmic translation (Figure 4B), as well as molecular functions, such as single-stranded DNA binding and ribonucleoprotein complex binding (Figure 4C). Hallmark pathway analysis showed enrichment of pathways related to the negative regulation of *MYC* target genes and cell cycle progression (Figure 4D).

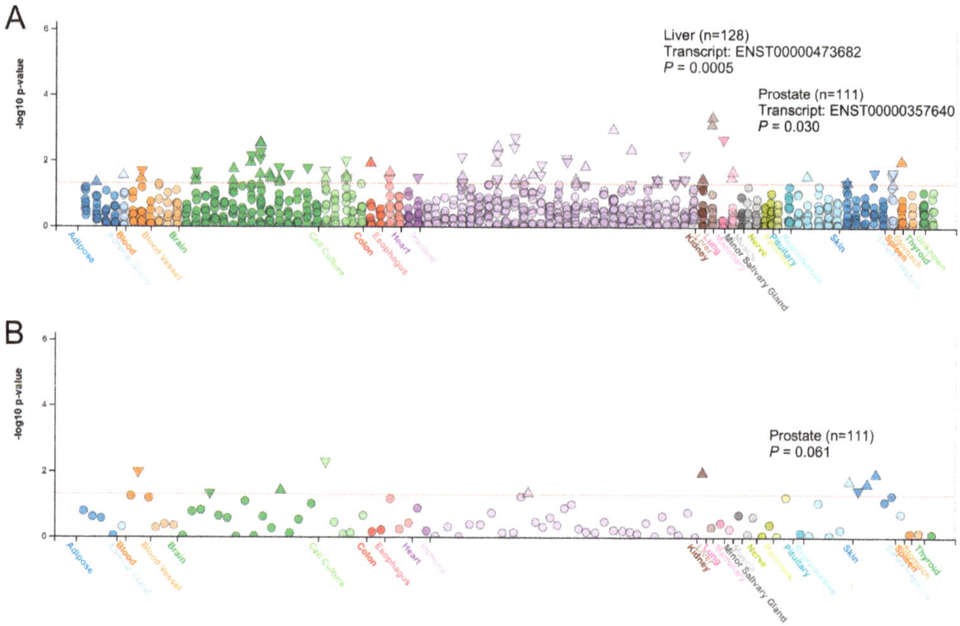

Figure 2. Functional implications of *DENND2D* rs610261: (**A**) Splicing quantitative trait loci and (**B**) expression quantitative trait loci analyses displaying the significant associations between rs610261 and *DENND2D* transcripts in multiple human tissues. The red horizontal line represents the nominal significance threshold (p = 0.05). Triangles indicate a positive effect of rs610261 on *DENND2D* expression, inverted triangles indicate a negative effect, and circles represent no significant effect.

GSEA identified "*MYC* targets v1" as the most significantly enriched pathway (normalized ES = -3.0371, FDR $< 2.2 \times 10^{-16}$), suggesting a link between *DENND2D* and *MYC* target genes. To validate this connection, we evaluated the correlation between *DENND2D* expression and the expression of genes within this highly enriched pathway. We discovered that *DENND2D* expression was inversely correlated with the expression of *MYC* target genes *MAD2L1*, *ERH*, and *CLNS1A* (Figure 5, left). Analysis of gene expression in prostate cancer tissues vs. normal tissues in the TCGA-PRAD dataset revealed significantly higher gene expressions in the prostate cancer tissues (Figure 5, middle). Moreover, their elevated expression levels were associated with poor survival outcomes, supporting

DENND2D's potential protective role through the suppression of *MYC* target genes in prostate cancer progression.

As *DENND2D* was also implicated in the activation of interferon and inflammatory pathways in the enrichment analysis, we explored its relationship with immune cell infiltration in prostate cancer. Additionally, the deep deletion of *DENND2D* was linked to the reduced B cell infiltration (Figure 6A). Conversely, higher *DENND2D* expression positively correlated with the infiltration of various immune cells, including B cells, $CD8^+$ T cells, $CD4^+$ T cells, macrophages, neutrophils, and dendritic cells (Figure 6B). Thus, *DENND2D* is essential to the regulation of immune cell infiltration in prostate cancer.

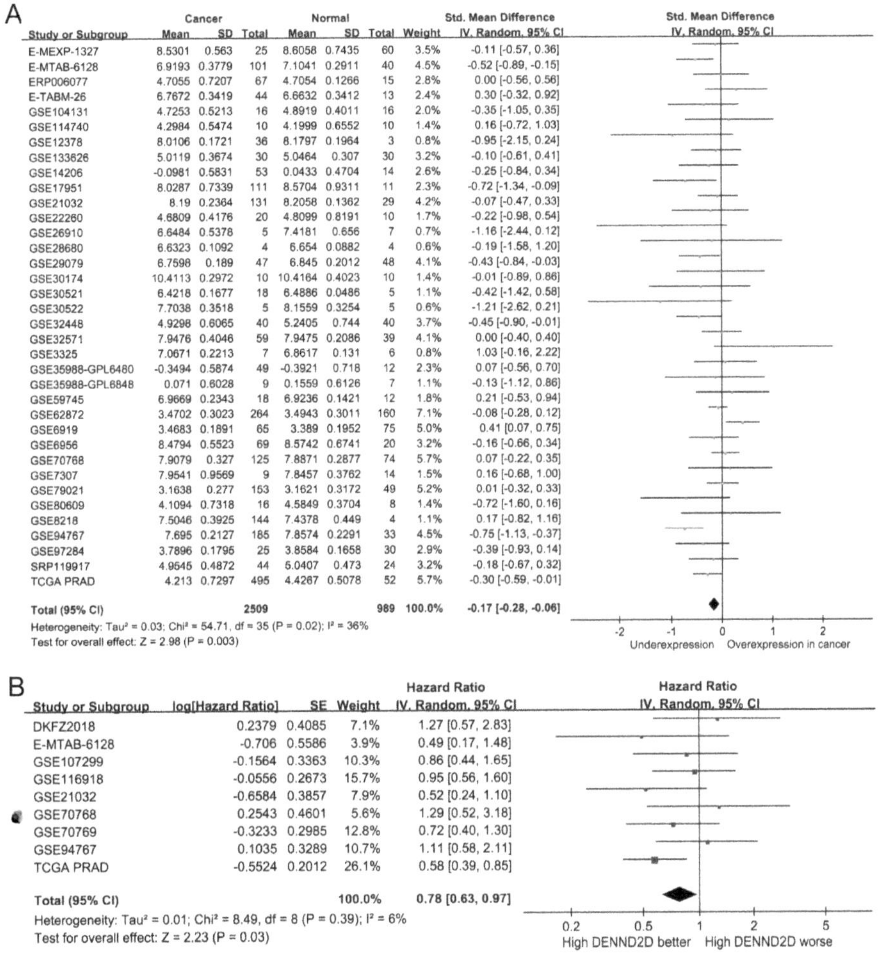

Figure 3. Clinical significance of *DENND2D* expression in prostate cancer: (**A**) *DENND2D* expression was significantly lower in prostate cancer tissues than in normal tissues using the analysis of 36 public datasets. (**B**) Pooled analysis revealed that higher *DENND2D* expression was associated with improved overall survival in patients with prostate cancer. Samples were stratified into low- and high-expression groups based on median expression values. SD, standard deviation. SE, standard error. IV, inverse variance. CI, confidence interval. Std, standardized. TCGA PRAD, The Cancer Genome Atlas Prostate Adenocarcinoma. df, degrees of freedom.

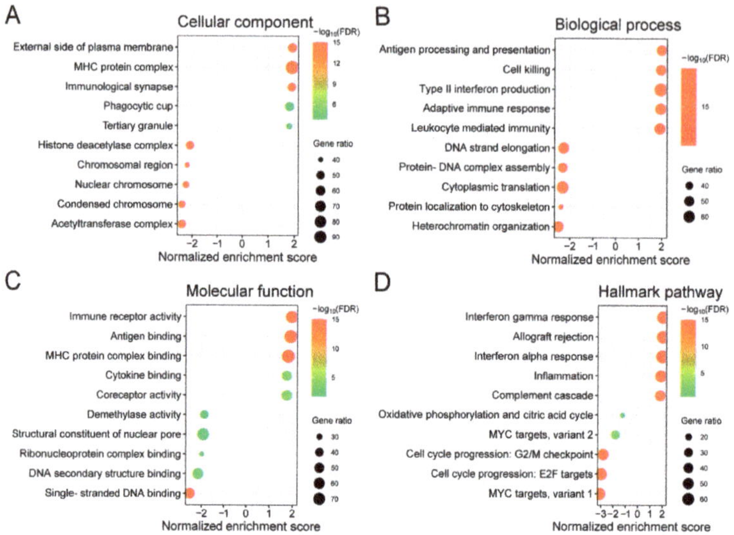

Figure 4. Gene Ontology and pathway analyses of genes correlated with *DENND2D* expression. Top 10 Gene Ontology terms in (**A**) cellular components, (**B**) biological processes, and (**C**) molecular functions. (**D**) Top 10 enriched Hallmark pathways. The size of the bubble indicates the number of enriched genes and color indicates the significance of the enrichment.

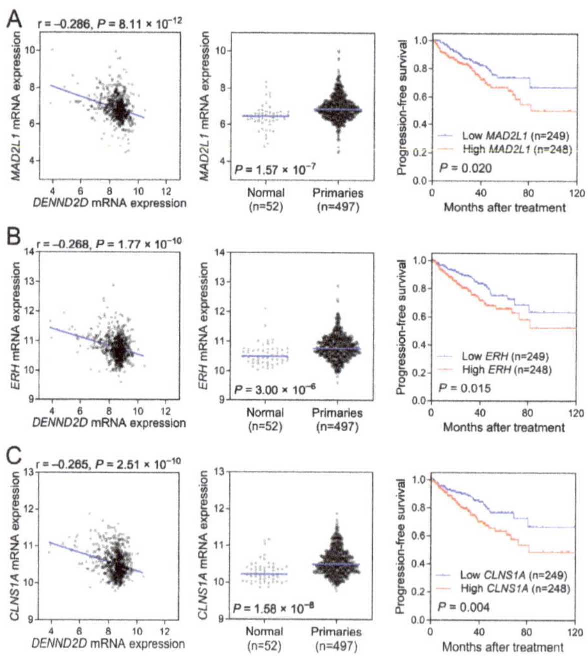

Figure 5. Association between *DENND2D* and *MYC* target gene expression in prostate cancer. The left panel illustrates the negative correlation between *DENND2D* and *MYC* target gene expression,

including (**A**) *MAD2L1*, (**B**) *ERH*, and (**C**) *CLNS1A*, in prostate cancer. The middle panel shows increased expression of these *MYC* target genes in prostate cancer tissues compared to normal tissues. The right panel shows that the higher expression levels of *MAD2L1*, *ERH*, and *CLNS1A* are associated with worse survival outcomes in patients with prostate cancer. Expression data were log2(x + 1) transformed RNA-Seq by Expectation-Maximization normalized count. Samples were stratified into low- and high-expression groups based on median expression values.

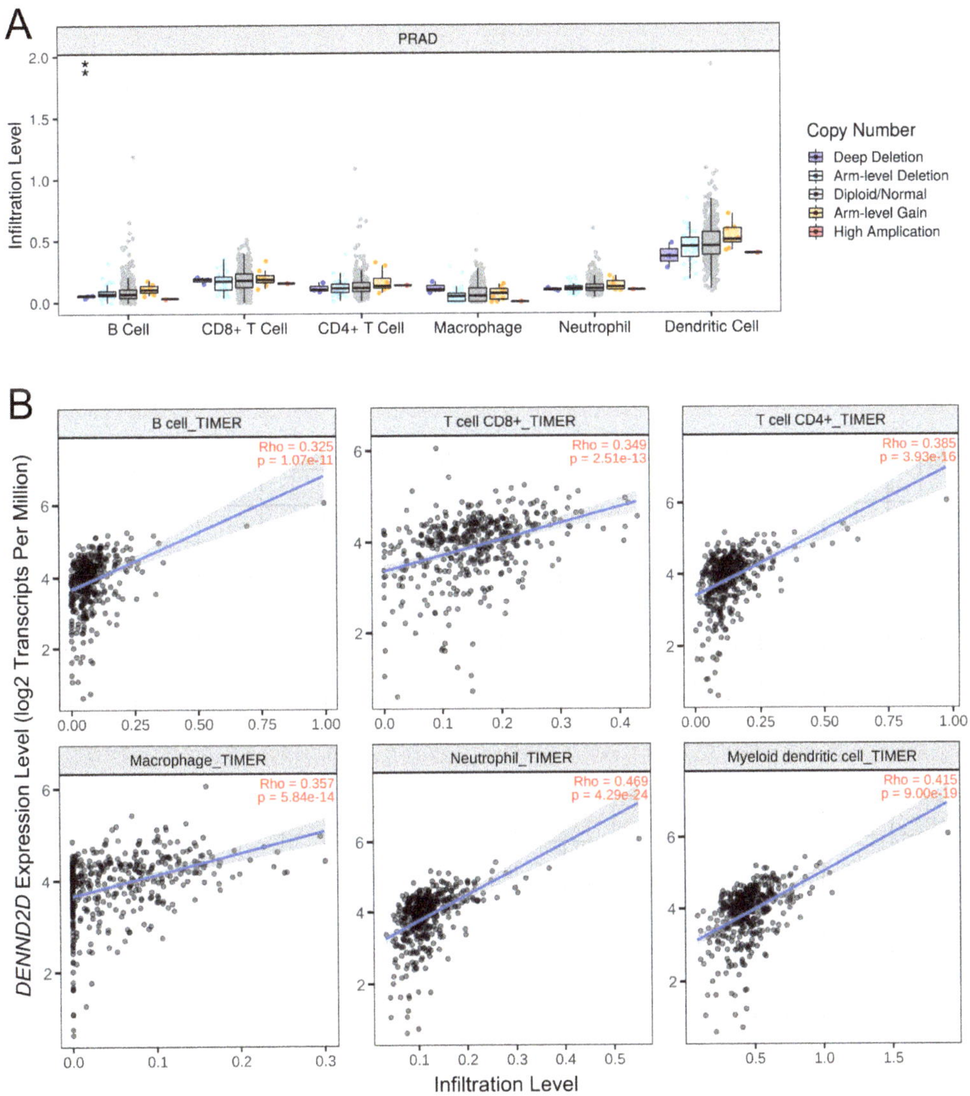

Figure 6. *DENND2D* expression and immune cell infiltration in prostate cancer: (**A**) The deep deletion of *DENND2D* correlated with reduced B-cell infiltration. The infiltration levels for each copy number category (deep deletion, n = 3; arm-level deletion, n = 34; diploid, n = 446; arm-level gain, n = 8; high amplification, n = 1) were compared to that of normal samples using a two-sided Wilcoxon rank-sum test. ** $p < 0.01$. (**B**) Higher *DENND2D* expression positively correlated with the infiltration of B cells, $CD8^+$ T cells, $CD4^+$ T cells, macrophages, neutrophils, and dendritic cells.

Table 1. Association of *DENND2D* rs610261 with biochemical recurrence after radical prostatectomy.

Genotype	Discovery				Replication				Combined			
	Patients	BCR	HR (95% CI)	p	Patients	BCR	HR (95% CI)	p	HR (95% CI)	p	HR (95% CI) [a]	p [a]
GG	366	118	1.00		170	88	1.00		1.00		1.00	
GA	86	19	0.66 (0.40–1.07)	0.089	17	4	0.33 (0.12–0.91)	0.032	0.56 (0.36–0.86)	0.008	0.42 (0.24–0.72)	0.002
AA	5	0	-	-	0	0	-	-	-	-	-	-
Trend			0.60 (0.38–0.95)	0.029			0.33 (0.12–0.91)	0.032	0.52 (0.34–0.80)	0.002	0.39 (0.23–0.66)	0.001

Abbreviations: BCR, biochemical recurrence; HR, hazard ratio; CI, confidence interval. [a] Adjustment for age, prostate-specific antigen at diagnosis, pathologic stage, Gleason score, surgical margin, and lymph node metastasis. -, Not estimated due to no event.

4. Discussion

This study identified *DENND2D* and its genetic variant rs610261 as significant contributors to BCR risk in prostate cancer. The rs610261 A allele was associated with improved BCR-free survival, likely mediated by enhanced *DENND2D* expression. Functional analyses revealed that *DENND2D* exerts tumor-suppressive effects, with reduced *DENND2D* expression correlating with prostate cancer progression and poor prognosis. In addition, *DENND2D* expression was inversely associated with the expression of *MYC* target genes and showed a positive correlation with immune cell infiltration. Thus, *DENND2D* is a promising prognostic biomarker and target for therapeutic intervention in prostate cancer.

SNP rs610261 is located within an intronic region characterized by promoter- and enhancer-like chromatin modification patterns along with overlapping DNase I-hypersensitive sites, suggesting a potential regulatory role in *DENND2D* expression. *DENND2D* was determined to exert significant tumor-suppressive effects by inhibiting tumor progression in various cancers [12,27,28]. *DENND2D* downregulation or silencing, frequently driven by promoter hypermethylation, has been implicated in the development of non-small cell lung cancer (NSCLC) [29], esophageal squamous cell carcinoma [30], hepatocellular carcinoma [8], and gastric cancer [10]. Promoter hypermethylation of *DENND2D* correlates with the advanced disease stage, early recurrence, and poor prognosis. Demethylation-based reactivation of *DENND2D* expression restores its tumor-suppressive function, positioning *DENND2D* as a potential biomarker for aggressive cancers [8,30]. Studies indicate that *DENND2D* inhibits tumor proliferation and metastasis primarily by inducing apoptosis and suppressing survival pathways in tumor cells. The overexpression of *DENND2D* in NSCLC significantly reduced proliferation and tumorigenicity by promoting apoptosis [29]. Notably, *DENND2D* has also been identified as a direct target of miR-522, linking its regulation to microRNA-mediated control of tumor proliferation and metastasis in NSCLC. This accentuates a novel axis for therapeutic intervention [31]. Herein, the clinical relevance and biological functions of *DENND2D* in prostate cancer were examined. Analysis of the pooled datasets revealed that *DENND2D* expression was significantly reduced in prostate tumors, and patients with elevated *DENND2D* levels demonstrated improved survival. The expression networks associated with *DENND2D* were analyzed using GSEA, revealing an inverse relationship between the expression of *MYC*-regulated genes, including *MAD2L1*, *ERH*, and *CLNS1A*. *MYC* is a proto-oncogene encoding a transcription factor that regulates the expression of numerous genes involved in cell growth, proliferation, metabolism, and apoptosis. Aberrant *MYC* expression, commonly through gene amplification, translocation, or increased transcription, drives tumorigenesis by promoting uncontrolled cell proliferation and survival. Given that *MYC* expression was inversely correlated with *DENND2D* expression (Pearson's $r = -0.127$, $p = 0.005$), the enrichment of *MYC* target pathways is expected. *MAD2L1* is a critical component of the spindle assembly checkpoint that ensures accurate chromosomal segregation during mitosis. *MAD2L1* dysregulation promotes tumorigenesis by inducing chromosomal instability and aneuploidy, and its overexpression has been linked to enhanced progression in various cancers [32]. Studies have demonstrated that *ERH*, a nuclear protein involved in cell cycle regulation and DNA replication, is frequently overexpressed in multiple cancer types wherein it modulates cell cycle checkpoints through interactions with mitotic kinases, thereby supporting the proliferation of rapidly dividing tumor cells [33]. *CLNS1A*, a chloride current regulator associated with the plasma membrane, interacts with various proteins to mediate diverse cellular functions, including the regulation of small nuclear ribonucleoprotein biosynthesis and cytoskeletal organization [34]. Additionally, *CLNS1A* amplification has been observed in malignant gliomas and breast cancer [35,36]. Notably, *CLNS1A* cooperates with the protein arginine methyltransferase 5, which functions as an epigenetic activator of androgen receptor transcription in castration-resistant prostate cancer [37]. Furthermore, the elevated expression of *DENND2D* was associated with the enhanced infiltration of immune cells, suggesting that *DENND2D* contributes to prostate cancer suppression through its combined effects on oncogenic pathways and immune modulation.

The advent of genomic tests has significantly enhanced the precision of prognostic tools in prostate cancer. By leveraging a 22-gene panel, Decipher has consistently demonstrated its ability to predict biochemical recurrence, metastasis, and cancer-specific mortality across multiple studies [38,39]. Although Decipher is a powerful classifier, its focus on a predefined gene set may overlook other relevant biomarkers or mechanisms involved in prostate cancer recurrence. *DENND2D* provides complementary insights into the molecular aggressiveness of prostate tumors, offering opportunities for refining treatment decisions and exploring novel therapeutic avenues. Nonetheless, further research is needed to elucidate the precise molecular mechanisms that underpin *DENND2D*'s tumor-suppressive functions in prostate cancer.

The strength of our study lies in its robust design, which combined genetic and functional analyses to comprehensively explore the role of *DENND2D* in prostate cancer. By integrating findings from discovery and replication cohorts, we ameliorated the validity of the association between rs610261 and improved BCR-free survival. Additionally, leveraging multiple datasets and conducting GSEA provided valuable insights into potential associations between *DENND2D* expression and tumor-suppressive mechanisms, including the regulation of *MYC* target genes and immune cell infiltration. This study has several limitations. The relatively small sample size reduced the statistical power of our results, particularly for less common genetic variants, and the exclusive inclusion of Taiwanese participants limited the generalizability of our data across ethnicities. Furthermore, the dependence on bioinformatic analyses for the functional interpretation of rs610261 necessitates experimental validation. The relatively short follow-up duration and focus on haplotype-tagged SNPs have restricted broader clinical implications. Although our findings reveal compelling associations between *DENND2D* and oncogenic processes, including *MYC* target gene regulation, cell cycle progression, and immune cell infiltration, our correlative analyses preclude definitive conclusions about causality. Future studies that address these limitations should strengthen our findings and their applicability.

5. Conclusions

In summary, this study highlights the clinical and biological significance of *DENND2D* in prostate cancer. Using a robust discovery–replication design, we provided compelling evidence that the *DENND2D* rs610261 G>A variant is a promising prognostic biomarker for prostate cancer recurrence. Moreover, the tumor-suppressive effects of *DENND2D*, which are mediated through *MYC* pathway regulation and immune cell infiltration, underscores its dual role in cancer control and immune modulation. While these findings advance our understanding of the role of *DENND2D* in prostate cancer, further research is needed to validate these results in larger cohorts and explore the therapeutic potential of targeting *DENND2D* in clinical settings.

Supplementary Materials: The following supporting information can be downloaded at: https://www.mdpi.com/article/10.3390/biomedicines13010025/s1. Table S1. Clinicopathologic characteristics of the study populations. Table S2. Association between *DENN* domain-containing gene polymorphisms and biochemical recurrence after radical prostatectomy. Table S3. Regulatory annotation of *DENND2D* rs610261.

Author Contributions: Conceptualization and methodology, C.-F.C., S.-P.H. and B.-Y.B.; resources and funding acquisition, C.-Y.H., C.-C.Y., V.C.L., S.-P.H. and B.-Y.B.; formal analysis and investigation, C.-F.C., T.-L.L., S.-P.H. and B.-Y.B.; data curation and visualization, L.-C.C., Y.-T.C. and T.-L.L. All authors have read and agreed to the published version of the manuscript.

Funding: This work was supported by the National Science and Technology Council of Taiwan (grant nos: 110-2314-B-002-113, 111-2314-B-002-240-MY3, 111-2320-B-039-021-MY3, 111-2218-E-037-001, and 112-2314-B-037-127), the Kaohsiung Medical University (grant nos: KMUH109-9R63, KMUH109-9R64, KMUH112-2R59 and NHRIKMU-111-I002), and the China Medical University (grant nos: CMU111-MF-09, and CMU112-MF-10, and CMU113-MF-11). The funders had no role in study design, data collection and analysis, decision to publish, or preparation of the manuscript.

Institutional Review Board Statement: The study was conducted in accordance with the Declaration of Helsinki and approved by the Research Ethics Committee of the Kaohsiung Medical University Hospital (approval no. KMUHIRB-2013132, 21 January 2014).

Informed Consent Statement: Written informed consent was obtained from all participants prior to the interviews and specimen collection.

Data Availability Statement: Data will be available on reasonable request.

Acknowledgments: The Authors thank Chao-Shih Chen for data analysis, and the National Centre for Genome Medicine, Taiwan, for technical support. The results published here are based in part on data generated by the HaploReg, 1000 Genomes, GTEx, and TCGA projects.

Conflicts of Interest: The authors declare no conflicts of interest.

References

1. Bray, F.; Ferlay, J.; Soerjomataram, I.; Siegel, R.L.; Torre, L.A.; Jemal, A. Global cancer statistics 2018: GLOBOCAN estimates of incidence and mortality worldwide for 36 cancers in 185 countries. *CA Cancer J. Clin.* **2018**, *68*, 394–424. [CrossRef] [PubMed]
2. Han, M.; Partin, A.W.; Zahurak, M.; Piantadosi, S.; Epstein, J.I.; Walsh, P.C. Biochemical (prostate specific antigen) recurrence probability following radical prostatectomy for clinically localized prostate cancer. *J. Urol.* **2003**, *169*, 517–523. [CrossRef] [PubMed]
3. Morgan, T.M.; Lange, P.H.; Porter, M.P.; Lin, D.W.; Ellis, W.J.; Gallaher, I.S.; Vessella, R.L. Disseminated tumor cells in prostate cancer patients after radical prostatectomy and without evidence of disease predicts biochemical recurrence. *Clin. Cancer Res.* **2009**, *15*, 677–683. [CrossRef] [PubMed]
4. Cullen, J.; Rosner, I.L.; Brand, T.C.; Zhang, N.; Tsiatis, A.C.; Moncur, J.; Ali, A.; Chen, Y.; Knezevic, D.; Maddala, T.; et al. A Biopsy-based 17-gene Genomic Prostate Score Predicts Recurrence After Radical Prostatectomy and Adverse Surgical Pathology in a Racially Diverse Population of Men with Clinically Low- and Intermediate-risk Prostate Cancer. *Eur. Urol.* **2015**, *68*, 123–131. [CrossRef] [PubMed]
5. Huang, S.P.; Huang, L.C.; Ting, W.C.; Chen, L.M.; Chang, T.Y.; Lu, T.L.; Lan, Y.H.; Liu, C.C.; Yang, W.H.; Lee, H.Z.; et al. Prognostic significance of prostate cancer susceptibility variants on prostate-specific antigen recurrence after radical prostatectomy. *Cancer Epidemiol. Biomark. Prev.* **2009**, *18*, 3068–3074. [CrossRef] [PubMed]
6. Liu, J.C.; Shen, W.C.; Shih, T.C.; Tsai, C.W.; Chang, W.S.; Cho, Y.; Tsai, C.H.; Bau, D.T. The current progress and future prospects of personalized radiogenomic cancer study. *Biomedicine* **2015**, *5*, 2. [CrossRef]
7. Marat, A.L.; Dokainish, H.; McPherson, P.S. DENN domain proteins: Regulators of Rab GTPases. *J. Biol. Chem.* **2011**, *286*, 13791–13800. [CrossRef]
8. Kanda, M.; Nomoto, S.; Oya, H.; Takami, H.; Hibino, S.; Hishida, M.; Suenaga, M.; Yamada, S.; Inokawa, Y.; Nishikawa, Y.; et al. Downregulation of DENND2D by promoter hypermethylation is associated with early recurrence of hepatocellular carcinoma. *Int. J. Oncol.* **2014**, *44*, 44–52. [CrossRef] [PubMed]
9. Efimova, E.V.; Al-Zoubi, A.M.; Martinez, O.; Kaithamana, S.; Lu, S.; Arima, T.; Prabhakar, B.S. IG20, in contrast to DENN-SV, (MADD splice variants) suppresses tumor cell survival, and enhances their susceptibility to apoptosis and cancer drugs. *Oncogene* **2004**, *23*, 1076–1087. [CrossRef] [PubMed]
10. Kanda, M.; Shimizu, D.; Nomoto, S.; Takami, H.; Hibino, S.; Oya, H.; Hashimoto, R.; Suenaga, M.; Inokawa, Y.; Kobayashi, D.; et al. Prognostic impact of expression and methylation status of DENN/MADD domain-containing protein 2D in gastric cancer. *Gastric Cancer* **2015**, *18*, 288–296. [CrossRef]

11. Cotterchio, M.; Lowcock, E.; Bider-Canfield, Z.; Lemire, M.; Greenwood, C.; Gallinger, S.; Hudson, T. Association between Variants in Atopy-Related Immunologic Candidate Genes and Pancreatic Cancer Risk. *PLoS ONE* **2015**, *10*, e0125273. [CrossRef] [PubMed]
12. Huang, C.C.; Tu, S.H.; Lien, H.H.; Jeng, J.Y.; Huang, C.S.; Huang, C.J.; Lai, L.C.; Chuang, E.Y. Concurrent gene signatures for han chinese breast cancers. *PLoS ONE* **2013**, *8*, e76421. [CrossRef]
13. Huang, E.Y.; Chang, Y.J.; Huang, S.P.; Lin, V.C.; Yu, C.C.; Huang, C.Y.; Yin, H.L.; Chang, T.Y.; Lu, T.L.; Bao, B.Y. A common regulatory variant in SLC35B4 influences the recurrence and survival of prostate cancer. *J. Cell. Mol. Med.* **2018**, *22*, 3661–3670. [CrossRef] [PubMed]
14. Freedland, S.J.; Sutter, M.E.; Dorey, F.; Aronson, W.J. Defining the ideal cutpoint for determining PSA recurrence after radical prostatectomy. Prostate-specific antigen. *Urology* **2003**, *61*, 365–369. [CrossRef] [PubMed]
15. Huang, S.P.; Levesque, E.; Guillemette, C.; Yu, C.C.; Huang, C.Y.; Lin, V.C.; Chung, I.C.; Chen, L.C.; Laverdiere, I.; Lacombe, L.; et al. Genetic variants in microRNAs and microRNA target sites predict biochemical recurrence after radical prostatectomy in localized prostate cancer. *Int. J. Cancer* **2014**, *135*, 2661–2667. [CrossRef] [PubMed]
16. Genomes Project, C.; Abecasis, G.R.; Auton, A.; Brooks, L.D.; DePristo, M.A.; Durbin, R.M.; Handsaker, R.E.; Kang, H.M.; Marth, G.T.; McVean, G.A. An integrated map of genetic variation from 1092 human genomes. *Nature* **2012**, *491*, 56–65. [CrossRef]
17. Li, C.Y.; Huang, S.P.; Chen, Y.T.; Wu, H.E.; Cheng, W.C.; Huang, C.Y.; Yu, C.C.; Lin, V.C.; Geng, J.H.; Lu, T.L.; et al. TNFRSF13B is a potential contributor to prostate cancer. *Cancer Cell Int.* **2022**, *22*, 180. [CrossRef] [PubMed]
18. Chang, H.H.; Lee, C.H.; Chen, Y.T.; Huang, C.Y.; Yu, C.C.; Lin, V.C.; Geng, J.H.; Lu, T.L.; Huang, S.P.; Bao, B.Y. Genetic Analysis Reveals the Prognostic Significance of the DNA Mismatch Repair Gene MSH2 in Advanced Prostate Cancer. *Cancers* **2022**, *14*, 223. [CrossRef] [PubMed]
19. Ward, L.D.; Kellis, M. HaploReg v4: Systematic mining of putative causal variants, cell types, regulators and target genes for human complex traits and disease. *Nucleic Acids Res.* **2016**, *44*, D877–D881. [CrossRef]
20. Kwong, A.; Boughton, A.P.; Wang, M.; VandeHaar, P.; Boehnke, M.; Abecasis, G.; Kang, H.M. FIVEx: An interactive eQTL browser across public datasets. *Bioinformatics* **2022**, *38*, 559–561. [CrossRef]
21. Li, R.; Zhu, J.; Zhong, W.-D.; Jia, Z. PCaDB-a comprehensive and interactive database for transcriptomes from prostate cancer population cohorts. *bioRxiv* **2022**. [CrossRef]
22. Park, S.J.; Yoon, B.H.; Kim, S.K.; Kim, S.Y. GENT2: An updated gene expression database for normal and tumor tissues. *BMC Med. Genom.* **2019**, *12*, 101. [CrossRef]
23. Vasaikar, S.V.; Straub, P.; Wang, J.; Zhang, B. LinkedOmics: Analyzing multi-omics data within and across 32 cancer types. *Nucleic Acids Res.* **2018**, *46*, D956–D963. [CrossRef] [PubMed]
24. Subramanian, A.; Tamayo, P.; Mootha, V.K.; Mukherjee, S.; Ebert, B.L.; Gillette, M.A.; Paulovich, A.; Pomeroy, S.L.; Golub, T.R.; Lander, E.S.; et al. Gene set enrichment analysis: A knowledge-based approach for interpreting genome-wide expression profiles. *Proc. Natl. Acad. Sci. USA* **2005**, *102*, 15545–15550. [CrossRef] [PubMed]
25. Mermel, C.H.; Schumacher, S.E.; Hill, B.; Meyerson, M.L.; Beroukhim, R.; Getz, G. GISTIC2.0 facilitates sensitive and confident localization of the targets of focal somatic copy-number alteration in human cancers. *Genome Biol.* **2011**, *12*, R41. [CrossRef] [PubMed]
26. Li, T.; Fan, J.; Wang, B.; Traugh, N.; Chen, Q.; Liu, J.S.; Li, B.; Liu, X.S. TIMER: A Web Server for Comprehensive Analysis of Tumor-Infiltrating Immune Cells. *Cancer Res.* **2017**, *77*, e108–e110. [CrossRef] [PubMed]
27. Mutalip, S.S.; Yunos, N.M.; Abdul-Rahman, P.S.; Jauri, M.H.; Osman, A.; Adenan, M.I. Mechanisms of action of 17betaH-neriifolin on its anticancer effect in SKOV-3 ovarian cancer cell line. *Anticancer Res.* **2014**, *34*, 4141–4151.
28. Sakha, S.; Muramatsu, T.; Ueda, K.; Inazawa, J. Exosomal microRNA miR-1246 induces cell motility and invasion through the regulation of DENND2D in oral squamous cell carcinoma. *Sci. Rep.* **2016**, *6*, 38750. [CrossRef]
29. Ling, B.; Zheng, H.; Fu, G.; Yuan, J.; Shi, T.; Chen, S.; Liu, Y.; Liu, Y.; Cao, Y.; Zheng, S.; et al. Suppression of non-small cell lung cancer proliferation and tumorigenicity by DENND2D. *Lung Cancer* **2013**, *79*, 104–110. [CrossRef] [PubMed]
30. Hibino, S.; Kanda, M.; Oya, H.; Takami, H.; Shimizu, D.; Nomoto, S.; Hishida, M.; Niwa, Y.; Koike, M.; Yamada, S.; et al. Reduced expression of DENND2D through promoter hypermethylation is an adverse prognostic factor in squamous cell carcinoma of the esophagus. *Oncol. Rep.* **2014**, *31*, 693–700. [CrossRef] [PubMed]
31. Zhang, T.; Hu, Y.; Ju, J.; Hou, L.; Li, Z.; Xiao, D.; Li, Y.; Yao, J.; Wang, C.; Zhang, Y.; et al. Downregulation of miR-522 suppresses proliferation and metastasis of non-small cell lung cancer cells by directly targeting DENN/MADD domain containing 2D. *Sci. Rep.* **2016**, *6*, 19346. [CrossRef] [PubMed]
32. Zhu, X.F.; Yi, M.; He, J.; Tang, W.; Lu, M.Y.; Li, T.; Feng, Z.B. Pathological significance of MAD2L1 in breast cancer: An immunohistochemical study and meta analysis. *Int. J. Clin. Exp. Pathol.* **2017**, *10*, 9190–9201. [PubMed]

33. Pang, K.; Li, M.L.; Hao, L.; Shi, Z.D.; Feng, H.; Chen, B.; Ma, Y.Y.; Xu, H.; Pan, D.; Chen, Z.S.; et al. ERH Gene and Its Role in Cancer Cells. *Front. Oncol.* **2022**, *12*, 900496. [CrossRef]
34. Chari, A.; Golas, M.M.; Klingenhager, M.; Neuenkirchen, N.; Sander, B.; Englbrecht, C.; Sickmann, A.; Stark, H.; Fischer, U. An assembly chaperone collaborates with the SMN complex to generate spliceosomal SnRNPs. *Cell* **2008**, *135*, 497–509. [CrossRef]
35. Braun, C.J.; Stanciu, M.; Boutz, P.L.; Patterson, J.C.; Calligaris, D.; Higuchi, F.; Neupane, R.; Fenoglio, S.; Cahill, D.P.; Wakimoto, H.; et al. Coordinated Splicing of Regulatory Detained Introns within Oncogenic Transcripts Creates an Exploitable Vulnerability in Malignant Glioma. *Cancer Cell* **2017**, *32*, 411–426.e11. [CrossRef] [PubMed]
36. Noblejas-Lopez, M.D.M.; Lopez-Cade, I.; Fuentes-Antras, J.; Fernandez-Hinojal, G.; Esteban-Sanchez, A.; Manzano, A.; Garcia-Saenz, J.A.; Perez-Segura, P.; La Hoya, M.; Pandiella, A.; et al. Genomic Mapping of Splicing-Related Genes Identify Amplifications in LSM1, CLNS1A, and ILF2 in Luminal Breast Cancer. *Cancers* **2021**, *13*, 4118. [CrossRef]
37. Beketova, E.; Fang, S.; Owens, J.L.; Liu, S.; Chen, X.; Zhang, Q.; Asberry, A.M.; Deng, X.; Malola, J.; Huang, J.; et al. Protein Arginine Methyltransferase 5 Promotes pICln-Dependent Androgen Receptor Transcription in Castration-Resistant Prostate Cancer. *Cancer Res.* **2020**, *80*, 4904–4917. [CrossRef]
38. Feng, F.Y.; Huang, H.C.; Spratt, D.E.; Zhao, S.G.; Sandler, H.M.; Simko, J.P.; Davicioni, E.; Nguyen, P.L.; Pollack, A.; Efstathiou, J.A.; et al. Validation of a 22-Gene Genomic Classifier in Patients With Recurrent Prostate Cancer: An Ancillary Study of the NRG/RTOG 9601 Randomized Clinical Trial. *JAMA Oncol.* **2021**, *7*, 544–552. [CrossRef]
39. Spratt, D.E.; Dai, D.L.Y.; Den, R.B.; Troncoso, P.; Yousefi, K.; Ross, A.E.; Schaeffer, E.M.; Haddad, Z.; Davicioni, E.; Mehra, R.; et al. Performance of a Prostate Cancer Genomic Classifier in Predicting Metastasis in Men with Prostate-specific Antigen Persistence Postprostatectomy. *Eur. Urol.* **2018**, *74*, 107–114. [CrossRef]

biomedicines

MDPI

Article

The Role of Sphingolipid Metabolism in Pregnancy-Associated Breast Cancer After Chemotherapy

Victor Blokhin [1,†], Tatiana Zavarykina [2,3,†], Vasily Kotsuba [4,5], Maria Kapralova [2], Uliana Gutner [2], Maria Shupik [2], Elena Kozyrko [3], Evgenia Luzina [3], Polina Lomskova [2], Darya Bajgazieva [3], Svetlana Khokhlova [3] and Alice Alessenko [2,*]

1 Koltzov Institute of Developmental Biology of the Russian Academy of Sciences, Moscow 119334, Russia; victor.blokhin@hotmail.com

2 Emanuel Institute of Biochemical Physics of Russian Academy of Sciences, Moscow 119334, Russia; tpalievskaya@yandex.ru (T.Z.); kapamariya97@gmail.com (M.K.); uliana.goutner@gmail.com (U.G.); mariashupik@gmail.com (M.S.); brenner123@mail.ru (P.L.)

3 B.I. Kulakov National Medical Research Center of Obstetrics, Gynecology and Perinatology of the Ministry of Health of the Russian Federation, Moscow 117997, Russia; lenochka525@gmail.com (E.K.); zhenyaluz@gmail.com (E.L.); ruzha88@mail.ru (D.B.); svkhokhlova@mail.ru (S.K.)

4 Federal Research Center "Fundamentals of Biotechnology" Russian Academy of Sciences, Moscow 119334, Russia; vasilyk@yandex.ru

5 Department of Theoretical and Applied Chemistry, Federal State University of Education, Moscow 105005, Russia

* Correspondence: alicealessenko@gmail.com; Tel.: +7-905-588-5066

† The authors contributed equally to the work.

Abstract: Background: The aim of our study was to determine the role of sphingolipids, which control proliferation and apoptosis, in the placenta of pregnant women with pregnancy-associated breast cancer (PABC) after chemotherapy compared with healthy patients. Methods: We analyzed (by the PCR method) the gene expression of key sphingolipid metabolism enzymes (sphingomyelinases (SMPD1 and SMPD3), acid ceramidase (ASAH1), ceramide synthases (CERS 1–6), sphingosine kinase1 (SPHK1), sphingosine-1-phosphate lyase 1 (SGPL1), and sphingosine-1-phosphate receptors (S1PR1, S1PR2, and S1PR3)) and the content of subspecies of ceramides, sphingosine, and sphingosine-1-phosphate in seven patients with PABC after chemotherapy and eight healthy pregnant women as a control group. Results: We found a significant increase in the expression of genes of acid ceramidase (ASAH1), sphingosine-1-phosphate lyase 1 (SGPL1), sphingosine kinase (SPHK1), and ceramide synthases (CERS 1-3, 5, 6) in the samples of patients with PABC during their treatment with cytostatic chemotherapy. The increase in the expression of the enzymes' genes was not accompanied by changes in the content of the studied sphingolipids. Such significant changes in the expression of genes controlling the level of CER, sphingosine, and S1P may indicate their ability to initiate the metabolism of pro-apoptotic and anti-apoptotic sphingolipids in the placenta of pregnant women with cancer undergoing chemotherapy in order to maintain levels typical of the placenta of healthy women. Conclusions: Our results may indicate the promising mechanism of placenta protection during chemotherapy for pregnant women with breast cancer and, consequently, of the newborn. This protective effect of the placenta and especially for the newborn has been discovered for the first time and requires more careful study.

Keywords: gene of sphingolipid metabolism; ceramides; sphingosine-1-phosphate; breast cancer; pregnancy; chemotherapy

1. Introduction

Sphingolipids are now recognized as multifaceted mediators in cancer biology and therapeutics [1–9]. Therefore, they may become novel targets for therapeutic applications.

Sphingolipids involved in the regulation of apoptosis and cell division, as well as enzymes and receptors that control their metabolism and functional activity are targets for anti-tumor therapy.

Some enzymes capable of enhancing ceramide synthesis and cleaving S1P have been shown to promote cancer cell death. These enzymes include the following sphingomyelinases (SMPD): lysosomal acid SMPD (SMPD1), magnesium-dependent neutral SMPD (SMPD2); ceramide synthase (CERS); sphingosine-1-phosphat kinase (SPHK); and sphingosine-1-phosphate lyase (SGPL) (Figure 1) [10–14].

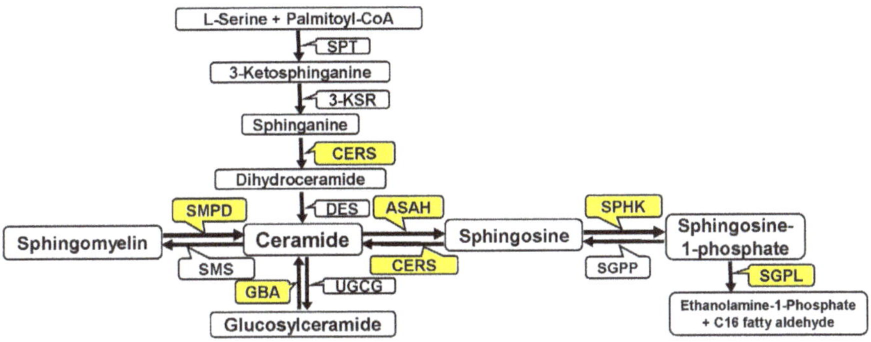

Figure 1. Abbreviated scheme of sphingolipid metabolism. SPT—serine palmitoyltransferase (the first step in the biosynthesis of sphingolipids; catalyzes the condensation of serine and palmitoyl-CoA); 3-KSR–3-ketosphinganine reductase (catalyzes the reduction of 3-ketodihydro sphinganine to sphinganine); CERS—(dihydro)ceramide synthase (key enzyme in the lipid metabolism of eukaryotic cells; there are six ceramide synthases (CERS1-6); each of which synthesizes ceramides de novo with distinct acyl chain lengths); DES—dihydroceramide desaturase (catalyzes the formation of double bond in C4–C5 positions in dihydroceramide); SMPD—sphingomyelinase (converts sphingomyelin to ceramide); SMS—sphingomyelin synthase (generates sphingomyelin and diacylglycerol from phosphatidylcholine and ceramide); ASAH—ceramidase (cleaves ceramides into sphingosine and fatty acids); GBA—glucosylceramidase (hydrolyzes glucosylceramide to form ceramide and glucose); UGCG—(catalyzes the transfer of glucose from UDP glucose to ceramide to produce glucosylceramide); SPHK—sphingosine kinase (converts sphingosine to sphingosine-1-phosphate); SGPP—sphingosine-1-phosphate phosphatase (dephosphorylates intracellular sphingosine-1-phosphate); and SGPL—sphingosine-1-phosphate lyase (the final step of S1P degradation; catalyzes the irreversible cleavage of sphingosine-1-phosphate to yield ethanolamine-1-phosphate and C16 fatty aldehyde).

Many studies have shown that SPHK1 activation can induce cancer cell migration and that the SPHK1/S1P axis enhances the metastatic potential of cancer cells [15–17]. The role of sphingolipids in pregnancy is also under active investigation [18–20]. Sphingosine-1-phosphate (S1P) is a multifunctional lipid that regulates numerous physiologic processes. S1P normally mediates protective cellular processes, whereas ceramide (CER) induces destructive processes in the placenta [18,20]. In normal pregnancy, these processes occur within their normal physiological balance, thus preserving the structure and function of the various cells that make up the placenta. Thus, the S1P/CER rheostat determines the fate and function of cells in the placenta [18]. Signaling by the bioactive sphingolipid S1P and its precursors are emerging areas in pregnancy research [20]. According to data from Fakhr et al. [18] circulating CER levels increase towards end of gestation, suggesting a physiological role in parturition, despite the maintenance of circulating S1P concentrations. Several studies have shown no changes in the expression of genes of sphingolipid metabolism during normal placental development [21–24]. However, high levels of circulating S1P and ceramides are correlated with pregnancy disorders such as mellitus, preeclampsia, diabetes, and cancer. The expression of placental and decidual enzymes metabolizing S1P, as well as S1P receptors, is impaired in pregnancy complications [18].

Current data indicate the promising potential of S1P and related sphingolipids to be considered potential candidates for both diagnostics and therapeutics in cancer and pregnancy disorder studies.

We also believe that determining the gene expression levels of the enzymes involved in the synthesis of CERs, sphingosines, and S1P, which control apoptosis, may be a tool for diagnosing obstetric complications and the efficacy of cancer treatment in pregnant patients.

It has now been established that the efficacy of many drugs used for cancer chemotherapy exhibit their therapeutic effects through effects on sphingolipid metabolism, in particular through the activation of enzymes that generate the proapoptotic metabolites CER and sphingosine, such as sphingomyelinases [25] and ceramidase [1,4,25–31]. For example, platinum + taxane-based chemotherapy is associated with high response rates initially, but later these patients develop chemotherapy-resistant disease. All of these results suggest that CER can enhance the antitumor activity of docetaxel (DTX) in a synergistic manner, and the sphingolipid pathway involved in cancer development has also been found to contribute to chemoresistance and metastasis in a wide range of malignancies. In particular, the interaction between SPHK1 and S1PR1 has been shown to be altered during ovarian and breast cancer development in a variety of ways and therefore may be an attractive therapeutic target [8,32]. Taxane-induced peripheral neuropathy (TIPN) is known to be a side effect that limits the effective dose of the drug in breast cancer treatment. Ganglioside monosialic acid (GM1) is known to have neuroprotective properties. The use of GM1 in combination with taxanes was found to reduce the severity and incidence of TIPN after four cycles of taxane-containing chemotherapy in breast cancer patients [33]. Currently, CER-based combination therapy is being used as a new therapeutic strategy. The synergistic effect of CER in combination with DTX (CER + DTX) and the mechanism of this synergism have been studied. It was shown that simultaneous administration of CER and DTX in a molar ratio of 0.5:1 could induce an optimal synergistic effect on murine malignant melanoma cells (B16, CI = 0.31) and human breast carcinoma cells (MCF-7, CI = 0.48), suggesting that combined application prospects of CER + DTX treatment are promising [34].

CER glycosylation, through glucosylceramide synthase (GCS), allows for cellular escape from ceramide-induced programmed cell death. This glycosylation event confers cancer cell resistance to cytotoxic anticancer agents. It has been shown that multidrug resistance can be increased over baseline and then completely reversed in human breast cancer cells by GCS gene targeting [34,35]. The S1P/S1PR axis is considered a therapeutic target for cancer, particularly for breast cancer [34–38]. New drugs that directly affect sphingolipid metabolism are currently attracting attention. The best known is fingolimod (FTY720). This drug is currently used for the treatment of multiple sclerosis. As a sphingosine analog, FTY720 has been shown to affect S1P metabolism. Due to this property, it has a protective effect in many preclinical models of breast cancer [36–38]. Treatment with FTY720 has potentiated the anticancer effects of doxorubicin in different mouse models. Sarah Spiegel's paper details the molecular mechanism of the antitumor action of FTY720 [39,40]. The protective effects of FTY720 are not limited to suppression of breast tumor development and progression only but are also seen in adjuvant therapy. In general, these studies show that FTY720 is a multifaceted drug that can work as an effective anticancer agent in its own right, as well as an adjuvant to hormonal therapy, conventional chemotherapy, and even radiation therapy for the treatment of not only estrogen-receptor-positive tumors but also more complex triple-negative breast cancer, as well as tumors that develop resistance to chemotherapeutic drugs [36–41].

2. Materials and Methods

2.1. Chemicals

All lipid analytical standards were obtained from Avanti (Avanti Polar Lipids, Birmingham, AL, USA). LCMS-grade acetonitrile and formic acid were from Fisher (Fisher

Chemicals, Pittsburgh, PA, USA). LCMS-grade methanol was provided by EVA Science (EVA Science, Saint Petersburg, Russia). LCMS-grade isopropanol was procured from Panreac (Panreac Quimica, Barcelona, Spain). Ultrapure water was produced by a Millipore (Merck Millipore, Burlington, MA, USA), Direct-Q 3 system.

2.2. Study Population

This study was conducted in compliance with the principles of voluntariness and confidentiality in accordance with the Federal Law "On the Fundamentals of Protecting the Health of Citizens in the Russian Federation" and the 1964 Declaration of Helsinki and its subsequent amendments. This study was approved by the Biomedical Research Ethics Committee of Kulakov National Medical Research Center of Obstetrics, Gynecology and Perinatology of the Ministry of Health of Russia. Informed consent was obtained from each of the participants included in this study. The studied biological samples of patients with pregnancy-associated breast cancer (PABC) and healthy pregnant persons were obtained from Kulakov National Medical Research Center of Obstetrics, Gynecology and Perinatology of the Ministry of Health of Russia.

The criteria for the inclusion of patients in this study were a morphologically confirmed diagnosis of PABC; satisfactory general condition; normal function of hematopoiesis, kidneys, and liver; and the absence of metastasis. The diagnosis was established by histological examination.

The patient group included 7 patients with breast cancer. Seven patients with PABC received cytostatic chemotherapy during pregnancy (Table 1). All patients had live births delivered by spontaneous labor or cesarean section. Pre-term labor was observed in two patients. The median week of gestation at cancer diagnosis was 20 (min 4–max 26). On average, 3 (min, 1; max, 7) cycles of chemotherapy were applied. In this work, the samples of placenta from 7 women with PABC and 8 samples of placenta from healthy women were studied. The median age in the control group (healthy pregnant women) was 27.5 years old (min 23–max 39). In patients with PABC, the following obstetric parameters were analyzed: neonatal weight and height, fetal percentile (ultrasound data), placental weight, placental weight percentile (ultrasound data), and their relations with the expression of sphingolipid metabolism genes using logistic regression and Spearman's rank correlation methods.

Table 1. Clinical characteristics of patients with pregnancy-associated breast cancer (PABC).

Parameter	Data
Age, median -Minimum–maximum	37 years old 31–43 years old
Stage of the disease: -II -III	-5 out of 7 (71.4%) -2 out of 7 (28.6%)
Luminal A Luminal B HER2-negative Luminal B HER2-positive Triple negative	-1 out of 7 (14%) -3 out of 7 (43%) -1 out of 7 (14%) -2 out of 7 (29%)
Chemotherapy: -Taxanes -Chloroethylamines, anthracyclines -Taxanes, chloroethylamines, anthracyclines -Taxanes, chloroethylamines	 -1 out of 7 (14.3%) -4 out of 7 (57.1%) -1 out of 7 (14.3%) -1 out of 7 (14.3%)

Samples of placenta were collected during labor in IntactRNA reagent (Evrogen, Moscow, Russia) for RNA protection. For lipid extraction, samples of placenta were collected in clear tubes. All samples were stored at −80 °C.

2.3. RNA Isolation, Reverse Transcription, and Real-Time PCR

RNA was isolated using Extract RNA reagent (Evrogen, Russia), and total RNA was subsequently cleaned by CleanRNA Standart Kit (Evrogen, Russia). Samples of RNA were stored with RNAse inhibitor RiboCare (Evrogen, Russia). For reverse transcription, an MMLV RT kit (Evrogen, Russia), random (dN)10 primer, and 1 μg of RNA were used. For the analysis of gene expression, real-time PCR was carried out using 5X qPCRmix-HS SYBR kit (Evrogen, Russia) on LightCycler96 (Roche, Vaud, Switzerland). Sequences of primers are presented in Table 2; primers were designed using Primer-BLAST. PCR conditions: denaturation phase—95.0 °C;—10 min; amplification phase—40 cycles; denaturation: 95.0 °C—10 s., amplification: Tann—annealing temperature—60.0 °C—60 s; melting curve: 95.0 °C—10 s., 65.0 °C—60 s., 97.0 °C—1 s. (single).

Table 2. Primers for analysis of gene expression.

Gene, Number in NCBI	Sequence	Length, b.p.
SPHK1 NM_001142602.2	F: GAGCAGGTCACCAATGAAG R: ATCAGCAATGAAGCCCCAG	150
SGPL1 NM_003901.4	F: TTCCATTCCCCATCTCAGG R: CACACACACACACACACAC	240
ASAH1 NM_001363743.2	F: AGTCAATAGCTTGTCTTCGTC R: GTGTTTACTGTCCCGTTACTC	265
SMPD1 NM_001365135.2	F: AGTCAATAGCTTGTCTTCGTC R: GTGTTTACTGTCCCGTTACTC	265
GBA1 NM_001171812.2	F: GCCACAGCATCATCACGAAC R: TAGCACGACCACAACAGCAG	293
SMPD3 NM_018667.4	F: CCTTCATACCCACCACCTAC R: CAGAAGAGAAAGCCGAGAAAC	145
CERS2 NM_022075.5	F: CACCCCATCCTCAATAACAAC R: CCTCTCACTTTCTCCTTTTTCC	148
CERS1 NM_001387444.1	F: CCCCAAGCCTACTCCAAAAC R: AACTACTCCTCACCACCCAC	216
CERS4 NM_024552.3	F: AGACCAGGAGGCAAGTGAAG R: CGAAGGAGGACAGGTAGAAGAG	225
CERS6 NM_203463.3	F: AGGACAGGAGTGGACAAAG R: AGGGGAAAAGCGAGATAGAG	154
CERS3 NM_001378789.1	F: GAAGAGGAAGAGGAAGAGGAAG R: TGGTGAGAAAGAGGGAAGGG	226
CERS5 NM_147190.5	F: GCCCTTCCCATATCTACTCTTC R: GCACAAACGCACATCAAC	179
S1PR1 NM_001400.5	F: AATTCAGCCGCAGCAAATC R: AACTCTACCCACCAACACCC	279
S1PR2 NM_004230.4	F: TGTATGGCAGCGACAAGAG R: ACAGGATGATGGAGAAGATGG	192
S1PR3 NM_005226.4	F: CCCACTCTTCATCCTCTTCC R: GCTGCTATTGTTGCTGCTG	268

Note: F—forward primer; R—reverse primer.

Calculation of relative expression was performed using the 2ΔΔCt method, normalized by housekeeping gene B2M.

2.4. Mass Spectrometry of Sphingolipids

Lipids were extracted from the placenta of healthy pregnant women and those with pregnancy-associated breast cancer after chemotherapy according to the Bligh and Dyer method [42]. Lipid analysis was performed by HPLC/MS on an Agilent 1290 Infinity system coupled to an Agilent 6460 triple quadrupole mass spectrometer (Agilent Technologies, Santa Clara, CA, USA).

A Phenomenex (Phenomenex Inc., Torrance, CA, USA) Luna Omega PS chromatographic column (50 × 2.1 mm, 1.6 μ) was used for the separation of lipids under the following conditions: 0.1% formic acid in water as mobile phase A; a mixture of methanol, acetonitrile, and isopropanol (4:1:1) containing 0.1% formic acid as mobile phase B; mobile phase flow–0.4 mL/min; and column temperature of 35 °C. The mobile phase gradient program was as follows: 60% B → 100% B in 8 min, hold at 100% B for 4 min, back to 60% B in 0.1 min, and re-equilibration for 2.9 min.

The electrospray ion source operated at a nebulizing gas pressure of 30 psi, whereas the drying gas flow and temperature were 10 L/min and 300 °C, respectively. The nebulizing gas, drying gas, and collision gas was nitrogen. Multiple reaction monitoring (MRM) mode was used for data acquisition. Positive ions only were detected. Ceramides exhibited two MRM transitions, resulting in a m/z 264.2 fragment, with the parent ions being $[M + H]^+$ (used as quantifier) and $[M - H_2O + H]^+$ (used as qualifier). Sphingosine and sphingosine phosphate exhibited only single MRM transitions; sphingosine molecules, like the ceramides, produced the m/z 264.2 product ions, whereas sphingosine phosphate predominantly underwent dehydration. The corresponding values of optimized fragmentor voltage, collision energy, dwell time, and capillary voltage for each MRM transition are listed in Table 3. The cell accelerator voltage was set to 5 V for all transitions.

Table 3. Optimized parameters for the MRM transitions of the studied lipids.

Sphingolipid	MRM Transition	Fragmentor Voltage, V	Collision Energy, V	Dwell Time, ms	Capillary Voltage, kV
C16 Cer (d18:1/16:0)	538.0→264.2 520.0→264.2	100 150	35 20	45	4000
C22 Cer (d18:1/22:0)	622.5→264.2 604.5→264.2	100 150	35 35	45	4000
C24 Cer (d18:1/24:0)	650.5→264.2 632.5→264.2	100 100	35 35	45	4000
C24:1 Cer (d18:1/24:1(15Z))	649.0→264.2 631.0→264.2	100 100	35 35	45	4000
Sph	305.5→264.2	150	5	55	3000
S1P	380.5→362.5	100	15	55	3000

Each lipid was quantified using the external standard method. Calibration curves were obtained for the following concentration ranges: 5–10,000 ng/mL.

2.5. Statistical Analysis

Statistical analysis was carried out using Statistica 8.0.360.0 (StatSoft). Comparative analysis of gene expression and mass spectrometric analysis of sphingolipids was carried out in groups of patients with PABC and healthy women. The nonparametric Mann–

Whitney test was used to compare the control and experimental groups. Differences were considered statistically significant at $p < 0.05$.

3. Results

3.1. Analysis of Gene Expression of Enzymes of Ceramide and Sphingoid Base Metabolism (Sphingosine and S1P) in Pregnancy-Associated Breast Cancer After Treatment

Breast cancer is the most common cancer in women, often leading to death. Because of this, intensive research is being conducted on causes, progression, and effective treatments for breast cancer. Sphingolipids have been found to be involved in many processes important in breast cancer, including growth, progression, transformation, and metastasis. PABC is the most common variant of cancer in pregnancy. In our study, we analyzed the gene expression of enzymes that are involved in the metabolism of ceramide and S1P, which largely determine apoptosis and cell division during breast cancer development.

We performed PCR analysis of the gene expression of enzymes involved in the generation of ceramides and S1P in placenta samples of patients with PABC after cytostatic chemotherapy with taxanes, chloroethylamines (cyclophosphamide), and anthracyclines in different combinations (Table 1). The results were compared to those of healthy pregnant patients.

3.1.1. Analysis of Sphingomyelinase Gene Expression in Pregnancy-Associated Breast Cancer After Treatment

In our study, the tendency to undergo activation of the acidic sphingomyelinase gene was observed (4.5 times, $p = 0.09$, Figure 2b), whereas the neutral sphingomyelinase gene was slightly activated (1.5 times, $p = 0.15$, Figure 2a) during pregnancy in the course of breast cancer treatment (Figure 2).

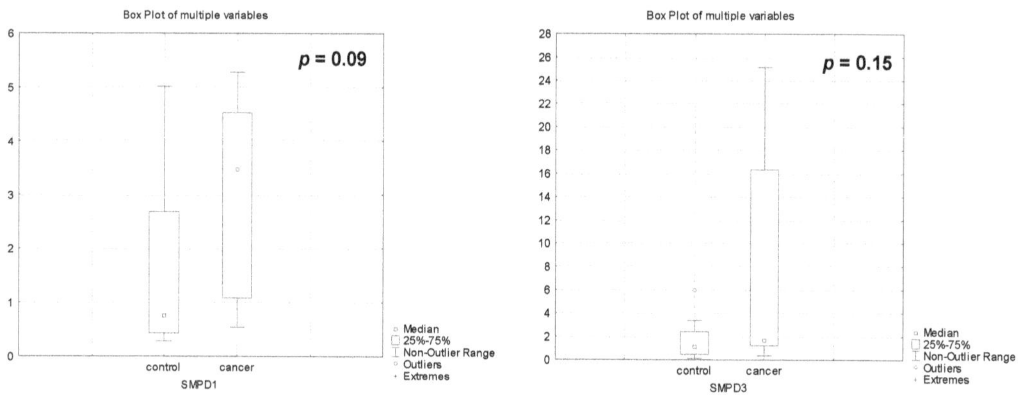

(a) (b)

Figure 2. Gene expression of (**a**) acid (*SMPD1*) and (**b**) neutral (*SMPD3*) sphingomyelinases in the placenta of healthy pregnant women (control) and women with pregnancy-associated breast cancer after chemotherapy (cancer).

3.1.2. Analysis of Ceramide Synthase Gene Expression in Pregnancy-Associated Breast Cancer After Treatment

When analyzing the expression of genes encoding different CERS isoforms, which are responsible for de novo synthesis of CER, we found a significant increase in the expression of the 0*CERS1*, *CERS2*, *CERS3*, and *CERS5* genes (*CERS1* (39.8-fold, $p = 0.001$), *CERS2* (3.9-fold, $p = 0.004$), *CERS3* (17.3-fold, $p = 0.001$), *CERS5* (5.1-fold, $p = 0.002$), *CERS6* (2.2-fold, $p = 0.006$)), except *CERS4* (no changes, $p > 0.05$), in the placenta of patients with PABC after their treatment compared to the results obtained for healthy pregnant women (Figure 3).

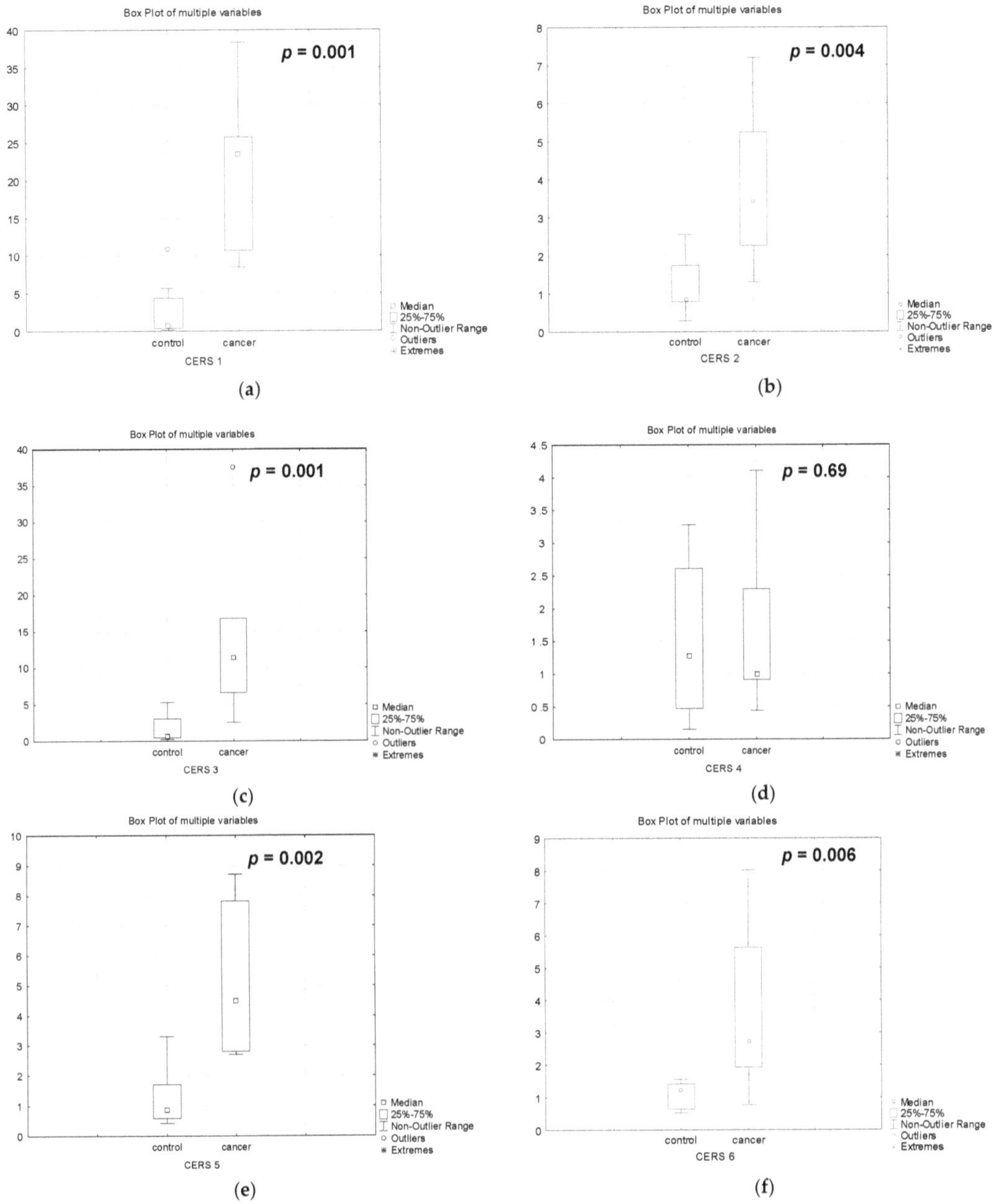

Figure 3. Gene expression of ceramide synthases in the placenta of healthy pregnant women (control) and women with pregnancy-associated breast cancer after chemotherapy: (**a**) *CERS1*, (**b**) *CERS2*, (**c**) *CERS3*, (**d**) *CERS4*, (**e**) *CERS5*, (**f**) *CERS6*.

Sphingomyelinases and ceramide synthases act in opposite directions, and, depending on their activity, the content of total CER can both accumulate and decrease. In cases of balanced activity of these enzymes, its content can remain within the normal range. To determine the final effect of the gene expression, we studied the changes in the content of molecular types of CERs in the placenta of healthy women and patients after breast cancer therapy.

3.1.3. Analysis of Acid Ceramidase (ASAH1) Gene Expression in Pregnancy-Associated Breast Cancer After Treatment

In our experiments, it was found that the expression of the acid ceramidase (*ASAH*) gene sharply increased during the chemotherapy of patients with PABC 3 times, $p = 0.09$ (Figure 4). This fact determined a possible decrease in the content of CER, which was formed by the degradation of sphingomyelin and its synthesis from sphingosine.

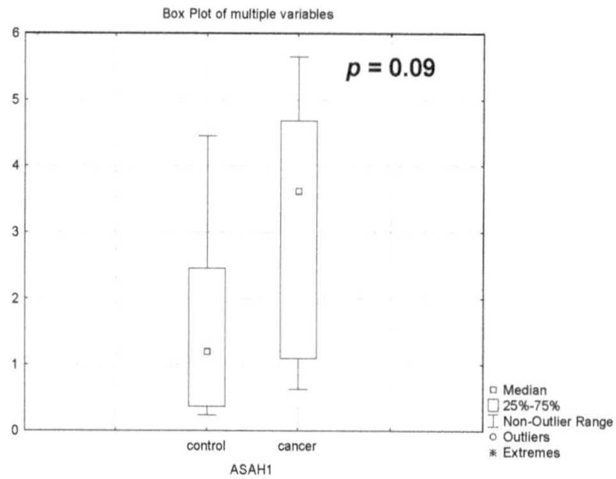

Figure 4. Gene expression of acid ceramidase (*ASAH1*) in the placenta of healthy pregnant women (control) and women with pregnancy-associated breast cancer after chemotherapy (cancer).

3.2. Analysis of Ceramide Species Level in the Placenta of Healthy Pregnant Women and Women with Pregnancy-Associated Breast Cancer After Chemotherapy

We analyzed long-chain CER (C16:0, C22:0, C24:0, and C24:1), which are generally cytotoxic and pro-apoptotic, in the placenta of healthy pregnant women and women with PABC after chemotherapy (Figure 5).

Cytostatic chemotherapy drugs are able to induce the accumulation of CERs that lead to cancer cell death. Their effectiveness due to the increase in CER levels by increasing the expression of ceramide synthase genes results in the increased content of proapoptotic products of sphingolipid metabolism, CER. This effect of cytostatic chemotherapy drugs has been confirmed in other studies [5,43].

But when this proapoptotic agent is destroyed as a result of the more active action of ceramidase—in our case, acidic ceramidase—there can be either a decrease in its content or it can remain within the control values. When analyzing the content of the most significant molecular CER species in the placenta of healthy pregnant women and patients with PABC after chemotherapy by mass spectrometry, we found the same level for almost all CER species in these two groups of patients. This may imply the existence of a molecular mechanism to protect the placenta, and consequently the fetus, from the toxic effects of chemotherapy.

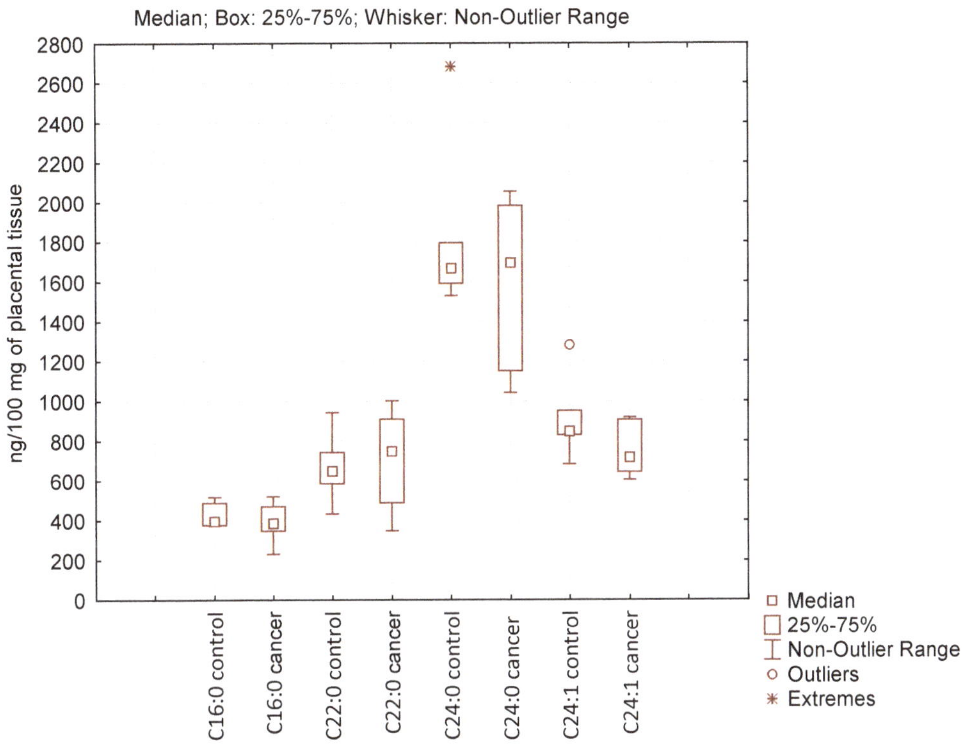

Figure 5. Level of ceramide species in the placenta of healthy pregnant women (control) and women with pregnancy-associated breast cancer after chemotherapy (cancer). Non-significant changes ($p > 0.05$) are not indicated.

3.3. Changes in the Expression of Genes Controlling S1P Metabolism and Level of Sphingosine-1-Phosphate in the Placenta of Healthy Pregnant Women and Women with Pregnancy-Associated Breast Cancer After Chemotherapy

In our work, we investigated the expression of sphingosine kinase 1 (SPHK1) and sphingosine phosphate lyase 1 (SGPL1) genes that determine the metabolism of S1P, which is involved in pregnancy and malignancy and determines the efficacy of chemotherapy.

Sphingosine can be converted under the action of sphingosine phosphate kinase into anti-apoptotic S1P, which has anti-apoptotic properties, promotes cell proliferation, survival and migration, and participates in differentiation, neurogenesis, and angiogenesis [43,44]. Two main SPHK isoforms, types 1 and 2, have been identified and described; these isoforms have a similar polypeptide structure but differ in cellular localization and physiological functions. SPHK1 is the most studied enzyme of S1P metabolism. The basal level of SPHK1 activity maintains the cellular balance of sphingosine and S1P under the action of several agonists on the cell, including proinflammatory cytokines, various growth factors, etc. By contrast, sphingosine phosphate lyase 1 (*SGPL1*) degrades S1P.

In our experiments, we found a dramatic increase in *SPHK1* gene expression in patients with PABC undergoing treatment compared to healthy patients (by 6.3 times, $p = 0.009$, Figure 5). Despite the fact that S1P generated by SPHK1 has anti-apoptotic properties, it can influence survival through its effects on drug resistance [12]. Simultaneously, there is a sharp activation of the expression of the sphingosine phosphate lyase gene (4 times, $p = 0.040$, Figure 6). This fact determines the possible degradation of S1P. Consequently, two opposing processes occur simultaneously that may maintain a stable level of S1P in the placenta. This fact determines the possible degradation of S1P.

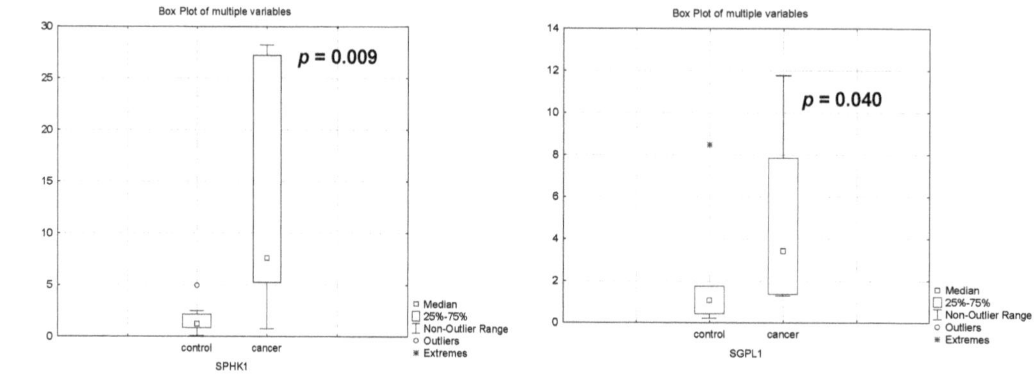

(a) (b)

Figure 6. Gene expression of sphingosine kinase 1 (*SPHK1*) (**a**) and sphingosine phosphate lyase 1 (*SGPL1*) (**b**) in the placenta of healthy pregnant women (control) and women with pregnancy-associated breast cancer after chemotherapy (cancer).

3.3.1. Analysis of Sphingosine and Sphingosine-1-Phosphate Level in the Placenta of Healthy Pregnant Women and Women with Pregnancy-Associated Breast Cancer After Chemotherapy

The analysis of sphingosine and sphingosine-1-phosphate (Figure 7) content in the placenta of healthy pregnant women and women with PABC after chemotherapy has shown that these sphingolipids, which have opposite properties in cell life, also remain stable after chemotherapy. Simultaneous activation of the gene expression of genes with opposite properties has a stabilizing effect on the content of these sphingolipids. These facts additionally confirm the possible existence of a very reliable mechanism of placental protection against the toxic effect of chemotherapy.

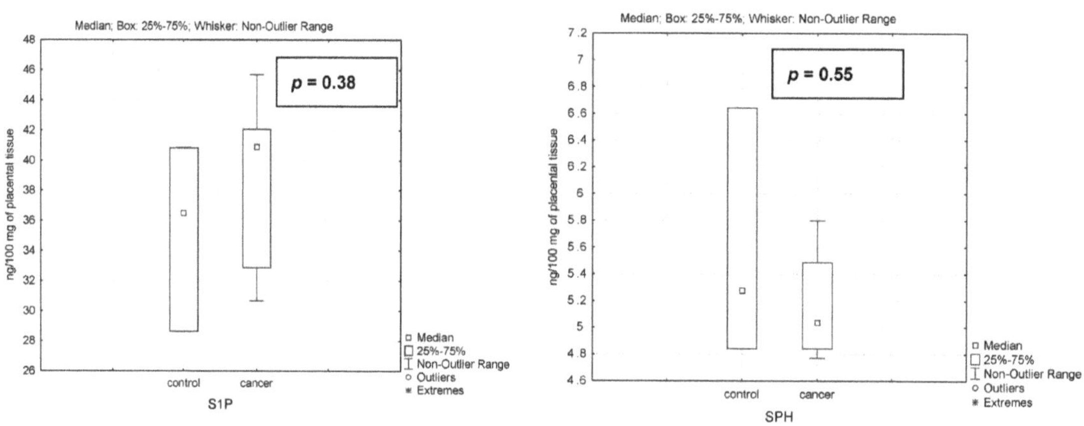

(a) (b)

Figure 7. Level of sphingosine-1-phosphate (S1P) (**a**) and sphingosine (SPH) (**b**) in the placenta of healthy pregnant women (control) and women with pregnancy-associated breast cancer after chemotherapy (cancer).

3.3.2. Analysis of Sphingosine-1-Phosphate Receptors (S1PR1, S1PR2 and S1PR3) Gene Expression in Pregnancy-Associated Breast Cancer After Treatment

S1P can bind to one of five specific G protein-coupled cell surface S1P receptors (S1PR1-5). S1PR1 and S1PR3 have been linked to breast cancer progression. The SPHK1-S1PR1 axis has been shown to be altered in different localizations of cancer in multiple ways and therefore represents an attractive therapeutic target [45–48].

Our experiments show that the gene expression of these two receptors is significantly higher in patients with PABC undergoing treatment than in controls: *S1PR1* 3 times, $p = 0.01$; *S1PR2* 2.6 times, $p = 0.04$; and *S1PR3* 3.3 times, $p = 0.002$ (Figure 8).

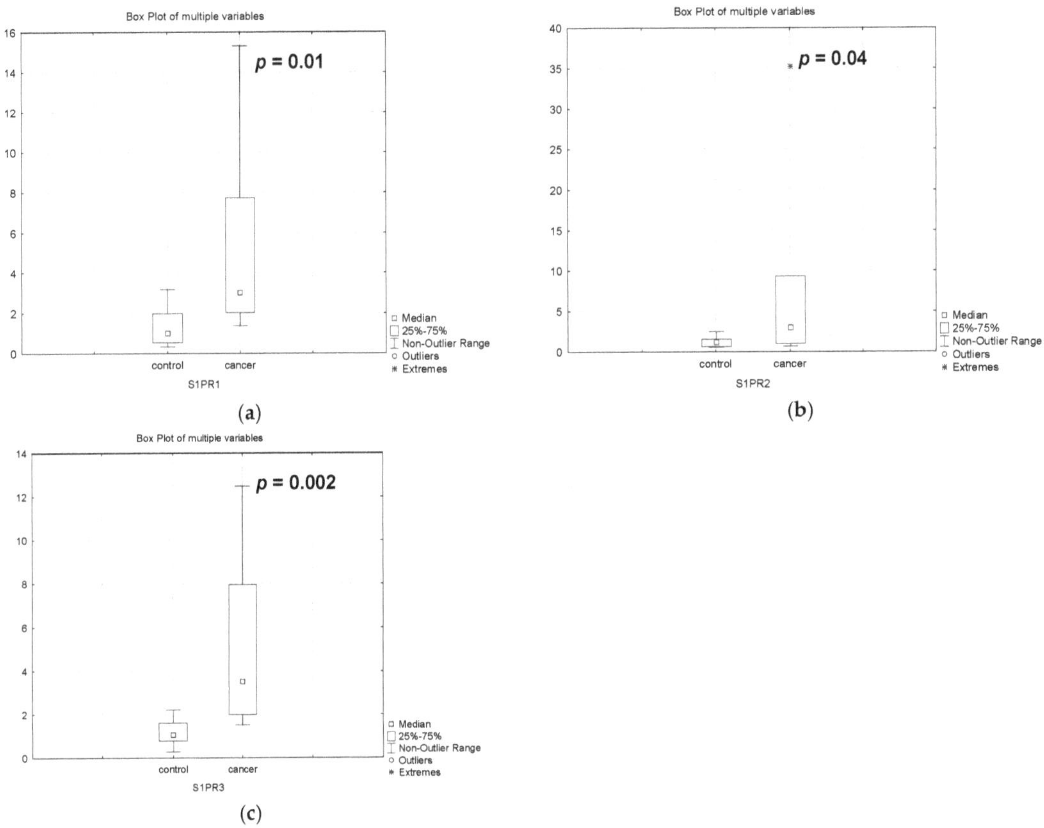

Figure 8. Gene expression of sphingosine-1-phosphate receptors in the placenta of healthy pregnant women (control) and women with pregnancy-associated breast cancer after chemotherapy (cancer): (**a**) *S1PR1*, (**b**) *S1PR2*, (**c**) *S1PR3*.

3.4. *The Effect of PABC and Therapy on the Newborn and Mother*

No differences were found between the healthy pregnant women and patients with PABC in the following obstetric parameters studied: newborn weight ($p = 0.23$), newborn height ($p = 0.28$), fetal percentile ($p = 0.54$), and placental weight ($p = 0.69$). Among the newborns in the group of patients with PABC, there was a higher frequency of pathological conditions in the early neonatal period; most newborns had a combination of several such conditions (5/7, 71.4%). However, no severe malformations were identified. Physiological birth tumor was observed in 3/7 (42.9%) newborns; jaundice in 2/7 (28.6%); anemia in 2/7 (28.6%); interatrial communication in 2/7 (28.6%) newborns; and thermoregulation disorder in 2/7 (28.6%). One of newborns in this group (1/7, 14.3%) was in a severe condition, accompanied by depression of the central nervous system and respiratory distress syndrome, anemia, the presence of a patent ductus arteriosus, and interatrial communication. This condition might have been due to premature labor at 36 weeks and 3 days. In children from women with PABC after chemotherapy in 1/7 (14.3%) cases, a "felt hat" type of ossification of the skull bones was recorded. In 1/7 (14.3%) cases, the newborn had rhinitis, otitis, and toxic erythema.

In children from the group of healthy pregnant women, only a birth tumor was observed in 2/7 (28.6%) newborns (Table 4). No differences were found in this parameter between the groups of newborns from healthy pregnant women and women with PABC ($p = 0.46$).

Table 4. Pathological conditions in newborns in groups of healthy pregnant women and patients with PABC (pregnancy-associated breast cancer).

Number of Patient	Pathological Condition	Number of Pathological Conditions in the Newborn
BC1		2
BC2	Physiological birth tumor, Rash on face	4
BC3	Toxic erythema, rhinitis, otitis, jaundice	4
BC4	Interatrial communication, thermoregulation disorder, asymmetry of the sizes of the lateral ventricles of the brain, birth tumor	1
	Ossification disorder of the skull bones	
BC5	Serious condition, respiratory distress syndrome, central nervous system depression, patent ductus arteriosus, interatrial communication, thermoregulation disorder, anemia	7
	No	
BC6	Jaundice, anemia, physiological birth tumor	0
BC7	No	3
C1	No	0
C2	No	0
C3	Physiological birth tumor	0
C4	No	1
C5	Physiological birth tumor	0
C6	No	1
C7	No	0
C8		0

Note: BC (breast cancer)—pregnancy-associated breast cancer (PABC) patients; C (control)—healthy pregnant women.

Thus, the frequency of pathological conditions differed in newborns of the PABC group (median M = three pathologies in the newborn) from newborns in the group of healthy pregnant women (median M = zero pathologies in the newborn, $p = 0.009$).

We excluded from the analysis physiological birth tumors as an insignificant condition, often considered a normal variant, and jaundice, which is characteristic of the physiological process of a child's adaptation to a new environment and is often observed in the neonatal period as a norm. Differences between groups in the frequency of pathological conditions in newborns remained, median M = 1 in women with PABC and M = 0 in healthy pregnant women, $p = 0.0001$.

It should be taken into account that healthy patients without any serious acute or chronic diseases before and during pregnancy were selected as the control group. In the general population of Russia, the incidence of neonatal pathological conditions is observed in 43.1% of children [49]. In our work, they were detected in 6/7 (86%) newborns in the PABC group. However, the spectrum of pathologies detected did not allow for their classification as severe conditions, with the exception of the child of patient BC5. According to the literature, children of patients with PABC are characterized by fetal growth restriction, premature labor, low birth weight, stillbirth, and increased neonatal mortality [50]. In our work, from the listed conditions above, only premature labor was observed in 3/7 patients with PABC (42.9%), which was not revealed in the group of healthy pregnant women, $p = 0.020$.

Thus, in the PABC group, no increase in the incidence of severe neonatal pathologies was detected, but an increase in the incidence of premature labor was observed. However, at this stage, it is impossible to assert if this was an effect of chemotherapy. More extensive studies are needed due to the fact that premature labor is a common obstetric complication of pregnancy [51,52].

During further follow-up over 12 months, the subsequent growth and development of children born from mothers with PABC proceeded without any special features. All of the children had no health problems at the time of the cut-off. Among the mothers in the PABC group, two of them (BC4, BC5) showed progression of the disease, whereas the rest were in remission after one year of follow-up. Patient BC4 had metastases in the brain. Patient BC5's had rapidly progressing, multiple distant metastases in the liver, lungs, and pleura, in addition to greater omentum.

The data available at this stage are insufficient to assess the association between the expression of sphingomyelin metabolism genes in the placenta and the effectiveness of the treatment of PABC. This requires clarifying the commonality of sphingolipid metabolism in the body of pregnant women and the admissibility of extrapolating expression data in the placenta to the body level.

In the PABC group, cytotoxic chemotherapy was used, with 5/7 (71.4%) patients receiving doxorubicin in the chemotherapy regimen. No association was found between the presence of doxorubicin in the chemotherapy regimen and the following obstetric parameters: newborn weight ($p = 0.28$), newborn height ($p = 0.18$), fetal percentile ($p = 0.74$), placental weight ($p = 0.73$), and placental percentile ($p = 0.20$). Patients who did not receive doxorubicin had lower levels of CERS4 and SMPD3 gene expression in the placenta. For the CERS4 gene, the median expression in the group receiving doxorubicin was two-fold higher compared to patients who did not receive this drug, $p = 0.021$. For the SMPD3 gene, expression in the doxorubicin group increased by 12.7 times; however, differences were observed at the trend level, $p = 0.071$.

4. Discussion

Since the aim of our study was to determine the role of sphingolipid metabolism genes and the products that control proliferation, apoptosis, and the efficacy of cancer chemotherapy by changing their expression level in the placenta of pregnant women against the background of malignant neoplasm development, we examined changes in the expression of key genes of CER and S1P metabolism and its level, which may play an important role both in the development of oncology and pregnancy. In addition, they reflect the efficacy of chemotherapy and signal the emergence of resistance to many drugs used to treat cancers of various localizations. The S1P/CER ratio determines cell fate because S1P is protective, as opposed to long-chain CERs (C16:0-C24:0) that are generally cytotoxic and pro-apoptotic [46].

The expression of acidic and neutral sphingomyelinase genes produces CERs from sphingomyelins. CERs are also produced through de novo synthesis in the endoplasmic reticulum. CERs can also be metabolized by acidic, alkaline, and neutral ceramidases to yield sphingosine [47], which is then phosphorylated by SPHK to produce S1P.

Since S1P is formed as a product of CER metabolism, the S1P/CER ratio is highly dependent on the level and activity of enzymes regulating S1P and CER turnover. The expression of enzymes synthesizing and degrading S1P controls its levels in the placenta, and decidua in normal pregnancy is positively correlated with increasing gestational age [18,20]. This suggests an increase in S1P turnover with the course of pregnancy, but whether S1P levels in the placenta change with increasing gestational age remains unknown. In complicated pregnancy, the expression of placental S1P-producing enzymes is decreased, and S1P-degrading enzymes is increased.

Because S1P acts in balance with CERs, their ratio determines cell fate and function in the placenta [18]. CERs induce apoptosis, and high levels of circulating CERs are often associated with pregnancy pathologies [18]. Current evidence suggests that S1P and CERs are promising for being considered strong candidates for both diagnosis and therapy in future studies. Sphingolipids also reflect the development of malignant neoplasms [4,6,7,26,36,45,48].

In our case, we paid special attention to patients with PABC, which is the most frequent of all pregnancy-associated cancers. Moreover, breast cancer is the first cause of cancer mortality and incidence among women. We found significant changes in the expression levels of genes controlling CER and S1P synthesis in pregnant patients treated with chemotherapy for breast cancer. The expression levels of sphingomyelinases and ceramide synthases, responsible for the level of CER content in the placenta, dramatically increased.

Mass-spectrometric analysis of CERs showed unchanged levels in groups of healthy pregnant women and patients with PABC. Activation of sphingomyelinase, sphingomyelin synthase, and ceramidase gene expression can lead to the synthesis of corresponding enzymes with opposite properties that can be activated. It is this process that may keep CER levels in patients with PABC at control levels. It is possible that through this mechanism the placenta protects the fetus from the toxic effects of chemotherapeutic agents. We plan to investigate this question in the future.

The expression of the *SGPL* gene is dramatically increased during chemotherapy of patients with PABC. However, we also found a dramatic increase in *SPHK1* gene expression in patients with PABC undergoing treatment compared to healthy patients. Thus, we showed that the genes of two enzymes with opposite properties in the process of S1P metabolism are activated in the placenta of pregnant women with breast cancer after chemotherapy compared to healthy pregnant women. It is these processes that can explain the maintenance of S1P content in these patients at the same level as in healthy women. In other words, our experiments show that in the placenta of pregnant women with breast cancer after chemotherapy, the balance of CERs and S1P, characteristic of healthy pregnant women, is preserved.

The special role of S1P is determined by the fact that it can bind to one of five specific S1P receptors on the cell surface. Two receptors, S1PR1 and S1PR3, are associated with breast cancer progression. The SphK1/S1P/S1PR axis in breast cancer cells promotes their growth, survival, dissemination and metastasis. It is also usually accompanied by increased chemotherapeutic resistance [31]. In our experiments, we found increased expression of *S1PR1* and *S1PR3* in the placenta of women with PABC after chemotherapy. These results may indicate the development of resistance to the drugs used to treat breast cancer. However, at this stage of our studies, which are pilot studies, we cannot answer this question. Nevertheless, such significant changes in the expression of genes controlling the level of CERs, sphingosine, and S1P may indicate their ability to initiate the metabolism of pro-apoptotic and anti-apoptotic sphingolipids in the placenta of pregnant women with cancer undergoing chemotherapy in order to maintain levels typical of the placenta of healthy women. This hypothesis is supported by the fact that in the PABC patient group, no increase in the incidence of severe neonatal pathologies was detected. During monitoring over 12 months, the subsequent growth and development of children born from mothers with PABC proceeded without any special features, and all children had no health problems.

In conclusion, we may note that our results may indicate the promising mechanism of protection by placenta during the chemotherapy of pregnant women with breast cancer and, consequently, of newborns. This effect of protection by the placenta, especially, for the newborn has been discovered for the first time and requires more careful study.

Author Contributions: Conceptualization, A.A. and T.Z.; methodology, T.Z. and V.B.; formal analysis, M.K., V.B., V.K., M.S. and U.G.; investigation, V.K., M.K., V.B., E.K., E.L., D.B., M.S., U.G. and P.L.; writing—original draft preparation, A.A. and T.Z.; writing—review and editing, T.Z.; visualization, T.Z., M.K., U.G. and M.S.; supervision, S.K. and A.A. All authors have read and agreed to the published version of the manuscript.

Funding: This research was supported by Ministry of Science and Higher Education of the Russian Federation (№ 122041400080-0).

Institutional Review Board Statement: This study was conducted in accordance with the Declaration of Helsinki and was approved by the Biomedical Research Ethics Committee of Kulakov National Medical Research Center of Obstetrics, Gynecology and Perinatology of the Ministry of Health of Russia (Protocol №4, 29 April 2021).

Informed Consent Statement: Informed consent was obtained from all the subjects involved in this study.

Data Availability Statement: The data presented in this study are available on reasonable request from the corresponding author.

Acknowledgments: The LC/MS analysis of lipids was carried out using the equipment of the Core Shared Research Facility «Industrial Biotechnologies» of Federal Research Center «Fundamentals of Biotechnology», Russian Academy of Sciences.

Conflicts of Interest: The authors declare no conflicts of interest.

Abbreviations

ASAH1	acid ceramidase
GBA	glucosylceramidase
CDase	ceramidase
CER	ceramide
CER + DTX	CER in combination with docetaxel
C1P	ceramide-1-phosphate
CERS 1–6	ceramide synthases
DTX	docetaxel
FTY720	fingolimod
GCS	glucosylceramide synthase
MCF-7	human breast carcinoma cell
MRM	multiple reaction monitoring
PABC	pregnancy-associated breast cancer
S1P	sphingosine-1-phosphate
SPH	sphingosine
SGPL1	sphingosine-1-phosphate lyase 1
SMPD1	acidic sphingomyelinase
SMPD3	neutral sphingomyelinase
SMS	sphingomyelin synthase
SPHK1	sphingosine kinase1

References

1. Alkafaas, S.S.; Elsalahaty, M.I.; Ismail, D.F.; Radwan, M.A.; Elkafas, S.S.; Loutfy, S.A.; Elshazli, R.M.; Baazaoui, N.; Ahmed, A.E.; Hafez, W.; et al. The Emerging Roles of Sphingosine 1-Phosphate and SphK1 in Cancer Resistance: A Promising Therapeutic Target. *Cancer Cell Int.* **2024**, *24*, 89. [CrossRef] [PubMed]
2. Li, R.-Z.; Wang, X.-R.; Wang, J.; Xie, C.; Wang, X.-X.; Pan, H.-D.; Meng, W.-Y.; Liang, T.-L.; Li, J.-X.; Yan, P.-Y.; et al. The Key Role of Sphingolipid Metabolism in Cancer: New Therapeutic Targets, Diagnostic and Prognostic Values, and Anti-Tumor Immunotherapy Resistance. *Front. Oncol.* **2022**, *12*, 941643. [CrossRef] [PubMed]
3. Liu, Y.; Han, T.; Giuliano, A.E.; Cabot, M.C. Ceramide Glycosylation Potentiates Cellular Multidrug Resistance. *FASEB J.* **2001**, *15*, 719–730. [CrossRef] [PubMed]
4. Lin, M.; Li, Y.; Wang, S.; Cao, B.; Li, C.; Li, G. Sphingolipid Metabolism and Signaling in Lung Cancer: A Potential Therapeutic Target. *J. Oncol.* **2022**, *2022*, 9099612. [CrossRef]
5. Noda, S.; Yoshimura, S.; Sawada, M.; Naganawa, T.; Iwama, T.; Nakashima, S.; Sakai, N. Role of Ceramide during Cisplatin-Induced Apoptosis in C6 Glioma Cells. *J. Neuro-Oncol.* **2001**, *52*, 11–21. [CrossRef]

6. Pherez-Farah, A.; López-Sánchez, R.D.C.; Villela-Martínez, L.M.; Ortiz-López, R.; Beltrán, B.E.; Hernández-Hernández, J.A. Sphingolipids and Lymphomas: A Double-Edged Sword. *Cancers* **2022**, *14*, 2051. [CrossRef]
7. Piazzesi, A.; Afsar, S.Y.; Van Echten-Deckert, G. Sphingolipid Metabolism in the Development and Progression of Cancer: One Cancer's Help Is Another's Hindrance. *Mol. Oncol.* **2021**, *15*, 3256–3279. [CrossRef]
8. Pitman, M.; Oehler, M.K.; Pitson, S.M. Sphingolipids as Multifaceted Mediators in Ovarian Cancer. *Cell. Signal.* **2021**, *81*, 109949. [CrossRef]
9. Zhou, S.; Sun, L.; Mao, F.; Chen, J. Sphingolipids in Prostate Cancer Prognosis: Integrating Single-Cell and Bulk Sequencing. *Aging* **2024**, *16*, 8031. [CrossRef]
10. Hannun, Y.A.; Obeid, L.M. Principles of Bioactive Lipid Signalling: Lessons from Sphingolipids. *Nat. Rev. Mol. Cell Biol.* **2008**, *9*, 139–150. [CrossRef]
11. Clarke, C.J. Neutral Sphingomyelinases in Cancer: Friend or Foe? In *Advances in Cancer Research*; Elsevier: Amsterdam, The Netherlands, 2018; Volume 140, pp. 97–119, ISBN 978-0-12-814223-3.
12. Datta, A.; Loo, S.Y.; Huang, B.; Wong, L.; Tan, S.S.L.; Tan, T.Z.; Lee, S.-C.; Thiery, J.P.; Lim, Y.C.; Yong, W.P.; et al. SPHK1 Regulates Proliferation and Survival Responses in Triple-Negative Breast Cancer. *Oncotarget* **2014**, *5*, 5920–5933. [CrossRef] [PubMed]
13. Hertervig, E.; Nilsson, A.; Nyberg, L.; Duan, R.D. Alkaline Sphingomyelinase Activity Is Decreased in Human Colorectal Carcinoma. *Cancer* **1997**, *3*, 448–453. [CrossRef]
14. Jacobi, J.; García-Barros, M.; Rao, S.; Rotolo, J.A.; Thompson, C.; Mizrachi, A.; Feldman, R.; Manova, K.; Bielawska, A.; Bielawska, J.; et al. Targeting Acid Sphingomyelinase with Anti-Angiogenic Chemotherapy. *Cell. Signal.* **2017**, *29*, 52–61. [CrossRef] [PubMed]
15. Nagahashi, M.; Miyoshi, Y. Targeting Sphingosine-1-Phosphate Signaling in Breast Cancer. Available online: https://www.mdpi.com/1422-0067/25/6/3354 (accessed on 4 September 2024).
16. Chen, H.; Haddadi, N.; Zhu, X.; Hatoum, D.; Chen, S.; Nassif, N.T.; Lin, Y.; McGowan, E.M. Expression Profile of Sphingosine Kinase 1 Isoforms in Human Cancer Tissues and Cells: Importance and Clinical Relevance of the Neglected 1b-Isoform. *J. Oncol.* **2022**, *2022*, 2250407. [CrossRef]
17. Gao, Y.; Gao, F.; Chen, K.; Tian, M.; Zhao, D. Sphingosine Kinase 1 as an Anticancer Therapeutic Target. *Drug Des. Dev. Ther.* **2015**, *9*, 3239–3245. [CrossRef]
18. Fakhr, Y.; Brindley, D.N.; Hemmings, D.G. Physiological and Pathological Functions of Sphingolipids in Pregnancy. *Cell. Signal.* **2021**, *85*, 110041. [CrossRef]
19. Huang, Q.; Hao, S.; Yao, X.; You, J.; Li, X.; Lai, D.; Han, C.; Schilling, J.; Hwa, K.Y.; Thyparambil, S.; et al. High-Throughput Quantitation of Serological Ceramides/Dihydroceramides by LC/MS/MS: Pregnancy Baseline Biomarkers and Potential Metabolic Messengers. *J. Pharm. Biomed. Anal.* **2021**, *192*, 113639. [CrossRef]
20. Yamamoto, Y.; Olson, D.M.; Bennekom, M.V.; Brindley, D.N.; Hemmings, D.G. Increased Expression of Enzymes for Sphingosine 1-Phosphate Turnover and Signaling in Human Decidua During Late Pregnancy1. *Biol. Reprod.* **2010**, *82*, 628–635. [CrossRef]
21. Apicella, C.; Ruano, C.S.M.; Thilaganathan, B.; Khalil, A.; Giorgione, V.; Gascoin, G.; Marcellin, L.; Gaspar, C.; Jacques, S.; Murdoch, C.E.; et al. Pan-Genomic Regulation of Gene Expression in Normal and Pathological Human Placentas. *Cells* **2023**, *12*, 578. [CrossRef]
22. Suryawanshi, H.; Max, K.; Bogardus, K.A.; Sopeyin, A.; Chang, M.S.; Morozov, P.; Castano, P.M.; Tuschl, T.; Williams, Z. Dynamic Genome-Wide Gene Expression and Immune Cell Composition in the Developing Human Placenta. *J. Reprod. Immunol.* **2022**, *151*, 103624. [CrossRef]
23. Saben, J.; Zhong, Y.; McKelvey, S.; Dajani, N.K.; Andres, A.; Badger, T.M.; Gomez-Acevedo, H.; Shankar, K. A Comprehensive Analysis of the Human Placenta Transcriptome. *Placenta* **2014**, *35*, 125–131. [CrossRef] [PubMed]
24. Mikheev, A.M.; Nabekura, T.; Kaddoumi, A.; Bammler, T.K.; Govindarajan, R.; Hebert, M.F.; Unadkat, J.D. Profiling Gene Expression in Human Placentae of Different Gestational Ages: An OPRU Network and UW SCOR Study. *Reprod. Sci.* **2008**, *15*, 866–877. [CrossRef] [PubMed]
25. Alexander, S.; Alexander, H. Lead Genetic Studies in Dictyostelium Discoideum and Translational Studies in Human Cells Demonstrate That Sphingolipids Are Key Regulators of Sensitivity to Cisplatin and Other Anticancer Drugs. *Semin. Cell Dev. Biol.* **2011**, *22*, 97–104. [CrossRef] [PubMed]
26. Gomez-Larrauri, A.; Das Adhikari, U.; Aramburu-Nuñez, M.; Custodia, A.; Ouro, A. Ceramide Metabolism Enzymes—Therapeutic Targets against Cancer. *Medicina* **2021**, *57*, 729. [CrossRef] [PubMed]
27. Lee, S.-C.; Xu, X.; Lim, Y.-W.; Iau, P.; Sukri, N.; Lim, S.-E.; Yap, H.L.; Yeo, W.-L.; Tan, P.; Tan, S.-H.; et al. Chemotherapy-Induced Tumor Gene Expression Changes in Human Breast Cancers. *Pharmacogenetics Genom.* **2009**, *19*, 181–192. [CrossRef] [PubMed]
28. Min, J.; Stegner, A.L.; Alexander, H.; Alexander, S. Overexpression of Sphingosine-1-Phosphate Lyase or Inhibition of Sphingosine Kinase in *Dictyostelium Discoideum* Results in a Selective Increase in Sensitivity to Platinum-Based Chemotherapy Drugs. *Eukaryot. Cell* **2004**, *3*, 795–805. [CrossRef] [PubMed]
29. Prinetti, A.; Millimaggi, D.; D'Ascenzo, S.; Clarkson, M.; Bettiga, A.; Chigorno, V.; Sonnino, S.; Pavan, A.; Dolo, V. Lack of Ceramide Generation and Altered Sphingolipid Composition Are Associated with Drug Resistance in Human Ovarian Carcinoma Cells. *Biochem. J.* **2006**, *395*, 311–318. [CrossRef] [PubMed]

30. Sattar, R.S.A.; Sumi, M.P.; Kumar, A.; Sharma, A.K.; Ahmad, E.; Ali, A.; Mahajan, B.; Saluja, S.S. S1P Signaling, Its Interactions and Cross-Talks with Other Partners and Therapeutic Importance in Colorectal Cancer. *Cell. Signal.* **2021**, *86*, 110080. [CrossRef] [PubMed]
31. Lifshitz, V.; Priceman, S.J.; Li, W.; Cherryholmes, G.; Lee, H.; Makovski-Silverstein, A.; Borriello, L.; DeClerck, Y.A.; Yu, H. Sphingosine-1-Phosphate Receptor-1 Promotes Environment-Mediated and Acquired Chemoresistance. *Mol. Cancer Ther.* **2017**, *16*, 2516–2527. [CrossRef] [PubMed]
32. Singh, S.K.; Spiegel, S. Sphingosine-1-Phosphate Signaling: A Novel Target for Simultaneous Adjuvant Treatment of Triple Negative Breast Cancer and Chemotherapy-Induced Neuropathic Pain. *Adv. Biol. Regul.* **2020**, *75*, 100670. [CrossRef] [PubMed]
33. Das, M. GM1 for Taxane-Induced Neuropathy in Breast Cancer. *Lancet Oncol.* **2019**, *20*, e348. [CrossRef] [PubMed]
34. Feng, L.-X.; Li, M.; Liu, Y.-J.; Yang, S.-M.; Zhang, N. Synergistic Enhancement of Cancer Therapy Using a Combination of Ceramide and Docetaxel. *Int. J. Mol. Sci.* **2014**, *15*, 4201–4220. [CrossRef] [PubMed]
35. Byrne, F.L.; Olzomer, E.M.; Lolies, N.; Hoehn, K.L.; Wegner, M.-S. Update on Glycosphingolipids Abundance in Hepatocellular Carcinoma. *Int. J. Mol. Sci.* **2022**, *23*, 4477. [CrossRef] [PubMed]
36. Saddoughi, S.A.; Gencer, S.; Peterson, Y.K.; Ward, K.E.; Mukhopadhyay, A.; Oaks, J.; Bielawski, J.; Szulc, Z.M.; Thomas, R.J.; Selvam, S.P.; et al. Sphingosine Analogue Drug FTY720 Targets I2PP2A/SET and Mediates Lung Tumour Suppression via Activation of PP2A-RIPK1-dependent Necroptosis. *EMBO Mol. Med.* **2013**, *5*, 105–121. [CrossRef] [PubMed]
37. Azuma, H.; Takahara, S.; Horie, S.; Muto, S.; Otsuki, Y.; Katsuoka, Y. Induction of Apoptosis in Human Bladder Cancer Cells In Vitro and In Vivo Caused by FTY720 Treatment. *J. Urol.* **2003**, *169*, 2372–2377. [CrossRef] [PubMed]
38. Azuma, H.; Takahara, S.; Ichimaru, N.; Wang, J.D.; Itoh, Y.; Otsuki, Y.; Morimoto, J.; Fukui, R.; Hoshiga, M.; Ishihara, T.; et al. Marked Prevention of Tumor Growth and Metastasis by a Novel Immunosuppressive Agent, FTY720, in Mouse Breast Cancer Models. *Cancer Res.* **2002**, *62*, 1410–1419.
39. Hait, N.C.; Avni, D.; Yamada, A.; Nagahashi, M.; Aoyagi, T.; Aoki, H.; Dumur, C.I.; Zelenko, Z.; Gallagher, E.J.; Leroith, D.; et al. The Phosphorylated Prodrug FTY720 Is a Histone Deacetylase Inhibitor That Reactivates ERα Expression and Enhances Hormonal Therapy for Breast Cancer. *Oncogenesis* **2015**, *4*, e156. [CrossRef]
40. Hait, N.C.; Allegood, J.; Maceyka, M.; Strub, G.M.; Harikumar, K.B.; Singh, S.K.; Luo, C.; Marmorstein, R.; Kordula, T.; Milstien, S.; et al. Regulation of Histone Acetylation in the Nucleus by Sphingosine-1-Phosphate. *Science* **2009**, *325*, 1254–1257. [CrossRef]
41. Lim, K.G.; Tonelli, F.; Li, Z.; Lu, X.; Bittman, R.; Pyne, S.; Pyne, N.J. FTY720 Analogues as Sphingosine Kinase 1 Inhibitors: Enzyme Inhibition Kinetics, Allosterism, Proteasomal Degradation, and Actin Rearrangement in MCF-7 Breast Cancer Cells. *J. Biol. Chem.* **2011**, *286*, 18633–18640. [CrossRef]
42. Bligh, E.G.; Dyer, W.J. A rapid method of total lipid extraction and purification. *Can. J. Biochem. Physiol.* **1959**, *37*, 911–917. [CrossRef]
43. Molino, S.; Tate, E.; McKillop, W.; Medin, J. Sphingolipid Pathway Enzymes Modulate Cell Fate and Immune Responses. *Immunotherapy* **2017**, *9*, 1185–1198. [CrossRef] [PubMed]
44. Pyne, N.J.; El Buri, A.; Adams, D.R.; Pyne, S. Sphingosine 1-Phosphate and Cancer. *Adv. Biol. Regul.* **2018**, *68*, 97–106. [CrossRef] [PubMed]
45. Pyne, N.J.; McNaughton, M.; Boomkamp, S.; MacRitchie, N.; Evangelisti, C.; Martelli, A.M.; Jiang, H.-R.; Ubhi, S.; Pyne, S. Role of Sphingosine 1-Phosphate Receptors, Sphingosine Kinases and Sphingosine in Cancer and Inflammation. *Adv. Biol. Regul.* **2016**, *60*, 151–159. [CrossRef] [PubMed]
46. Pettus, B.J.; Chalfant, C.E.; Hannun, Y.A. Ceramide in Apoptosis: An Overview and Current Perspectives. *Biochim. Biophys. Acta* **2002**, *1585*, 114–125. [CrossRef]
47. Hannun, Y.A.; Obeid, L.M. Many Ceramides. *J. Biol. Chem.* **2011**, *286*, 27855–27862. [CrossRef]
48. Pyne, N.J.; Tonelli, F.; Lim, K.G.; Long, J.S.; Edwards, J.; Pyne, S. Sphingosine 1-Phosphate Signalling in Cancer. *Biochem. Soc. Trans.* **2012**, *40*, 94–100. [CrossRef]
49. Healthcare in Russia. *Statistical Book*; Rosstat: Moscow, Russia, 2023.
50. Margioula-Siarkou, G.; Margioula-Siarkou, C.; Petousis, S.; Vavoulidis, E.; Margaritis, K.; Almperis, A.; Haitoglou, C.; Mavromatidis, G.; Dinas, K. Breast Carcinogenesis during Pregnancy: Molecular Mechanisms, Maternal and Fetal Adverse Outcomes. *Biology* **2023**, *12*, 408. [CrossRef]
51. Ohuma, E.O.; Moller, A.-B.; Bradley, E.; Chakwera, S.; Hussain-Alkhateeb, L.; Lewin, A.; Okwaraji, Y.B.; Mahanani, W.R.; Johansson, E.W.; Lavin, T.; et al. National, Regional, and Global Estimates of Preterm Birth in 2020, with Trends from 2010: A Systematic Analysis. *Lancet* **2023**, *402*, 1261–1271. [CrossRef]
52. Perin, J.; Mulick, A.; Yeung, D.; Villavicencio, F.; Lopez, G.; Strong, K.L.; Prieto-Merino, D.; Cousens, S.; Black, R.E.; Liu, L. Global, Regional, and National Causes of under-5 Mortality in 2000–19: An Updated Systematic Analysis with Implications for the Sustainable Development Goals. *Lancet Child Adolesc. Health* **2022**, *6*, 106–115. [CrossRef]

biomedicines

Article

Prognostic Significance and Treatment Response Associations of Genetic Mutations in Chronic Myelomonocytic Leukemia: A Retrospective Cohort Study

Jing Di [1,*], Leonard N. Yenwongfai [1,2], Talal Arshad [1], Bin Huang [3,4], Jaclyn K. McDowell [4], Eric B. Durbin [5], Reinhold Munker [6,†] and Sainan Wei [1,*]

1 Department of Pathology & Laboratory Medicine, University of Kentucky, Lexington, KY 40536, USA
2 Department of Pathology, The Johns Hopkins University School of Medicine, Baltimore, MD 21205, USA
3 Division of Cancer Biostatistics, University of Kentucky, Lexington, KY 40536, USA
4 Markey Cancer Center, Cancer Research Informatics Shared Resource Facility, University of Kentucky, Lexington, KY 40536, USA
5 Kentucky Cancer Registry, Lexington, KY 40504, USA
6 Division of Hematology, Blood and Marrow Transplantation, University of Kentucky, Lexington, KY 40536, USA; rmunker@uky.edu
* Correspondence: jingdi2015@gmail.com (J.D.); swe253@uky.edu (S.W.)
† Senior author.

Abstract: Background: This retrospective cohort study investigates the prognostic significance of genetic mutations in Chronic Myelomonocytic Leukemia (CMML) and their association with treatment responses among patients treated at a single institution, juxtaposed with a statewide dataset from Kentucky. **Methods:** The study includes 51 patients diagnosed with CMML under the World Health Organization criteria from January 2005 to December 2023. It examines their genomic profiles and subsequent survival outcomes. The analysis also categorizes patients into CMML-1 and CMML-2 subtypes and assesses survival differences between transformed and non-transformed cases. **Results:** Mutations in TET2, ASXL1, and SRSF2 were found to significantly influence survival, establishing their roles as critical prognostic markers. Additionally, the cohort from the University of Kentucky exhibited distinct survival patterns compared to the broader Kentucky state population, suggesting that demographic and treatment-related factors could underlie these variances. **Conclusions:** This research underscores the pivotal role of targeted genetic profiling in deciphering the progression of CMML and refining therapeutic strategies. The findings emphasize the necessity for advanced genetic screening in managing CMML to better understand individual prognoses and optimize treatment efficacy, thereby offering insights that could lead to personalized treatment approaches.

Keywords: chronic myelomonocytic leukemia; genetic profiling; prognostic biomarkers; survival analysis

1. Introduction

Chronic Myelomonocytic Leukemia (CMML) is an enigmatic clonal hematopoietic disorder that bridges myelodysplastic syndromes (MDS) and myeloproliferative neoplasms (MPN), manifesting a considerable risk of progression to acute myeloid leukemia (AML) within one and three years of diagnosis. Recent advancements in the diagnostic criteria of CMML have increasingly recognized the importance of molecular features in determining the prognosis of affected patients [1]. CMML is notably challenging due to its varied clinical presentations and outcomes, which are profoundly influenced by genetic abnormalities and the demographic characteristics of the patient population [1,2].

CMML is typically categorized into two subtypes based on the percentage of bone marrow blasts: CMML-1, which has less than 10% blasts, and CMML-2, which has 10–19% blasts or evidence of transformation to AML. Further stratification considers the disease's proliferative and dysplastic features [1]. The "proliferative" variant is characterized by higher white blood cell counts and an elevated risk of leukemic transformation, while the "dysplastic" variant exhibits more features of bone marrow failure. At the molecular level, mutations in genes such as TET2, ASXL1, and SRSF2 are frequently observed, and their presence is often linked to prognosis [3]. For instance, the ASXL1 mutation is associated with poorer outcomes and a higher risk of transformation to AML [1]. Understanding these variants is critical for personalized treatment strategies and improving patient outcomes.

Globally, research into CMML has revealed a spectrum of survival outcomes and responses to treatment, highlighting the role of geographic and ethnic factors in disease progression and management efficacy. Studies conducted across different regions—ranging from the United States to Europe and Asia—have documented significant disparities in median survival rates, which can be as varied as the populations themselves [3,4]. Such variations underscore the necessity for a deeper understanding of the biological and social determinants influencing CMML.

Kentucky, particularly the Appalachian region, is identified as a high-risk area for various cancers [2], suggesting a potential unique environmental or genetic interplay affecting disease characteristics and patient outcomes. Despite the progress in understanding the molecular underpinnings of CMML, patient outcomes remain dismal, with a median overall survival (OS) of only 17 months, as reported in a comprehensive population-based study from 2007–2011 [3].

Our study posits that Kentucky's distinct socio-environmental and genetic backdrop might influence both the mutation spectrum and survival outcomes in CMML. Focusing on a cohort from this high-risk region, our single-center study aims to delineate the correlation between specific gene mutations, overall survival, and the risk of AML transformation. Through this focused exploration, we seek to uncover potentially divergent disease phenotypes and inform targeted therapeutic strategies that could enhance patient outcomes in specific subpopulations.

2. Materials and Methods

2.1. Patient Population

This retrospective cohort study included 51 patients diagnosed with CMML at a single institution between January 2005 and December 2023. Patients were eligible if they met the World Health Organization's (WHO's) fifth edition of diagnostic criteria for CMML, had comprehensive testing, and had follow-up data available. The study was approved by the Institutional Review Board of the University of Kentucky.

2.2. Data Collection

Clinical data, including patient demographics, disease characteristics, treatment regimens, and clinical outcomes, were extracted from electronic medical records. The key variables collected were age at diagnosis, sex, white blood cell count, percentage of peripheral blood monocytes, hemoglobin levels, platelet count, bone marrow blast percentage, and cytogenetic abnormalities. Treatment regimens were classified into broad categories, including azacitidine-based, decitabine-based, hydroxyurea-based, combination therapy, and supportive care.

2.3. Genomic Profiling

Genomic DNA was extracted from bone marrow aspirates or peripheral blood samples at diagnosis. Next-generation sequencing (NGS) was performed using a panel of 97 genes, including 50 common myeloid focus genes such as TET2, ASXL1, SRSF2, EZH2, and TP53, known to be mutated in CMML. Variants were identified and annotated using standard bioinformatics pipelines, and only variants with a variant allele frequency (VAF) of $\geq$5% were considered for analysis.

2.4. Survival Analysis

Survival data, including overall survival (OS) and progression-free survival (PFS), were collected. OS was defined as the time from diagnosis to death from any cause, and PFS was defined as the time from diagnosis to disease progression. Patients were censored at the last follow-up if neither event had occurred. Kaplan–Meier survival curves were generated to estimate OS and PFS, and differences between groups were assessed using the log-rank test.

The survival analysis also includes Kaplan–Meier survival estimates from a broader statewide cohort of 254 CMML cases from the Kentucky Cancer Registry from 2012 to 2021. This enhancement allows for a direct comparison of localized hospital-based outcomes with broader statewide trends, offering insights into the generalizability and applicability of our findings.

2.5. Statistical Analysis

The impact of specific gene mutations on survival was analyzed using Kaplan–Meier estimates and log-rank tests to compare the survival distributions of patients with and without these mutations. To control the false discovery rate (FDR) across multiple hypothesis testing scenarios in our genetic analyses, we employed the Benjamini–Hochberg procedure. This method adjusts for multiple comparisons by controlling the FDR at a threshold of 5%, providing a robust means to limit type I error. This is especially pertinent given our study's extensive analysis of numerous genetic variants, ensuring that the reported associations are statistically significant and reducing the likelihood of false positives. A p-value of less than 0.05 was considered statistically significant. All statistical analyses were performed using Python (version 3.8) with relevant statistical libraries.

3. Results

3.1. Patient Demographics and Clinical Characteristics

A total of 51 patients with CMML from our center were included in this study. The cohort was divided into two groups: CMML-1 (n = 34) and CMML-2 (n = 17). A further category of patients (included in the group of 51 patients) undergoing AML transformation was analyzed (n = 14). The median age at diagnosis was 71 years (range: 35–88 years), with a predominance of male patients (71%). A previous or concomitant malignancy was diagnosed in 39% of the patients. Leukemic transformations occurred in 28% of the cohort. The median OS was significantly different between the groups, with 129 months for CMML-1, 29 months for CMML-2, and a significantly shorter survival for patients with CMML who went on to develop leukemic transformation ($p = 0.0077$) (Table 1).

3.2. Cytogenetic Analysis

The cytogenetic analysis revealed the following common abnormalities: monosomy 7, deletion 5q, trisomy 8, and complex karyotype (defined as three or more chromosomal abnormalities). Patients with monosomy 7 had a significantly shorter median OS than those without this abnormality. The median OS for patients with monosomy 7 was 14 months, while it was 42 months for those without ($p < 0.05$). Deletion 5q was observed in two patients. One patient had a survival of 15 months, and the other had a survival of 5 months. Both cases involved additional cytogenetic abnormalities. Due to the low number of cases, statistical analysis was not performed specifically for 5q deletions alone. Trisomy 8 was associated with significantly longer OS. The median OS for patients with trisomy 8 was 129.5 months compared to 44 months for those without ($p < 0.05$). Patients with a complex karyotype had the poorest survival outcomes. The median OS for these patients was 5 months compared to 45 months for patients with a normal karyotype or less complex abnormalities ($p < 0.01$).

Table 1. Clinical and genetic features and subsequent events in 51 patients with CMML.

Variable	CMML (n = 51)	CMML-1 (n = 34)	CMML-2 (n = 17)	*p*-Value
Age in years; median (range)	71 (35–88)	73 (35–88)	66 (53–80)	0.0647
Male; *n* (%)	36 (71)	25 (74)	11 (65)	0.532
Other malignancies; *n* (%) [a]	20 (39)	14 (41)	6 (35)	0.7672
Leukemic transformations; *n* (% LT)	14 (28)	4 (12)	10 (59)	0.0008
Overall survival; median months	42	129	29	0.0077
Genetic Analysis	**CMML (n = 36)**	**CMML-1 (n = 23)**	**CMML-2 (n = 13)**	**AML (n = 14)**
Epigenetic regulation analysis; n (%)				
TET2	16 (44)	12 (52)	4 (31)	3 (21)
ASXL1	15 (42)	8 (35)	7 (54)	8 (57)
DNMT3A	5 (14)	2 (9)	3 (23)	2 (14)
BCOR	2 (6)	0 (0)	2 (15)	2 (14)
EZH2	1 (3)	1 (4)	0 (0)	0 (0)
Spliceosome mutational analysis; n (%)				
SRSF2	10 (28)	6 (26)	4 (31)	4 (29)
ZRSR2	7 (19)	5 (22)	2 (15)	2 (14)
U2AF1	1 (3)	1 (4)	0 (0)	0 (0)
Cellular signaling analysis; n (%)				
NRAS	5 (14)	2 (9)	3 (23)	4 (29)
KRAS	3 (8)	1 (4)	2 (15)	2 (14)
CBL	1 (3)	1 (4)	0 (0)	0 (0)
FLT3	2 (6)	0 (0)	2 (15)	1 (7)
PTPN11	2 (6)	1 (4)	1 (8)	2 (14)
Other; n (%)				
RUNX1	12 (33)	7 (30)	5 (38)	6 (43)
SETBP1	2 (6)	0 (0)	2 (15)	2 (14)
NPM1	3 (8)	1 (4)	2 (15)	2 (14)

[a] Patients with other cancers: prostate cancer (3), breast cancer (3), non-Hodgkin lymphoma (2), multiple cancers (2), and treatment-related cancers (2). Note on treatment: no treatment (11 patients), hydroxyurea (11 patients), decitabine (12 patients), azacitidine (11 patients), venetoclax with demethylating agents (2 patients), and various other protocols (4 patients). Special cases include 2 patients with treatment-related CMML and 5 who underwent allogeneic transplantation.

3.3. Genetic Mutation Analysis

The analysis of genetic mutations related to epigenetic regulation revealed significant variability across the patient groups. The TET2 mutation was present in 44% of the overall CMML cohort, with the highest frequency observed in CMML-1 patients (52%), followed by CMML-2 (31%). Patients who later transformed had a lower rate of TET2 mutations (21%). ASXL1 mutations were found in 42% of the total cohort, showing notable frequencies of 35% in CMML-1, 54% in CMML-2, and 57% in the transformation cohort. DNMT3A mutations were detected in 14% of patients, with similar occurrences across CMML-1 (9%), CMML-2 (23%), and AML transformation (14%). EZH2 mutations were rare, observed in only 3% of the total cohort, and exclusively found in CMML-1 patients (4%) (see Table 1 and Figure 1).

Mutations affecting the spliceosome machinery also showed distinct patterns. The SRSF2 mutation was the most common spliceosome-related mutation, found in 28% of the overall cohort, with 26% in CMML-1, 31% in CMML-2, and 29% in AML transformation. The ZRSR2 mutation was present in 19% of patients, with frequencies of 22% in CMML-1, 15% in CMML-2, and 14% in AML transformation. U2AF1 mutations were rare, detected in only 3% of patients and exclusively in the CMML-1 group (4%) (see Table 1 and Figure 1).

The analysis of mutations in cellular signaling pathways and other genes revealed further variability. NRAS mutations were present in 14% of patients, with higher frequencies in CMML-2 (23%) and AML transformation (29%) compared to CMML-1 (9%). KRAS mutations were found in 8% of the cohort, with 4% in CMML-1, 15% in CMML-2, and 14%

in AML transformation. Other notable mutations included CBL (3% overall, detected only in CMML-1), FLT3, and PTPN11 (each 6% overall with variable frequencies). Among other genes, RUNX1 mutations were highly prevalent, detected in 33% of the total cohort, with higher frequencies in CMML-2 (38%) and cases that later transformed (43%) compared to CMML-1 (30%). SETBP1 mutations were found in 6% of patients across all groups. NPM1 mutations were present in 8% of the cohort, with similar frequencies across all groups (see Table 1 and Figure 1).

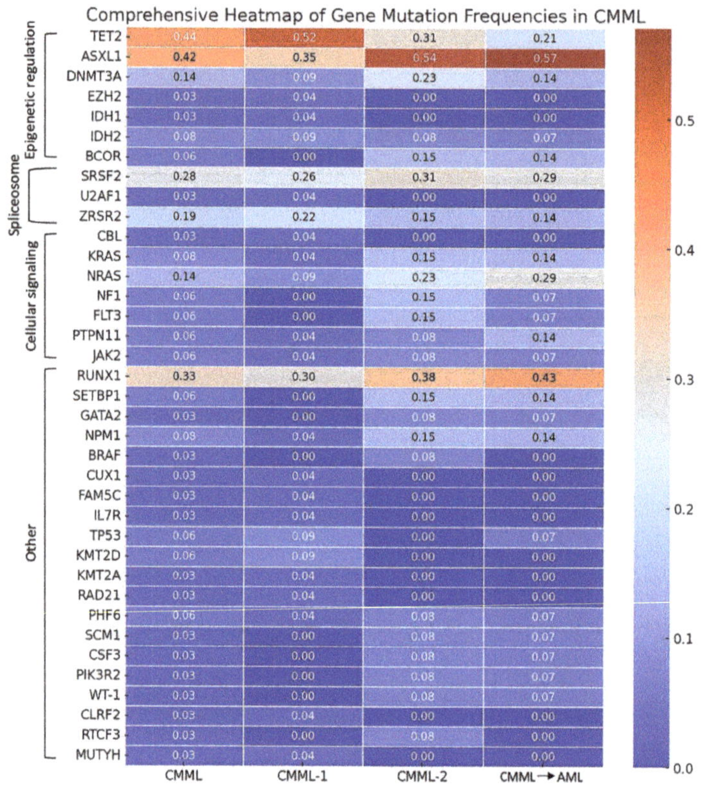

Figure 1. Heatmap of gene mutation frequencies in CMML. This heatmap illustrates the prevalence of various gene mutations across different stages and transformations of CMML. The data are categorized into three groups: CMML-1 (n = 23), CMML-2 (n = 13), and CMML, which later underwent transformation (n = 14), representing the progression stages of the disease.

3.4. Statistical Analysis of Mutation Frequencies

The statistical analysis comparing mutation frequencies between CMML-2 and the other stages (CMML-1 and AML transformation) revealed that the TET2 mutation showed a trend towards significance when compared with CMML-1 (p = 0.065). No gene mutations showed significant differences compared to CMML-2 and AML transformation stages. These results indicate the potential role of TET2 in transitioning from CMML-1 to CMML-2. However, further research with larger datasets is needed to confirm this trend and validate these findings.

3.5. Survival Analysis and Outcomes in CMML Patients as Retrieved from the Kentucky Cancer Registry

We expanded our analysis by incorporating statewide population data to construct Kaplan–Meier plots and life table estimates, examining survival probabilities within a geographically and demographically diverse patient cohort. This statewide data from 2012 to 2021 offers insights into potential variations in treatment outcomes and survival rates, stratified by gender and race, thereby enriching our understanding beyond our hospital-specific dataset (Figure 2A). The mean age in this cohort was 74 years (ranging from 47 to 97). The broader dataset revealed no significant differences in survival when stratified by gender, with a log-rank p-value of 0.0813, suggesting marginal disparities between male and female patients in survival times across Kentucky. Racial analysis indicated slight variances in survival probabilities between Black and White/other racial groups, though these differences were not statistically significant (log-rank $p = 0.0991$) (Figure 2B,C). Furthermore, analysis considering Appalachian status showed no significant survival difference between Appalachian and non-Appalachian populations (log-rank $p = 0.8042$), reinforcing the need to explore other social and biological determinants that may influence disease outcomes (Figure 2D). Finally, the age-adjusted incidence of CMML in Kentucky (0.49/100,00) was not different from that of the rest of the United States (0.50/100,000, $p = 0.596$), as estimated based on SEER 17 registry data [4].

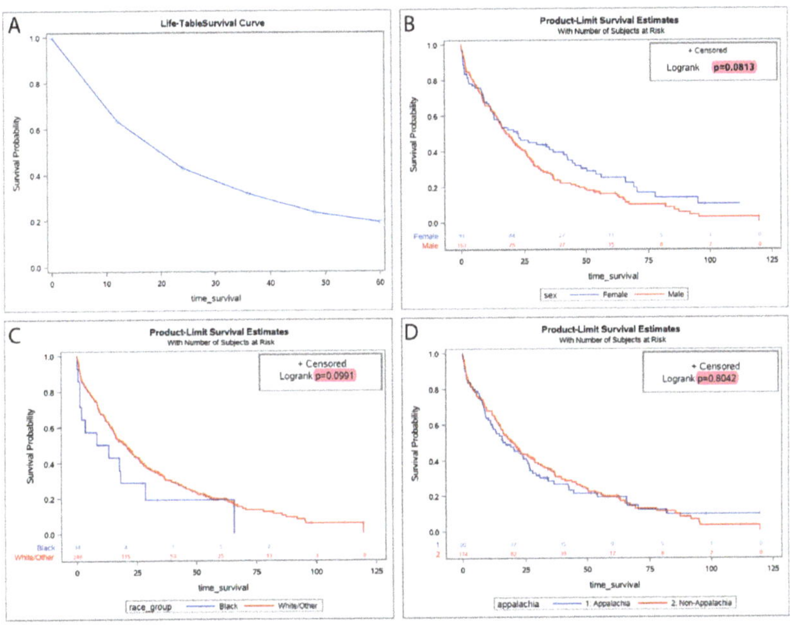

Figure 2. Kaplan–Meier survival estimates for CMML patients stratified by demographic and geographic variables. (**A**) Statewide Kaplan–Meier survival curves comparing localized hospital-based outcomes with broader statewide trends. (**B**) Survival analyses stratified by gender, highlighting potential differences in outcomes. (**C**) Survival analyses stratified by race provide insights into demographic influences on CMML outcomes. (**D**) Comparison of survival probabilities between patients in Appalachian versus non-Appalachian regions, assessing regional disparities in treatment outcomes.

Contrasting these findings with the Kaplan–Meier survival curves for CMML patients at the University of Kentucky, we observed pronounced differences in survival outcomes by clinical factors. The median OS for the University of Kentucky cohort was 42 months. Notably and not unexpectedly, there was a significant survival discrepancy between CMML-1 and CMML-2 subtypes, with median OS rates of 129 months and 29 months, respectively ($p = 0.0077$) (Figure 3A). Additionally, non-transformed patients at our institution displayed a median survival of 129 months, indicating superior outcomes compared to patients who later transformed, who had a median survival of 22 months ($p = 0.0006$) (Figure 3B). This disparity underscores the variance in disease progression and treatment response between the subtypes.

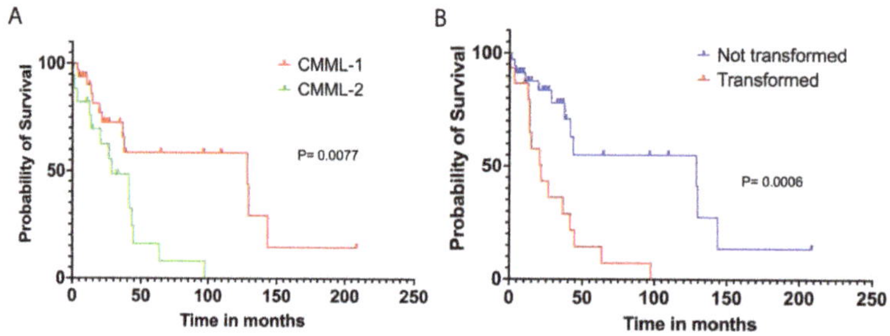

Figure 3. Kaplan–Meier survival curves for CMML patients at the University of Kentucky. (**A**) Survival probabilities between CMML-1 patients (red line) and CMML-2 patients (green line). (**B**) Survival probabilities for CMML patients, comparing those who have transformed (red line) versus those who have not (blue line). The p-values indicate the statistical significance of the differences in survival distributions ($p = 0.0006$ for transformation comparison, $p = 0.0077$ for subtype comparison).

In addition, the Kaplan–Meier survival analysis was employed to elucidate the impact of selected significant gene mutations on the survival outcomes of patients diagnosed with CMML. The analysis demonstrated that mutations in EZH2, TET2, ASXL1, SRSF2, RUNX1, TP53, NRAS, and FLT3 are associated with significantly decreased patient survival probabilities. Specifically, mutations in EZH2 ($p = 6.40 \times 10^{-8}$, TET2 ($p = 1.28 \times 10^{-3}$), ASXL1 ($p = 9.80 \times 10^{-8}$), SRSF2 ($p = 3.47 \times 10^{-5}$), RUNX1 ($p = 2.48 \times 10^{-7}$), TP53 ($p = 7.10 \times 10^{-8}$), NRAS ($p = 2.76 \times 10^{-9}$), and FLT3 ($p = 4.62 \times 10^{-8}$) were all linked to poorer survival outcomes compared to their respective wild-type counterparts (Figure 4). These findings suggest that these genetic alterations may serve as important prognostic markers in the studied cohort.

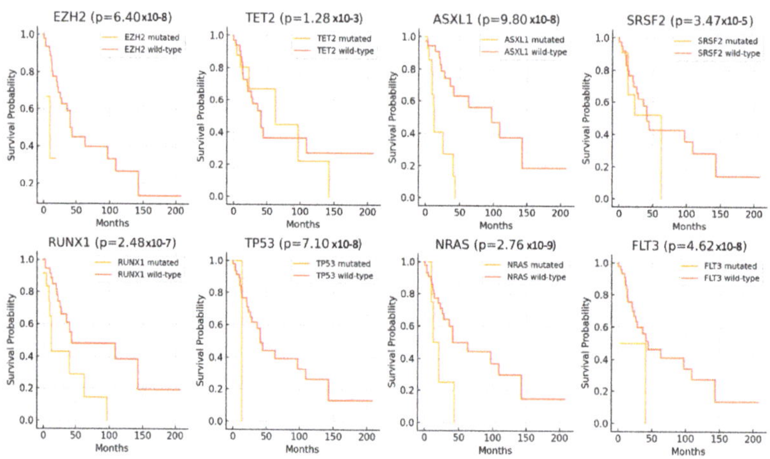

Figure 4. Kaplan–Meier survival curves for significant gene mutations in CMML patients. Kaplan–Meier survival curves for selected gene mutations significantly associated with survival outcomes in patients with CMML. Each panel represents a different gene, comparing survival probabilities over time between patients with mutations (yellow line) and wild-type (orange line) alleles.

4. Discussion

CMML presents significant heterogeneity, both in clinical manifestation and in outcomes, predominantly affecting an older, primarily male population. Our study confirms these demographics, with median ages of 71 and 74 years in our institution and the broader Kentucky cohort, respectively. These findings are consistent with global research, which shows similar age and gender distributions. However, our data also highlight unique regional characteristics that may influence disease progression and treatment responses, underscoring the complexity of managing CMML.

A noteworthy aspect of our study is the examination of the referral patterns and their impact on patient characteristics and survival. Approximately 39% of our cohort had a history of other malignancies, a common feature among older populations, which, intriguingly, did not alter prognostic outcomes in our research. This aspect raises questions about the underlying mechanisms that may insulate survival outcomes from the impacts of comorbidities, suggesting a potential area for deeper investigation.

Survival rates at our institution are on par with or better than those reported by other academic centers and the state cancer registry, which could be attributed to the strategic use of demethylating agents and allogeneic transplantation. These therapies, while effective, highlight the need for tailored treatment approaches to further improve patient outcomes. The transformation rate into a blast phase or acute myelogenous leukemia in our cohort was 28%, comparable to 24% in Barcelona [5] and varying between 13% and 39% in Vienna [6], depending on the age at diagnosis. This transformation significantly shortens patient lifespans and underscores the urgency of developing strategies to mitigate this risk.

In the realm of genetic insights, our study brings to light the utility and limitations of current prognostic scores. Published scores incorporating mutations in RUNX1, NRAS, SETBP1, and ASXL1 provide a framework for assessing prognosis in CMML patients [7]. Additionally, similar analytical methodologies have been applied to evaluate outcomes post-allogeneic transplantation [8]. However, these prognostic scores often lack the precision necessary to guide treatment decisions for individual patients, reflective of the intrinsic variability within CMML pathogenesis.

This heterogeneity is further underscored by our genetic findings, where the mutation patterns within our Kentucky cohort revealed lower frequencies of TET2 mutations (44% vs. 60–73%) and higher frequencies of RUNX1 mutations (33% vs. 15–27%) compared to global data [1,5,9]. These discrepancies may stem from varying sensitivities of NGS technologies, differences in referral patterns, or inherent biological differences within the Kentucky population. Such variability suggests that while global data provide valuable benchmarks, local contextualization is crucial for optimal patient management.

Moreover, the confirmatory role of ASXL1 and NRAS mutations in influencing CMML prognosis, consistent with broader literature, emphasizes the potential of targeted therapies and highlights the need for enhanced predictive tools. Despite advancements, the prognosis for CMML has not seen substantial improvement over the past few decades. The adoption of treatments such as Venetoclax, though promising, underscores an ongoing need for novel therapeutic approaches and more refined prognostic tools [10–12].

The findings from the recent study on p53 mutations can be directly correlated with the clinical implications of TP53 mutations in CMML. In both solid and hematologic malignancies, including CMML, TP53 mutations are associated with poor prognosis, reduced overall survival, and a higher risk of progression to AML. The study's demonstration of thermal instability in mutant p53 proteins, such as R248Q, R248W, and R273H, highlights a mechanism that contributes to oncogenesis by promoting the unfolding and aggregation of the p53 protein [13]. This results in the loss of its tumor-suppressive functions, consistent with the observed effects of TP53 mutations in CMML. The reduced DNA-binding ability of mutant p53 and its tendency to form aggregates may further explain the impaired tumor suppression in CMML, leading to more aggressive disease progression and resistance to therapeutic interventions.

The introduction of artificial intelligence (AI) in prognostication, incorporating a broad spectrum of biological, social, and clinical data, presents a significant opportunity. Recent advancements, as shown in myelodysplastic syndromes, suggest that AI could substantially improve the accuracy of risk stratification [14], potentially revolutionizing treatment paradigms in CMML.

Our findings resonate with those reported by Coston et al., who observed suboptimal response rates to hypomethylating agent therapy in CMML at a single institution (Table 2) [15]. This underscores the challenge of treating CMML and the urgent need for developing more effective therapeutic strategies responsive to the unique genetic profiles of different patient subgroups. Furthermore, the work by Pleyer et al. offers a broader view by detailing the outcomes of CMML patients treated with non-curative therapies in a retrospective cohort study. Their findings highlight the limited efficacy of current treatment modalities and the variability in patient survival, which parallels our observations of diverse clinical outcomes within our cohort [16].

Table 2. Recent single- and multi-center institution studies for CMML.

Study Location	# of Patients	Median Age at Diagnosis (Years)	% Male	Timeframe	Median Survival (Months)	NGS Performed	Ref.
Lexington, KY (USA)	51	71	71	2005–2023	42	70.6%	This manuscript
Kentucky (USA)	254	73.9	64.2	2012–2022	23	NA	This manuscript
Rochester, MN	121	68	63	NA	~19	62%	[15]
38 centers worldwide	949	72	66	1981–2018	18.5	NA	[16]
Barcelona, SP	219	74.1	65.8	1997–2021	34	32.9%	[5]
Wuhan, CN	66	~65	63.0	2011–2020	10–18	25.8%	[17]
Bordeaux, FR	131	74	60	1999–2019	30–36	100%	[9]
Houston, TX (USA)	532	70	67%	2005–2022	35.9	70%	[18]

NA, not available.

While our findings provide valuable insights into the genetic underpinnings of CMML, the generalizability of these results may be limited by the study's single-institution nature and the relatively small sample size. Future research could benefit from multi-center studies that include larger and more diverse patient populations. Such studies would not only validate our findings, but also potentially reveal additional insights that could be obscured in smaller, less varied cohorts.

5. Conclusions

In summary, while our study affirms several established characteristics of CMML, it also provides new insights into the genetic and clinical diversity within specific populations like Kentucky. These insights advocate for continued research into the molecular mechanisms of CMML and the development of advanced, precise treatment modalities that can profoundly enhance patient care and outcomes. Future studies should aim to further these findings, leveraging local and global data to foster a more nuanced understanding of CMML's complex landscape.

Author Contributions: Conceptualization: R.M., S.W., and J.D.; data collection: L.N.Y., R.M., T.A., and J.D.; resources: B.H., J.K.M. and E.B.D. (Kentucky Cancer Registry data). All authors have read and agreed to the published version of the manuscript.

Funding: Drs. Bin Huang and Eric Durbin are supported by the NCI Cancer Center Support Grant (P30 CA177558).

Institutional Review Board Statement: This study was conducted according to the ethical standards of the Medical Institutional Review Board (IRB) at the University of Kentucky (approval code: 89748 on 29 August 2023), along with the 1964 Helsinki Declaration and its later amendments or comparable ethical standards.

Informed Consent Statement: Not applicable.

Data Availability Statement: The datasets generated and analyzed during the current study are available from the corresponding author upon reasonable request. Additional data supporting this study's findings are included within the article. All relevant data are contained within the manuscript, and high-resolution data are stored securely by the corresponding research institution and are available under specific conditions to researchers who meet the criteria for confidential data access.

Acknowledgments: Thanks to Shengyi Zhang, who performed statistical analysis on the University of Kentucky cohort. Markey Cancer Center's Biostatistics and Bioinformatics Shared Resource Facility and the Cancer Research Informatics Shared Resource Facility assisted with the data analysis. The Markey Cancer Center's Research Communications Office review is gratefully acknowledged.

Conflicts of Interest: The authors have no conflicts of interest to declare that are relevant to the content of this article.

References

1. Patnaik, M.M.; Tefferi, A. Chronic myelomonocytic leukemia: 2024 update on diagnosis, risk stratification and management. *Am. J. Hematol.* **2024**, *99*, 1142–1165. [CrossRef] [PubMed]
2. Hudson, L.; Burus, T.; Park, L.; Huang, B.; Hull, P.C.; Vanderford, N.L. Cancer disparities in Appalachian Kentucky. *J. Rural Health* **2024**, *40*, 87–95. [CrossRef] [PubMed]
3. Zeidan, A.M.; Hu, X.; Long, J.B.; Wang, R.; Ma, X.; Podoltsev, N.A.; Huntington, S.F.; Gore, S.D.; Davidoff, A.J. Hypomethylating agent therapy use and survival in older patients with chronic myelomonocytic leukemia in the United States: A large population-based study. *Cancer* **2017**, *123*, 3754–3762. [CrossRef] [PubMed]
4. National Cancer Institute. SEER*Stat Databases: SEER November 2023 Submission (2020–2021). Available online: https://seer.cancer.gov/data-software/documentation/seerstat/nov2023/ (accessed on 1 July 2024).
5. Castaño-Díez, S.; López-Guerra, M.; Bosch-Castañeda, C.; Bataller, A.; Charry, P.; Esteban, D.; Guijarro, F.; Jiménez-Vicente, C.; Castillo-Girón, C.; Cortes, A.; et al. Real-World Data on Chronic Myelomonocytic Leukemia: Clinical and Molecular Characteristics, Treatment, Emerging Drugs, and Patient Outcomes. *Cancers* **2022**, *14*, 4107. [CrossRef] [PubMed]
6. Machherndl-Spandl, S.; Jäger, E.; Barna, A.; Gurbisz, M.; Marschon, R.; Graf, T.; Graf, E.; Geissler, C.; Hoermann, G.; Nösslinger, T.; et al. Impact of age on the cumulative risk of transformation in patients with chronic myelomonocytic leukaemia. *Eur. J. Haematol.* **2021**, *107*, 265–274. [CrossRef] [PubMed]
7. Elena, C.; Gallì, A.; Such, E.; Meggendorfer, M.; Germing, U.; Rizzo, E.; Cervera, J.; Molteni, E.; Fasan, A.; Schuler, E.; et al. Integrating clinical features and genetic lesions in the risk assessment of patients with chronic myelomonocytic leukemia. *Blood* **2016**, *128*, 1408–1417. [CrossRef] [PubMed]
8. Mei, M.; Pillai, R.; Kim, S.; Estrada-Merly, N.; Afkhami, M.; Yang, L.; Meng, Z.; Abid, M.B.; Aljurf, M.; Bacher, U.; et al. The mutational landscape in chronic myelomonocytic leukemia and its impact on allogeneic hematopoietic cell transplantation outcomes: A Center for Blood and Marrow Transplantation Research (CIBMTR) analysis. *Haematologica* **2023**, *108*, 150–160. [CrossRef]
9. Dussiau, C.; Dupuy, H.; Bidet, A.; Sauvezie, M.; De-Grande, A.-C.; Boureau, L.; Riviere, E.; Forcade, E.; Bonnet, F.; Dumas, P.-Y.; et al. Impact of Mutational Status and Prognostic Factors on Survival in Chronic Myelomonocytic Leukemia with Systemic Inflammation and Autoimmune Disorders. *HemaSphere* **2023**, *7*, e847. [CrossRef]
10. Molina, J.C.; Asare, J.M.; Tuschong, L.; West, R.R.; Calvo, K.R.; Persky, R.; Boyce, A.M.; Hammoud, D.A.; Holland, S.M.; Hickstein, D.; et al. Venetoclax/decitabine for a pediatric patient with chronic myelomonocytic leukemia. *Pediatr. Blood Cancer* **2021**, *68*, e28865. [CrossRef] [PubMed]
11. Montalban-Bravo, G.; Hammond, D.; DiNardo, C.D.; Konopleva, M.; Borthakur, G.; Short, N.J.; Ramos-Perez, J.; Guerra, V.; Kanagal-Shamanna, R.; Naqvi, K.; et al. Activity of venetoclax-based therapy in chronic myelomonocytic leukemia. *Leukemia* **2021**, *35*, 1494–1499. [CrossRef] [PubMed]
12. Rezazadeh, A.; Deininger, M.; Atallah, E. Proposals for Clinical Trials in Chronic Myelomonocytic Leukemia. *Curr. Treat. Options Oncol.* **2023**, *24*, 1036–1051. [CrossRef] [PubMed]
13. Khadiullina, R.; Mirgayazova, R.; Davletshin, D.; Khusainova, E.; Chasov, V.; Bulatov, E. Assessment of Thermal Stability of Mutant p53 Proteins via Differential Scanning Fluorimetry. *Life* **2022**, *13*, 31. [CrossRef] [PubMed]
14. Orgueira, A.M.; Encinas, M.M.P.; Varela, N.A.D.; Mora, E.; Díaz-Beyá, M.; Montoro, M.J.; Pomares, H.; Ramos, F.; Tormo, M.; Jerez, A.; et al. Machine Learning Improves Risk Stratification in Myelodysplastic Neoplasms: An Analysis of the Spanish Group of Myelodysplastic Syndromes. *HemaSphere* **2023**, *7*, e961. [CrossRef] [PubMed]
15. Coston, T.; Pophali, P.; Vallapureddy, R.; Lasho, T.L.; Finke, C.M.; Ketterling, R.P.; Carr, R.; Binder, M.; Mangaonkar, A.A.; Gangat, N.; et al. Suboptimal response rates to hypomethylating agent therapy in chronic myelomonocytic leukemia; a single institutional study of 121 patients. *Am. J. Hematol.* **2019**, *94*, 767–779. [CrossRef] [PubMed]
16. Pleyer, L.; Leisch, M.; Kourakli, A.; Padron, E.; Maciejewski, J.P.; Cirici, B.X.; Kaivers, J.; Ungerstedt, J.; Heibl, S.; Patiou, P.; et al. Outcomes of patients with chronic myelomonocytic leukaemia treated with non-curative therapies: A retrospective cohort study. *Lancet Haematol.* **2021**, *8*, e135–e148. [CrossRef] [PubMed]

17. Wang, C.; Wang, Z.; Meng, F.; Luo, L.; Liu, X.; Shi, J.; Huang, L. Treatment Outcomes and Prognostic Factors in 66 Patients with Chronic Myelomonocytic Leukemia (CMML) in a Single Center. *Int. J. Gen. Med.* **2022**, *15*, 7843–7854. [CrossRef] [PubMed]
18. Bataller, A.; Gener-Ricos, G.; Almanza-Huante, E.; Chien, K.S.; Urrutia, S.; Bazinet, A.; Rodriguez-Sevilla, J.J.; Hammond, D.; Sasaki, K.; Takahashi, K.; et al. Therapy-related chronic myelomonocytic leukemia does not have the high-risk features of a therapy-related neoplasm. *Blood Adv.* **2024**, *8*, 2695–2706. [CrossRef] [PubMed]

biomedicines MDPI

Article

ABCG2 Gene Expression in Non-Small Cell Lung Cancer

Agnieszka Jeleń [1,2,*], Marta Żebrowska-Nawrocka [1,2], Mariusz Łochowski [3], Dagmara Szmajda-Krygier [1,2] and Ewa Balcerczak [1,2]

1 Department of Pharmaceutical Biochemistry and Molecular Diagnostics, Medical University of Lodz, Muszynskiego 1, 90-151 Lodz, Poland; marta.zebrowska@umed.lodz.pl (M.Ż.-N.); dagmara.szmajda@umed.lodz.pl (D.S.-K.); ewa.balcerczak@umed.lodz.pl (E.B.)

2 Laboratory of Molecular Diagnostics, BRaIn Laboratories, Medical University of Lodz, Czechoslowacka 4, 92-216 Lodz, Poland

3 Department of Thoracic Surgery, Copernicus Memorial Hospital, Medical University of Lodz, Pabianicka 62, 93-513 Lodz, Poland; mariusz.lochowski@umed.lodz.pl

* Correspondence: agnieszka.jelen@umed.lodz.pl

Abstract: Background/Objectives: ATP-binding cassette subfamily G member 2 [ABCG2/breast cancer resistance protein (BCRP)] contributes to mechanisms of multidrug resistance (MDR) and is a marker of side population (SP) cells in human cancers. The primary objective of this study was to investigate the impact of *ABCG2* gene expression on the non-small cell lung cancer (NSCLC) development, course of cancer disease, and patient prognosis using publicly available data. Obtained results were supplemented with assessment of *ABCG2* expression in blood of NSCLC patients. **Methods:** The dataset of lung cancer was analyzed utilizing the TIMER 2.0, UALCAN, TNMplot, MEXPRESS, cBioPortal, MethSurv, KM Plotter, STRING, and ShinyGO 0.80 databases. Blood samples from 50 patients were assessed using the real-time PCR method. **Results:** The *ABCG2* gene was expressed at a low level in NSCLC, and did not correlate with clinical aggressiveness of lung cancer. Higher *ABCG2* expression improved overall survival, but only in LUAD. In addition, CpG sites located on the CpG island affecting the NSCLC patient's prognosis were indicated. In the case of our own laboratory results, the study did not reveal any changes in the *ABCG2* expression levels in blood collected from patients at different time points during the diagnostic–therapeutic procedure. In the in silico analysis, most ABCG2 protein interactors were associated with the development of drug resistance. **Conclusions:** ABCG2 appears to have a particularly significant impact on the survival of patients with lung cancer and on the effect of immunotherapy related to immune cell infiltration. Presented findings may support personalized medicine strategies based on bioinformatics findings.

Keywords: ABCG2; BCRP; cancer biomarker; DNA methylation; gene expression; LUAD; lung cancer; LUSC

1. Introduction

Lung cancer is the most common cancer among men and the second most common in women worldwide. This type of cancer is also the leading cause of cancer-related deaths among over 30 groups of neoplasms in half of the regions analyzed worldwide (among both, men, and women). While tobacco smoking remains the most important factor predisposing to the development of the disease [1,2], up to a quarter of all lung cancer cases occur in lifelong never-smokers. The incidence of lung cancer is decreasing as smoking rates decline; however, the incidence of lung cancer in never-smokers remains stable or is increasing, and may depend on gender, age, or ethnicity. In addition to the effects of smoking, increasing attention is being paid to the indoor/workplace exposure to radon, asbestos, arsenic, cooking oil, or exhaust fumes and level of other pollutants in the air we live in. Other related factors are family lung cancer history, diet, and infectious and inflammatory diseases [3,4].

NSCLC is the most commonly diagnosed histological type of lung cancer. The constant rate of non-smokers developing NSCLC highlights the important role of non-modifiable factors that are associated with carcinogenesis in lung tissue. Differences between smokers and non-smokers with NSCLC concern features such as gene expression patterns or germline polymorphisms [5–7]. Moreover, the major obstacles to the successful management of lung cancer are diagnoses at advanced or locally advanced stages, a limited number of markers to predict the response to applied therapy and monitoring its efficacy, and the development of resistance to therapy, leading to nonresponse or insufficient response. Therefore, in this study, we analyze a promising molecular factor that may be important for the development of NSCLC and bring benefits in clinical practice.

The members of the ATP-binding cassette (ABC) transporter superfamily are primarily known to significantly alter the pharmacokinetics of most anticancer drugs, including traditional chemotherapeutics, as well as molecularly targeted therapeutic agents. However, according to our previous study, the gene encoding the best-known ABC transporter—ABCB1—may also be a promising indicator of carcinogenesis and a disease prognostic factor, which could contribute to the alteration of the cancer progression and survival of patients [8]. The second factor of similar importance may be ABCG2 (ATP-binding cassette superfamily member G 2). The overexpression of ABCG2 associated with drug efflux may be among mechanisms of multidrug resistance (MDR), leading to failure in cancer therapy. The efficacy of the targeted inhibition of ABCG2-mediated transport has been investigated in various cancers such as colon cancer [9], breast cancer [10], and leukemia [11]. After the first disappointing results, it was necessary to continue the search for new strategies, promising multipotential MDR modulators and further preclinical tests. In lung cancer, an association was found between the ABCG2 transporter and the frequency of osimertinib adverse events [12], the risk of resistance to platinum therapy [13], or the adagrasib penetration of target tissues [14]. New MDR modulators such as tazemetostat [15], an I-CBP112-CBP/EP300 bromodomain inhibitor [16], or sonidegib [17] may increase the tumor cells' sensitivity to anticancer agents by the functional inhibition of ABCG2. However, these new drugs could bring the most benefits in the clinical management of NSCLC patients with high ABCG2 expression.

Under normal physiological conditions, members of the ABCG subfamily are responsible for the regulation of cholesterol and bile acid homeostasis, steroid hormone transport, heme metabolism, and hypoxic signaling. Their presence at the strategic sites in the body along with the results of studies conducted on animals and in human cancer samples suggest that ABCG members play an important role in tumor formation and several other cancer-related processes. In addition, ABCG2 is a marker of the side population (SP) cells, representing pluripotent cancer stem cells. According to more recent data, the features of cancer that are significantly associated with activity of ABCG2 include genomic instability, resistance to cell death, plasticity of the cancer stem cell phenotype, sustaining proliferative signaling/ability to evade growth suppression, epigenetic reprogramming, and polymorphic differences in the microbiomes [18,19].

ABCG2 seems to be an important element of defense against carcinogens and factors that can stimulate inflammation. This was proven in a mouse model where the knockout of the gene analog caused toxic reactions and carcinogen accumulation [20,21]. ABCG2 also has the ability to pump out some of the polycyclic aromatic hydrocarbons contained in tobacco smoke. Therefore, it protects both normal lung cells and cancer cells from the effects of carcinogenic toxicity [22].

One of the biological effects of prolonged exposure to carcinogens and/or substances that affect the immune system is the production of reactive oxygen species (ROS), which may induce, e.g., genomic instability, epigenetic modifications, immunomodulation, or chronic inflammation, any of which can initiate carcinogenesis. The results obtained in a human colorectal adenocarcinoma cell line indicated that ROS promoted inflammation, which was more intense when *ABCG2* expression was decreased. It is likely that the downregulation of the ABCG2 contributes to the activation of the NF-κB signaling pathway, which controls multiple aspects of the immune response [23]. At the same time, molecular changes in ABC transporters (including ABCG2) may have an effect on the transport of chemical compounds affecting the microbiome and/or produced by them [24]. Similarly to colorectal cancer, inflammation in the respiratory tract may be preceded by an altered lung microbial community composition and microbiome outside the lungs [25]. The diet, environmental factors, and ABC transporters mutually influence the complex network of interaction between the lung, oropharynx, and gut microbiome. For example, a significantly increased risk of lung cancer has also been observed in patients with lower respiratory tract infections or a *H. pylori* presence [26,27].

Cancer tissue is organized in hierarchical heterogeneous cell populations that exhibit distinct phenotypes and function within the tumor. Among them and of particular interest are cancer stem cells (CSCs), which are derived from the initiated normal stem/progenitor cells and have the ability for self-renewal and differentiation into multiple cell types. ABCG2 plays an important role in the enhancement in CSC tumorigenic potential. SP cells isolated from lung cancer cell lines demonstrated a higher level of ABCG2 at the mRNA and protein levels, providing them a broad spectrum of drug/xenobiotics resistance [28,29]. The expression of ABCG2, which is responsible for phenotypic characteristics of SP cells, is also involved in the WNT/β-Catenin, Hedgehog, Hippo, and PI3K/Akt/mTOR signaling pathways [30–32]. Therefore, ABCG2 status has a significant impact on tumor initiation and progression, the risk of local recurrence and metastasis to another part of the body, and patient survival.

This study involves the analysis of molecular and phenotypic datasets collected by The Cancer Genome Atlas (TCGA) and other bioinformatics databases. Using massive amounts of data from multiple studies and centers can yield more robust results and more reliable findings. Cancer bioinformatics plays an important role in the preliminary identification and/or authentication of promising biomarkers, which are revealed from individual clinical-case research. An in-depth study of *ABCG2* gene expression becomes possible with the selection and processing of transcriptomic and epigenomic data collected during multiomics studies in non-small cell lung cancer [33,34].

Here, we primarily investigate the impact of *ABCG2* gene expression on the NSCLC development, course of cancer disease, and patient prognosis using data collected in databases. Analyses conducted using bioinformatics tools are additionally supplemented with the results of our own wet research. In this study, we also explore the metabolic pathways in which ABCG2 is involved and its interactions with other proteins. The obtained results were compared with the available literature and discussed thoroughly.

2. Materials and Methods

2.1. Description of Data Collection Methods and Bioinformatic Tools

2.1.1. A Pan-Cancer Analysis of the Expression of *ABCG2*

TIMER 2.0 (http://timer.cistrome.org, accessed on 4 May 2024) and TNMplot (https://tnmplot.com/analysis/, accessed on 4 May 2024) databases were used to analyze and present the differences in mRNA levels of *ABCG2* between normal and tumor tissue in different types of cancers. In the TIMER 2.0 tool, the Gene_DE module was chosen. This allowed for the identification of TCGA tumors in which the investigated gene was up- or down-regulated. The statistical significance computed by the Wilcoxon test was indicated by the number of asterisks displayed above the box plots [35,36]. The similar analysis in the TNMplot tool included not only samples from TCGA but also data from Gene Expression Omnibus (GEO), The Genotype-Tissue Expression Project (Gtex), and Therapeutically Applicable Research to Generate Effective Treatments (TARGET) databases. The differences in *ABCG2* expression were determined using the Mann–Whitney U test. The assessment of differences in the *ABCG2* mRNA level between lung cancer tissue (LUAD and LUSC) and adjacent normal tissues were performed using RNA-Seq data [37].

2.1.2. Association between *ABCG2* Expression and Clinicopathological Characteristics

The expression levels of *ABCG2* in lung cancer tissues were further analyzed using two tools: UALCAN (https://ualcan.path.uab.edu, accessed on 18 May 2024) and MEXPRESS (https://mexpress.be, accessed on 20 May 2024). The aim of this step was to indicate the potential association between the investigated gene expression level and clinicopathological as well as demographic features of lung cancer patients. The analyzed features included, e.g., the cancer stage; pathologic tumor, node, and metastasis (TNM) status; age; gender; ethnicity; mutation status in selected genes, and tobacco smoke exposure characteristics. In the UALCAN tool, the statistical significance of differences in *ABCG2* expression between lung cancer patients grouped according to selected feature was determined using Welch's *t*-test [38,39]. For the same purpose, the MEXPRESS tool was used, in which the gene expression was analyzed based on more detailed clinicopathological data from TCGA. Data were sorted according to the *ABCG2* expression level, and then the appropriate statistical test was performed (ANOVA, t test, or Pearson correlation coefficient calculation). All presented p values are Benjamini–Hochberg-adjusted p values [40,41].

2.1.3. *ABCG2* DNA Methylation Analysis

Using both UALCAN and MEXPRESS, a preliminary comparison of the *ABCG2* promoter methylation level (sum of data from CpG probes located up to 1500 bp upstream of gene's start site) between cancer and normal lung cells was made, and correlation between the expression of this gene and DNA methylation data in relation to its genomic location was estimated. The association between the *ABCG2* mRNA expression level and methylation beta-value (HM27 and HM450 merge) was analyzed using the cBioPortal platform (https://www.cbioportal.org, accessed on 2 September 2024). A total of 508 LUAD patients/samples and 483 LUSC patients/samples from the TCGA PanCancer Atlas with complete RNA-seq data were included in the analysis. Spearman's and Pearson's correlation coefficients were calculated [42]. The MethSurv tool (https://biit.cs.ut.ee/methsurv/, accessed on 25 July 2024) was used to characterize the DNA methylation level of all CpG islands located in *ABCG2* LUAD- and LUSC-TCGA samples [43].

2.1.4. Survival Analysis of *ABCG2*

Two survival databases, the Kaplan–Meier plotter (https://kmplot.com/analysis/, accessed on 30 May 2024) and above-mentioned MethSurv, were used to analyze the effect of *ABCG2* expression and methylation on patients' prognosis. The gene expression data obtained by gene chips from The European Genome-phenome Archive (EGA), GEO, and TCGA databases were analyzed. Overall survival (OS), first-progression survival (FP), and post-progression survival (PPS) were compared between two groups of lung cancer patients (high vs. low expression level) split by the "auto select best cutoff" option. The selected follow-up threshold was 60 months, and the biased arrays were excluded for array quality control. Similar analyses were performed in subgroups restricted to the histological type of lung cancer, cancer stage, tumor grade, chemotherapy reception, or smoking status. For each analysis, the hazard ratio (HR) with 95% confidence intervals (CIs) and p value by the log-rank test were calculated [44]. A survival analysis based on DNA methylation levels for any CpG site was performed using the MethSurv tool. The output visualized by the Kaplan–Meier plot presents the differences in survival between groups of patients with higher and lower methylation levels split by the "best" option. The p value of HR with 95% CI, derived from Cox fitting and the log-likelihood ratio (LR) test, was calculated for each analysis [43].

2.1.5. Immune Infiltration Analysis

We used the Gene module in the TIMER2.0 database to correlate *ABCG2* expression with the immune infiltration level in lung cancer tissue. B cells, CD8+T cells, CD4+T cells, macrophages, neutrophils, and dendritic cells were assessed by the TIMER algorithm. Cancer-associated fibroblasts were evaluated by MCP-COUNTER, XCELL, and TIDE algorithms. The "Purity adjusted" option was selected for all analyses. Spearman's RHO coefficient and statistical significance value were presented on scatter plots. $p < 0.05$ was considered as significantly different [35,36].

2.1.6. Gene Mutation and Copy Number Alteration Analyses

The *ABCG2* mutations and their location were detected using cBioPortal (http://www.cbioportal.org/; accessed on 10 September 2024) [42,45,46]. The web tool enabled generating the graphical visualization of mutation and copy number alterations in selected cancer via Oncoprint and MutationMapper modules. The chosen dataset for graphical visualization was the TCGA and PanCancer Atlas, with selected mutations, Structural Variant, and putative copy number alterations from GISTIC and mRNA Expression Genomic Profiles.

2.1.7. Analysis of ABCG2-Related Proteins and Gene Set Enrichment Analysis

To predict potential protein–protein functional interaction related to ABCG2, the STRING tool was used (https://string-db.org/; accessed on 7 September 2024) [47]. In the analysis, 20 interactions with a minimum confidence at level 0.7 and PPI enrichment p value of $p < 9.26 \times 10^{-9}$ were predicted. The k-means clustering of the generated PPI networks for ABCG2 was performed with a preset of three clusters (marked as red, green, and blue). A gene enrichment analysis was undertaken using the ShinyGO 0.80 tool (http://bioinformatics.sdstate.edu/go/; accessed on 7 September 2024), in order to identify the most important functions of particular clusters of correlated genes [48].

2.2. *Sample Collection*

The material was peripheral blood collected from patients hospitalized in the Department of Thoracic Surgery, Memorial Copernicus Hospital, in Lodz, and diagnosed with NSCLC. Blood samples were collected in the years 2022–2023. The study was conducted in accordance with the principles of the Declaration of Helsinki, and all patients provided informed consent prior to enrollment. The research protocol was approved by the Ethical Committee of the Medical University of Lodz (no. RNN/85/20/KE and no. KE/649/23).

This study involved 50 patients (13 females; 37 males; median age of the group: 67 years), of which 1 patient was excluded before the publication of results. Blood samples were collected before surgical removal of lung tumors, in all patients. In the case of 6 study participants, blood was also collected 100 days and one year after the surgical removal of the tumor. Basic clinical data (gender, age, smoking status, histological type of cancer, TNM stage, histological grade, and type of treatment, if implemented) were obtained from each patient. Detailed characteristics of the study group are presented in Table 1.

2.2.1. RNA Isolation

Total RNA from peripheral blood was isolated according to the "Total RNA Mini" protocol (A&A Biotechnology, Gdansk, Poland). The purity and concentration of RNA samples were assessed spectrophotometrically. RNA samples until analyses were stored at −80 °C.

2.2.2. Real-Time Polymerase Chain Reaction (RT-qPCR)

Isolated RNA was transcribed into complementary DNA (cDNA) in accordance with the "High-Capacity cDNA Reverse Transcription Kit" with the RNase Inhibitor protocol (Applied Biosystems by Thermo Fisher Scientific Baltics, UAB, Vilnius, Lithuania). The final concentration of RNA in the reaction mixture was 0.005 µg/µL. After that, quantification assessment of *ABCG2* mRNA was performed by the real-time PCR method using the Rotor-GeneTM6000 (Corbet Research, Qiagen GmbH, Hilden, Germany) according to the "iTaq Universal SYBR Green Supermix" (Bio-Rad, Hercules, CA, USA) protocol. *GAPDH* was used as the reference gene. The reaction mixture for both investigated and reference genes consisted of 5 µL of 2x concentrated master mix, 0.5 µL of each primer (10 mM) (*ABCG2* gene: F 5′-ATG TCA ACT CCT CCT TCT AC-3′, 5′-AAT GAT CTG AGC TAT AGA

GGC-3′; *GAPDH* gene: 5′-ACA GTT GCC ATG TAG ACC-3′, R 5′-TTG AGC ACA GGG TAC TTT A-3′), and 1 μL of cDNA or distilled water for a negative control (NTC) up to a final volume of 10 μL. All testing was performed in technical triplicates. The final Ct value for each sample was calculated as a mean of 3 replicates. In each experiment, NTC was included. To define the level of relative *ABCG2* gene expression, the ΔΔ Ct method was used.

Table 1. Characteristics of the investigated group.

Variable	No. of Patients
Age (range, years)	67 (32–82)
Gender:	
Male	37
Female	12
Tobacco smoking status:	
Non-smokers	22
smokers	27
Histological type of cancer:	
LUAD	19
LUSC	30
Cancer stage:	
I	22
II	16
III	11
IV	0
Grade of histological malignancy:	
G1	2
G2	35
G3	12
Chemotherapy:	
Yes	13
No	36

2.2.3. Statistical Analysis

To evaluate the correlation between the relative levels of investigated gene expression and age of patients, Spearman's rank correlation coefficient was calculated. To identify the potential differences in *ABCG2* expression between the lung cancer patients grouped according to clinicopathological features, the U Mann–Whitney test was used. Friedman's ANOVA was applied to compare the median of the *ABCG2* expression between the patients "before surgery", "100 days after surgery", and "one year after surgery". All statistical analyses were performed using STATISTICA 13.1. (StatSoft Inc., Tulsa, OK, USA). In all conducted analyses, a $p < 0.05$ was assumed as significant.

3. Results

3.1. *ABCG2 Gene Expression Pattern*

The results of the pan-cancer analysis demonstrated that the level of *ABCG2* gene expression differed significantly between tumor and normal tissue in more than half of the cancer types (16 out of 23). For 15 types of cancer, including lung cancer, a reduction in expression was observed in tumor tissue. Kidney renal cell carcinoma (KIRC) was an exception (Figure 1A). When samples deposited in databases other than TCGA were included in the analysis, there were no significant changes in outcomes (Figure 1B). Similarly, *ABCG2* expression was down-regulated in both LUAD (Figure 1C) and LUSC (Figure 1D) compared with adjacent normal tissue.

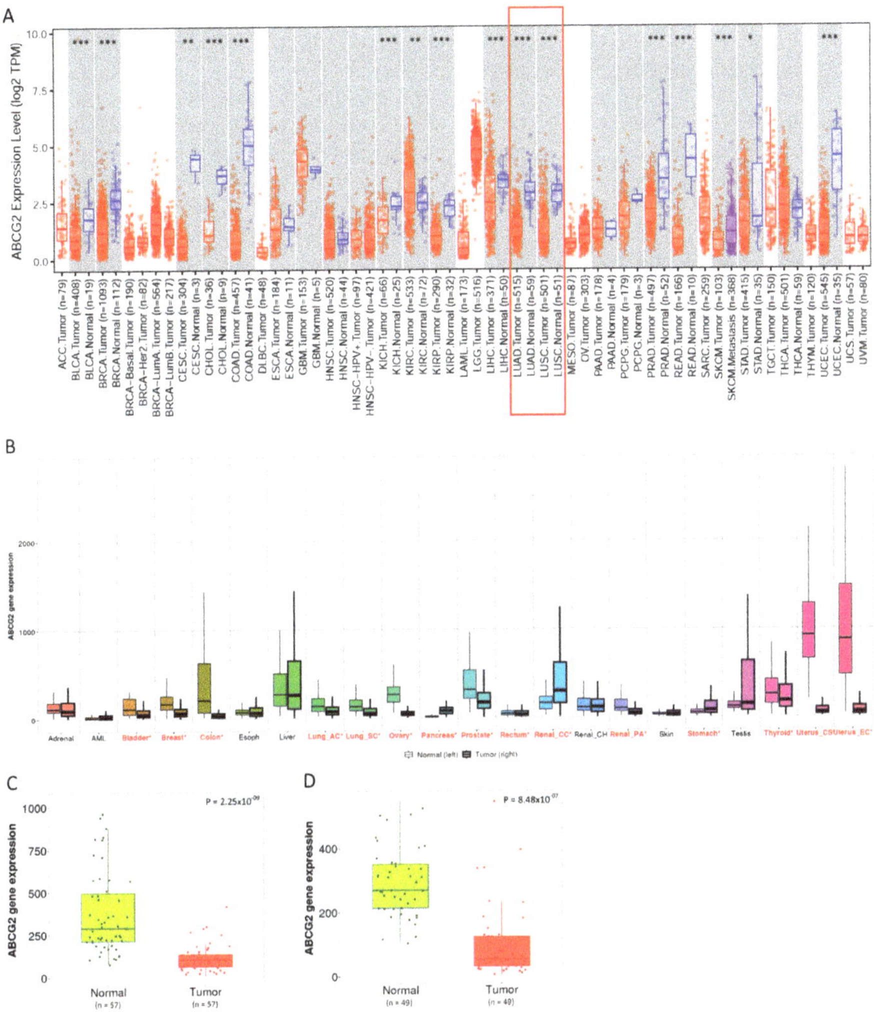

Figure 1. *ABCG2* expression in human pan-cancer and lung cancers. (**A**,**B**) The mRNA level in a panel of tumors (**A**) from the TIMER2.0 database (p value codes: $0 \leq$ *** $< 0.001 \leq$ ** $< 0.01 \leq$ * < 0.05); the red box mark the box plots for lung cancer, which is the focus of this study (**B**) and TNMplot database (significant differences in expression between cancer and normal tissue are indicated by a red asterisk; $p < 0.01$); a red * marks those tissues for which the differences in the expression levels were statistically significant. (**C**,**D**) The down-regulation of *ABCG2* in (**C**) LUAD and (**D**) LUSC in comparison with adjacent normal tissue (RNA-seq data, TNMplot).

Furthermore, the associations of *ABCG2* expression with clinicopathological and demographic features in lung cancer were evaluated. The investigated gene expression was significantly higher in LUSC stage 4 than 3 ($p < 0.05$; Figure S1A). For LUAD, the pathologic N stage was correlated with *ABCG2* expression ($p = 0.0190$; Figure S2A). Additionally, this gene expression was higher in Caucasians than African Americans, for both LUAD ($p = 0.0150$, Figure S2A) and LUSC ($p = 0.0480$, Figure S3A). No associations were observed between the *ABCG2* mRNA level and other characteristics, including cigarette smoking, *EGFR*, *KRAS* and *TP53* mutation status, pathologic T stage, and M stage.

3.2. Hypomethylated *ABCG2* Gene in Lung Cancer

To explore the reasons for the down-regulation of *ABCG2* expression in lung cancer, the methylation level of the investigated gene was analyzed in three ways. As shown in Figures 2A and 3A, in both LUAD and LUSC samples, the hypomethylated *ABCG2* promoter region was significantly less methylated in cancer samples than normal samples ($p < 0.001$). As is known, DNA methylation is a crucial epigenetic mark that influences gene expression. However, neither in LUAD (Figure 2B,C) nor in LUSC (Figure 3B,C) was there an association between the *ABCG2* gene expression and DNA methylation level in the analyzed regions. Furthermore, we found that cg02016771 was the most methylated (hypermethylated) site in this gene, in both LUAD (Figure 2D) and LUSC (Figure 3D). Most regions of the *ABCG2* gene remain hypomethylated. It is worth noting that an abnormal DNA methylation pattern as one of the hallmarks of cancer may correlate with the patient prognosis.

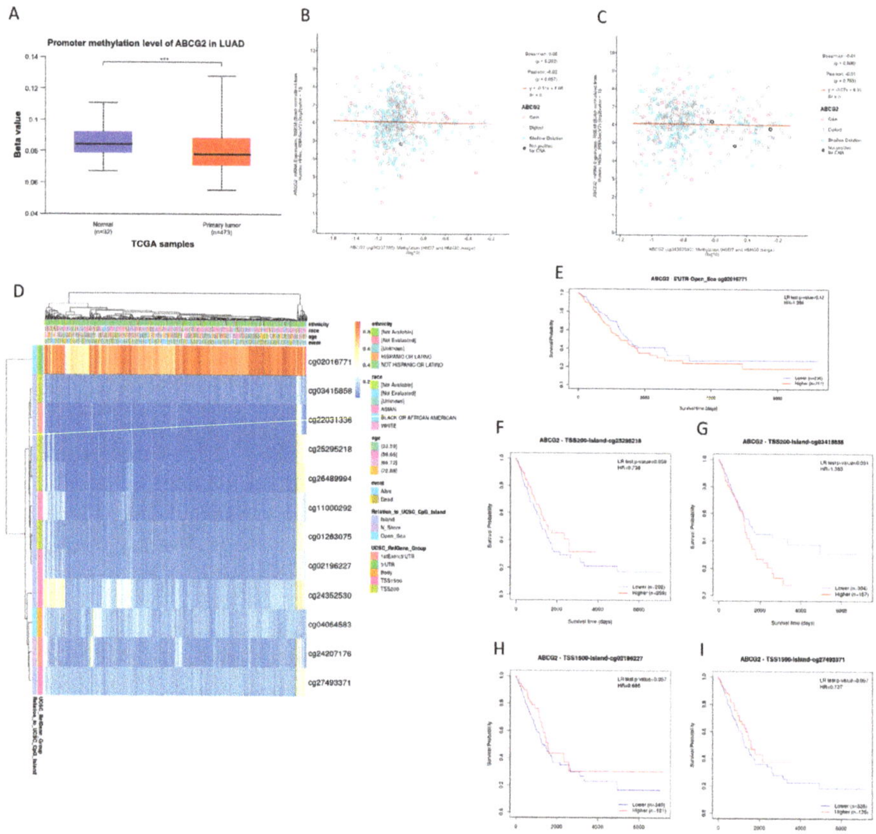

Figure 2. The DNA methylation analysis of the *ABCG2* gene in LUAD. (**A**) Comparison between the promoter methylation level between LUAD and normal lung tissue (*** $p < 0.001$; UALCAN). Correlation between the gene expression level and methylation of two *ABCG2* regions in LUAD samples ((**B**) cg24207176 and (**C**) cg24352530 probes; cBioPortal). (**D**) The heat map showing twelve methylated CpG sites of *ABCG2* (1 = fully methylated/red color; 0 = fully unmethylated/blue color; MethSurv). (**E**–**I**) Survival curves based on selected CpG methylation sites (MethSurv).

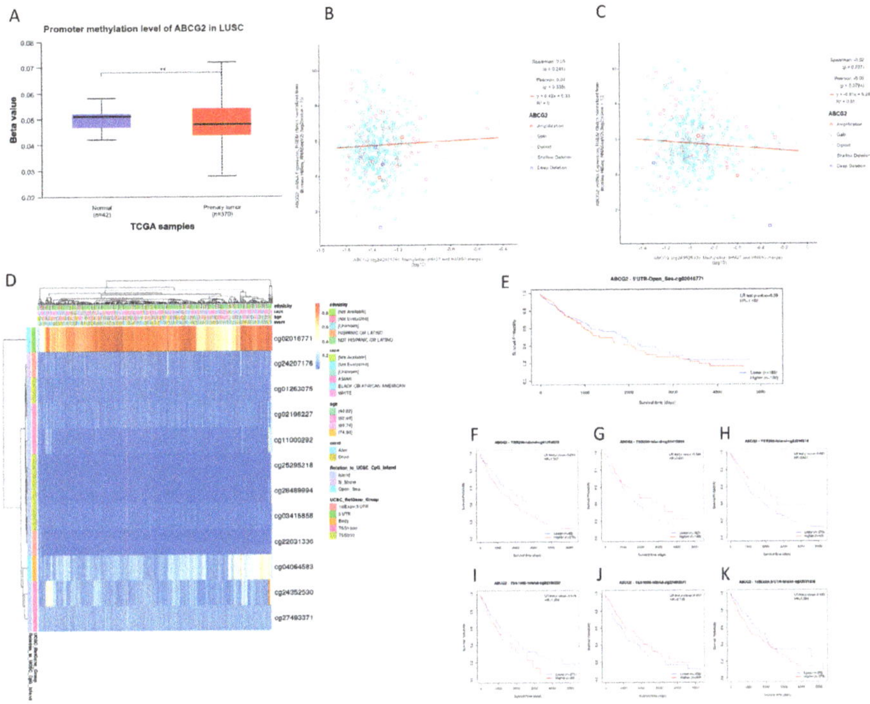

Figure 3. The DNA methylation analysis of the *ABCG2* gene in LUSC. (**A**) Comparison between the promoter methylation level between LUSC and normal lung tissue (** $p < 0.01$; UALCAN). Correlation between the gene expression level and methylation of two *ABCG2* regions in LUSC samples ((**B**) cg24207176 and (**C**) cg24352530 probes; cBioPortal). (**D**) The heat map showing twelve methylated CpG sites of *ABCG2* (1 = fully methylated/red color; 0 = fully unmethylated/blue color; MethSurv). (**E–K**) Survival curves based on selected CpG methylation sites (MethSurv).

3.3. Prognostic Value of ABCG2 Gene Expression and Methylation

To evaluate the prognostic significance of *ABCG2* gene expression in patients with lung cancer, Kaplan–Meier curves for OS, FP, and PPS were generated and analyzed. A higher expression of *ABCG2* in LUAD patients was associated with improved OS ($p = 0.0190$, Figure 4B) and FP ($p = 0.0034$, Figure 4E). In contrast, a higher *ABCG2* mRNA level was significantly associated with poorer FP ($p = 0.0200$, Figure 4F) and PPS ($p = 0.0130$, Figure 4I) in the LUSC group. It is worth noting that the number of participants involved in the analysis of PPS in LUAD was relatively small. Therefore, there is most likely no significant correlation between the expression of the investigated gene and PPS in lung cancer. The *ABCG2* gene expression level appears to have the greatest impact on the prognosis of LUAD patients (Figure 4).

Next, all LUAD cases were divided into two or three subgroups based on tumors' clinical/pathologic features and patient demographics. The OS analysis was performed for each of these subgroups (Figure S4). In this type of cancer, improved OS was correlated with high *ABCG2* expression only in early-stage cancer disease (stage 1) ($p < 0.001$, Figure S4A), in high-grade tumors (G3) ($p = 0.0.340$, Figure S4F), in patients who never smoked ($p = 0.0220$, Figure S4K), and regardless of gender ($p = 0.0400$, $p = 0.0021$, Figure S4I,J). In contrast, higher *ABCG2* expression was significantly associated with poorer OS in patients treated with chemotherapy ($p = 0.0270$, Figure S4G).

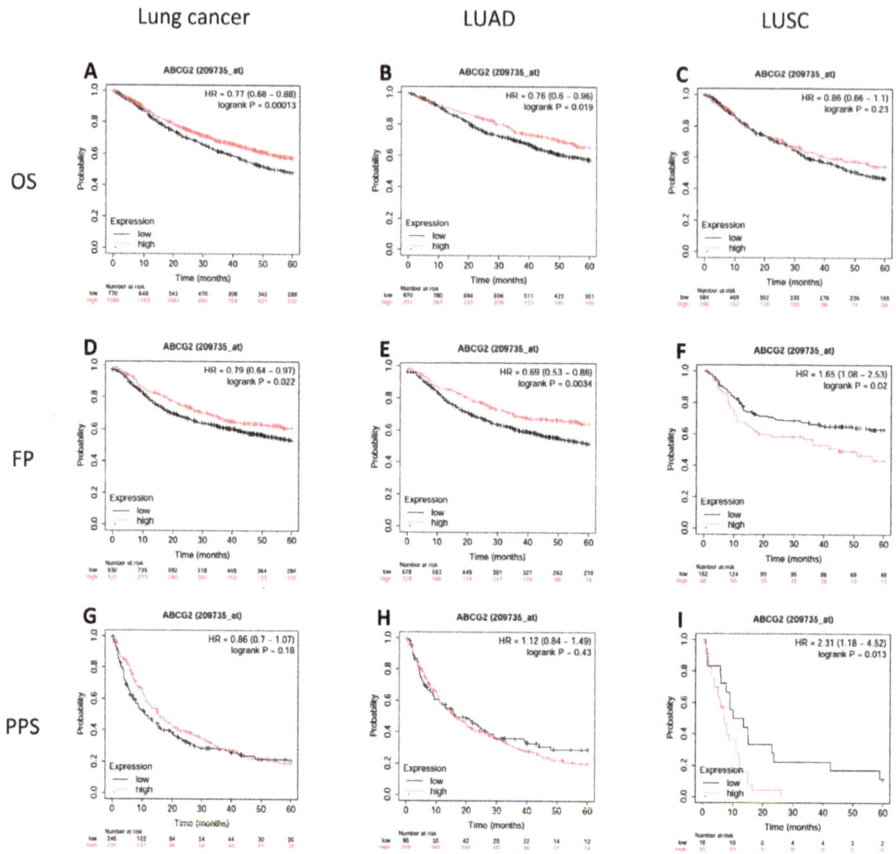

Figure 4. Kaplan–Meier survival curves of *ABCG2* (low vs. high expression level) overall (**A**,**D**,**G**) in non-small cell lung cancer, (**B**,**E**,**H**) in LUAD, and (**C**,**F**,**I**) in LUSC ($p < 0.05$; Kaplan–Meier plotter). OS, overall survival; FP, first-progression survival; PPS, post-progression survival; HR, hazard ratio; red: high expression; black: low expression.

Finally, we explored the prognostic value of DNA methylation levels of the *ABCG2* gene. The status of the only hypermethylated region (cg02016771, 5′UTR, Open_Sea) had no effect on OS of lung cancer patients (Figures 2E and 3E). Of the most poorly methylated CpG sites, the higher methylated cg03415858_TSS200, cg02196227_TSS1500, or cg27493371_TSS1500 slightly improved LUAD patients' survival. However, these observations were not statistically significant (Figure 2G–I). In the case of LUSC, CpG sites located on the CpG island, which influence the patient's prognosis, were successfully selected. Low methylated cg01263075_TSS200 has better survival statistics ($p = 0.038$, Figure 3F). On the other hand, a higher methylation of two CpG sites (cg03415858 and cg25295218) located up to 200 bp upstream from the transcription start site in the *ABCG2* gene was associated with better OS ($p = 0.026$, Figure 3G, and $p = 0.023$, Figure 3H, respectively). This suggests that unmethylated *ABCG2* takes part in lung squamous cell carcinoma progression.

3.4. The Associations between Immune Infiltrates and ABCG2 Gene Expression

The expression of the ABCG2 transporter can be regulated by diverse signaling molecules derived from immune cells. On the other hand, cytokines are transported and controlled by various ABC family proteins [49,50]. This indicates a link between the presence of immune infiltration cells and the function of transporters. The close correlation between the expression of *ABCG2* and macrophages, neutrophils, dendritic cells, and CD8+ T cells was found in LUAD based on the TIMER algorithm (Figure 5A). In the LUSC subtype, *ABCG2* expression showed positive correlations with the same immune cell types, except neutrophils (Figure 5B). Furthermore, the level of infiltration with cancer-associated fibroblasts was a distinguishing feature of the investigated histological subtypes of lung cancer. Based on the MCP-COUNTER, XCELL, and TIDE algorithms, a significant positive correlation between *ABCG2* expression and cancer-associated fibroblast infiltration was observed in LUAD, but not in LUSC (Figure 5C,D).

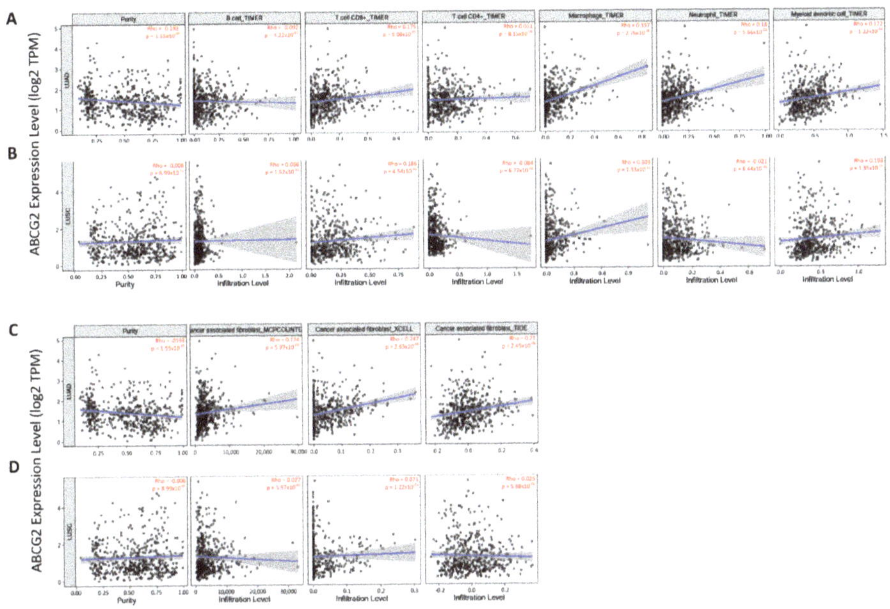

Figure 5. The association between *ABCG2* and tumor immune infiltration (B cells, CD8+ and CD4+ T cells, macrophages, neutrophils, myeloid dendritic cells) in (**A**) LUAD and (**B**) LUSC based on the TIMER algorithm. The correlation of the cancer-associated fibroblast infiltration level with (**C**) LUAD and (**D**) LUSC based on MCP-COUNTER, XCELL, and TIDE algorithms (TIMER2.0).

3.5. *ABCG2 Expression in the Blood of Lung Cancer Patients Based on Our Wet Analysis*

After analyzing the data available in online databases, we decided to check whether similar associations could be identified in the blood of patients with lung cancer. In the study group, the differences in relative expression of *ABCG2* in the blood samples were observed (median: 1.01; min–max: 0.03–6.92). Next, it was assessed whether there was a correlation between the clinicopathological features of investigated subjects and the level of *ABCG2* gene expression in peripheral blood. There was no association between *ABCG2* mRNA in blood of NSCLC patients and the age at diagnosis ($p = 0.1995$, Figure S5A), histological type of the cancer ($p = 0.2638$, Figure S5B), grade of histological malignancy ($p = 0.6334$, Figure S5C), cancer stage ($p = 0.8486$, Figure S5D), gender ($p = 0.8433$, Figure S5E), and cigarette smoking ($p = 0.3604$, Figure S5F). Additionally, we checked whether the expression of the investigated gene changes after tumor removal/as a result of the applied therapy. However, there were no differences in the *ABCG2* gene expression between the groups of patients before surgery and 100 days and one year after the surgery ($p = 0.8187$). Since it is the first such investigation, performed in a restricted study group, the unequivocal exclusion of the surgical tumor removal effect (and/or chemotherapy) on gene expression in patients with lung cancer is impossible. Data are summarized in Figure S5.

3.6. Analysis of ABCG2 Gene Mutations and Copy Number Variations in LUAD and LUSC

ABCG2 gene alterations were studied using the cBioPortal database utilizing the TCGA PanCancer Atlas set. Of the total samples queried (503 for LUAD and 466 for LUSC), the *ABCG2* gene was altered in 2% and 3%, respectively (Figures 6A and 7A), while the somatic mutation frequency was 2.4% for both subtypes (Figures 6B and 7B). In both, the missense variants dominate (10 in LUAD and 8 in LUSC). Then, the association between the *ABCG2* expression level and mutation as well as copy number alteration status was evaluated for LUAD (Figure 6C,D) and LUSC (Figure 7C,D). No significant differences were found, apart from lower levels of mRNA expression z-scores compared to normal tissue in the case of LUSC samples with deep deletion ($p < 0.01$).

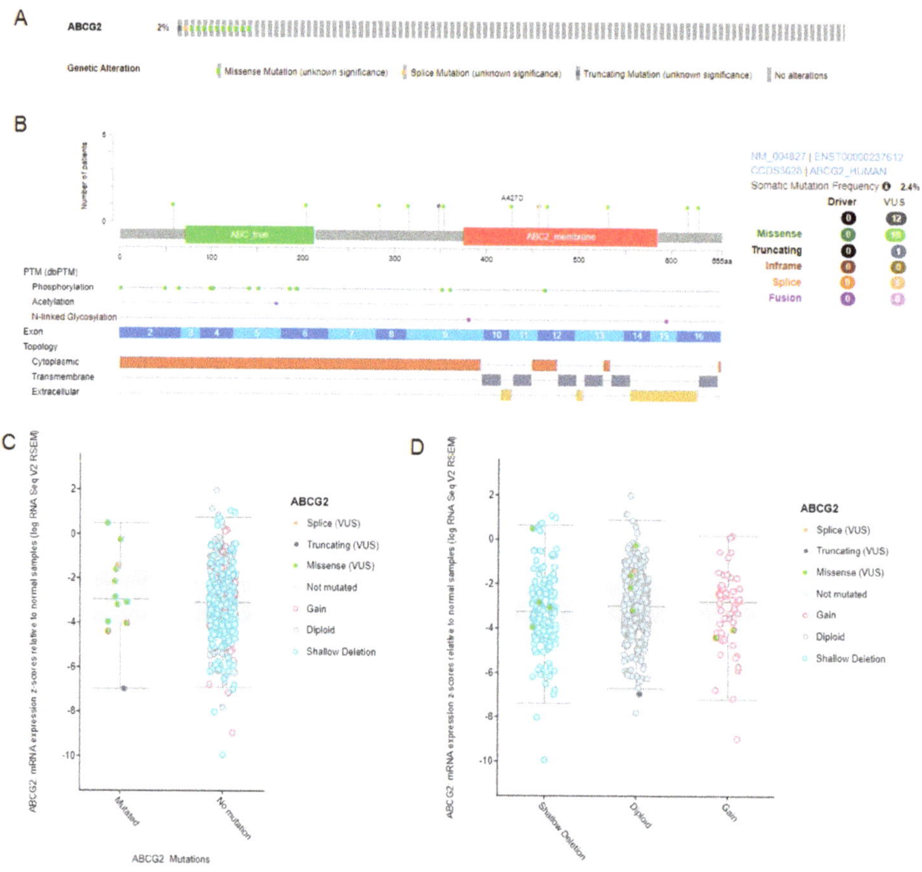

Figure 6. The graphical representation and analysis of mutations and copy number alterations in the *ABCG2* gene for LUAD samples, using cBioPortal. (**A**) The Oncoprint of overall genetic alterations. (**B**) The distribution of mutations and their effect on the protein, exon, and topology spans. (**C**) Association between mutations and mRNA expression z-scores relative to normal samples. (**D**) Association between copy number alterations and mRNA expression z-scores relative to normal samples.

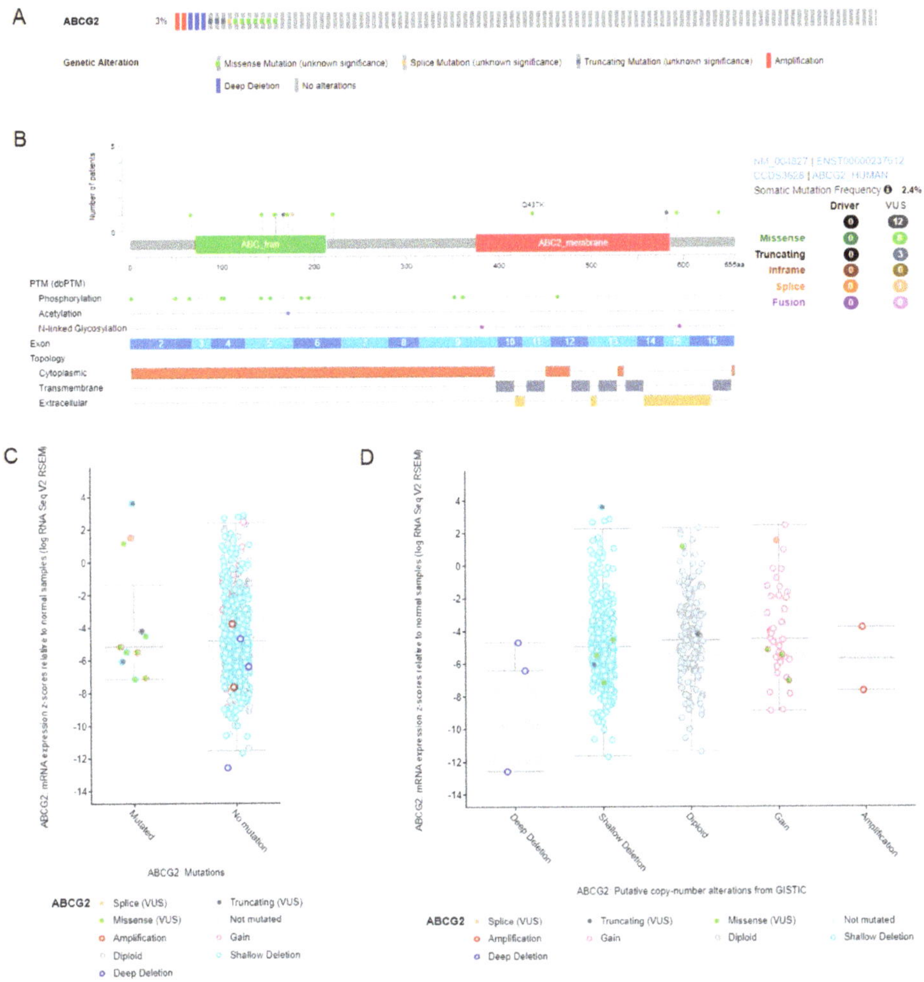

Figure 7. The graphical representation and analysis of mutations and copy number alterations in the ABCG2 gene for LUSC samples, using cBioPortal. (**A**) The Oncoprint of overall genetic alterations. (**B**) The distribution of mutations and their effect on the protein, exon, and topology spans. (**C**) Association between mutations and mRNA expression z-scores relative to normal samples. (**D**) Association between copy number alterations and mRNA expression z-scores relative to normal samples.

3.7. ABCG2 Functional Enrichment and Pathway Analysis

The in silico analysis showed the protein–protein interaction of the ABCG2-centered network. According to obtained results, ABCG2 functional partners, with a confidence score of at least 0.7, were ABCC2; ABCC1; SLCO1B1; SLC2A9; SLC22A12; BSG; MRPS7; SLC22A; SLC22A8; ALB; SLC17A1; CYP3A4; SLCO1B3; PROM1; SLCO2B1; SLCO1A2; NR1I2; SLC47A1; SLC22A11; and ERBB2. See Figure 8.

Within the generated PPI network, three clusters of interaction proteins were identified: red, green, and blue. In the red and green clusters, interactions indicate that members of these clusters are mostly transporters, for example, of organic cations (SLC22A1) or the excretion/detoxification of endogenous and exogenous organic anions (SLC22A1), phosphate into cells via Na^{+} cotransport, urate transport in the kidney (SLC17A1), etc. (Figure 8A). In the case of a blue cluster, it consists of three proteins involved in the metabolism of sterols, steroid hormones, retinoids, and fatty acids (CYP3A4); activation of transcription factors, involved in the metabolism and secretion of xenobiotics, drugs, and endogenous compounds (NR1I2); mediation of the Na^{+}-independent uptake of organic anions; and clearance of bile acids and organic anions from the liver (SLCO1B1). The analysis of gene enrichment revealed the most important pathways modulated by the *ABCG2* gene and its product. A notable enrichment of gene clusters composed primarily of transporters (red and green) in bile secretion, transmembrane transport via ATP-dependent proteins, and platinum drug resistance pathways was identified (Figure 8B). In addition, the blue cluster contained genes associated with linoleic acid and retinol metabolism, steroid hormone biosynthesis, chemical carcinogenesis, and the metabolism of drugs and xenobiotics via cytochrome P450 and other enzymes (Figure 8C).

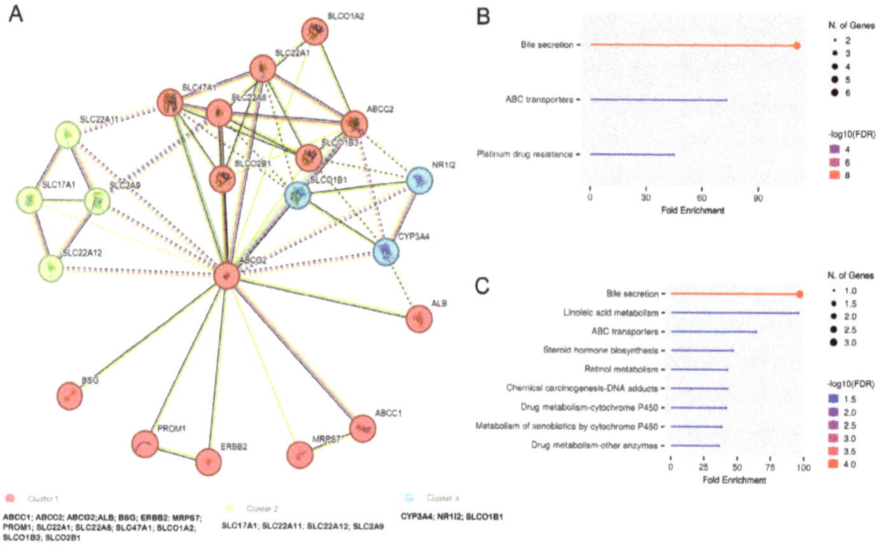

Figure 8. The protein–protein interaction (PPI) network and functional enrichment of ABCG2. (**A**) PPI networks of 20 interacting proteins correlated with ABCG2 using the STRING tool (dashed-lines represents the inter-cluster edges). (**B**,**C**) The analysis of pathways associated with gene clusters indicated in PPI networks: (**B**) cluster 1 and 2, (**C**) cluster 3 (ShinyGO 0.80).

4. Discussion

ABCG2 is highly expressed in placental syncytiotrophoblasts, the cerebral endothelium, and epithelial cells in the intestine and kidney [51] but can also be found in cells localized in lung tissue. A small amount of this protein is identified in the epithelial layer, in seromucinous glands, and in small endothelial capillaries of lung tissue. Simultaneously, high ABCG2 levels were found in many cell lines of a pulmonary origin [52]. The unambiguous identification of lung cells that express this protein remains difficult and controversial because the up-regulation of ABCG2 is mainly drug-induced, resulting in a multidrug-resistant cell phenotype Therefore, in some types of cancer, e.g., myeloid leukemia [51] or lung cancer [53], a high expression of the ABCG2 is associated with a negative patient prognosis. However, this transporter has particular relevance in the lung, where its activity may be critical not only for drug distribution but also in providing protection against inhaled toxins, and other xenobiotics.

ABCG2 is expressed at a low level in most TCGA cancers. This indicates an activation of common molecular mechanisms that are responsible for reduction in cellular *ABCG2* expression, which is associated with the ongoing process of carcinogenesis [54]. However, the mechanisms by which the *ABCG2* gene becomes underexpressed in cancers remain unknown, as well as relatively little being known about the mechanisms that physiologically regulate the expression of this gene. A possible mechanism might be DNA methylation, regulation through miRNA, or cytokine and growth factor activation in the lung cell environment. On the other hand, ABCG2 expression is high in SP cells isolated from lung cancer cell lines and other tumor cell lines. This subtype of cells has been identified as promoting carcinogenesis. However, the fraction of these cells is so small that it should not significantly influence the results of the assessment of the *ABCG2* mRNA level in tumor tissue.

ABCG2 expression levels were shown to be significantly lower in lung tumors than in normal tissues. It is consistent with other findings in primary tumor tissues from LUAD patients [55]. A significant correlation between pathological cancer stages and *ABCG2* expression was shown; its expression was higher in stage 4 in comparison with stage 3 of LUSC. However, the group of patients in the last stage of lung cancer was small, which could have influenced the obtained result. Overall, the *ABCG2* gene expression level did not correlate significantly with the age at the time of diagnosis, pathological cancer stage, cigarette smoking, ethnicity, or gender of lung cancer patients. Therefore, *ABCG2* expression most likely does not affect the processes related to clinical aggressiveness of the disease in this type of cancer.

The therapeutic approach in NSCLC depends on the presence or absence of specific mutations, which in this type of cancer occur most frequently in the *EGFR* or *KRAS* gene. Since LUAD and LUSC are characterized by different mutations, we hypothesized that the expression of the investigated gene would correlate with driver mutations' status of *EGFR* or *KRAS*. However, the results obtained from analyses in the MEXPRESS and UALCAN web tools did not confirm this hypothesis. It was shown that the mutations in one of three genes (*EGFR*, *KRAS*, and *TP53*) did not significantly change the *ABCG2* expression level, while some associations were observed in the study by Jaromi et al. Generally, in the *KRAS* mutant cell line, *ABCG2* expression was higher than in the *EGFR* mutant cell line. Furthermore, it was dependent on the expression of genes from the Wnt signaling pathway [55]. Nevertheless, it should be emphasized that the expression profile of the *ABCG2* in primary tumor tissues differs significantly from that observed in cell cultures [52]. It seems that cellular processes and strings of signaling pathways regulating activity of ABC transporters are complex and strongly dependent on environmental conditions; therefore, the best material for research may be primary patient samples, not subjected to prior manipulations or passages.

Next, we divided the lung cancer patients according to the histological subtype and investigated the correlation of *ABCG2* expression with the prognosis of patients within LUAD, LUSC, and both subtypes combined. The overexpressed *ABCG2* gene showed a protective effect, but only in LUAD. This result is in contradiction with a lot of reports indicating a poor prognosis of patients whose cancer cells are rich in the ABCG2 protein [53,56–58]. However, the surface ABC protein levels do not always correlate with its transcript levels, suggesting that the mechanism responsible for control of ABCG2 concentration may affect the amount of protein, without changing the mRNA level [59]. Additionally, according to Liang et al., the cellular localization of the ABCG2 protein also includes the mitochondrial membrane and inside the cell nucleus. They found that nuclear ABCG2 may serve as a transcription regulator for the factors related to epithelial cell adherence and their polarization and differentiation [60]. We hypothesized that the ability of ABCG2 to shuttle between the cytoplasm and nucleus, or interaction between this protein and DNA, may be modified by the presence/level of the *ABCG2* transcript. Further analyses would be necessary to clarify the mechanism of interaction between ABCG2 protein and its transcript.

Promoter methylation is one of the important mechanisms for the regulation of gene expression. So far, the knowledge about the mechanisms of the transcriptional regulation of *ABCG2* expression remains limited in most types of human cancers. In lung cancer, knowledge on this subject is extremely poor. In this study, a low level of *ABCG2* gene promoter methylation was found in lung cells. In addition, in both LUAD and LUSC, the hypomethylated *ABCG2* promoter region was significantly less methylated in cancer samples than normal samples. The hypomethylation of *ABCG2* was also confirmed in most cases of gallbladder cancer [61] or breast cancer [62]. Additionally, the hypomethylation of this gene may show significant correlation with its increased expression [61]. Methylation status may also be significantly associated with response to chemotherapy [62]. In our analysis, we did not show any correlation between the *ABCG2* gene expression and DNA methylation level in the promoter region. In this regard, lung cancer appears to differ from gallbladder cancer. Moreover, according to our best knowledge, this study is the first to explore the prognostic value of DNA methylation levels of this gene. CpG sites located on the CpG island, which influence the patients' prognosis, were selected, and it included cg01263075, cg03415858, and cg25295218 located up to 200 bp upstream from the transcription start site in *ABCG2*. Thus, an altered methylation of the defined gene region may be one of the important prognostic markers in lung cancer.

Cancer-associated fibroblasts are the dominant cell population in the tumor microenvironment. These cells promote tumorigenesis by initiating the extracellular matrix remodeling and secreting multiple growth factors and cytokines [63]. A positive correlation between cancer-associated fibroblast infiltration and *ABCG2* expression was observed in LUAD, but not in LUSC. Therefore, a higher expression of *ABCG2* could have a potential role in the prediction of tumorigenesis process activation in lung cells, especially in LUAD patients. Further analyses demonstrated a significant positive correlation between *ABCG2* expression and levels of multiple immune cells, which is consistent with the results of other research [64]. In summary, *ABCG2* is strongly involved in immunoinfiltration in lung cancer and therefore remains a promising target for immunotherapy related to immune cell infiltration.

The infiltration of immune cells, particularly macrophages, may be the result of EPHB2 overexpression, which is characteristic for LUAD. Eph receptor B2 (EphB2), an important member of the ephrin receptor family, can stimulate ABCG2 expression in other types of cancer cells, which can explain the correlation observed in our study [65]. In the case of other members of this superfamily, their overexpression has also been observed during the development of lung cancer. An example is EphB4, which has been linked to tumor angiogenesis, growth, and metastasis [66]. Assessment of the interaction between Eph receptors and ABCG2 requires further research.

In our study, the expression of the *ABCG2* gene was additionally evaluated in blood samples taken from patients at three times points (at NSCLC diagnosis and 100 days and one year after surgery). Unfortunately, there were no differences in the *ABCG2* gene expression between these time points. This means that the evaluation of *ABCG2* mRNA in the peripheral blood cells is most likely not suitable for assessing the effectiveness of therapeutic interventions in lung cancer patients. Due to the small number of analyzed samples, this statement should be verified in future research. It is the first such investigation, and thus the unequivocal exclusion of correlation between the *ABCG2* expression in blood and general effectiveness of anticancer treatment in patients with lung cancer is impossible.

The exploration of gene alterations can help to elucidate the gene function and role in lung cancer development and progression. cBioPortal was used to examine the frequency as well as the alteration layout across the *ABCG2* gene. The alteration frequency was rather low across LUSC and LUAD samples (less than or close to 3%), with missense variant domination. Overall, the observed mutations and copy number alterations did not have influence on the mRNA expression z-scores relative to normal samples. In their study, Wang et al. suggested that the mutation pattern of the *ABCG2* gene can be an independent risk factor for the NSCLC prognosis [67], although it remains unclear how this can influence gene interactions, and which mutation is characteristic for the chosen cancer type.

As indicated by the analysis using the STRING tool, the ABCG2 protein interacts mainly with other transporters. Available publications connected with this issue indicate that this protein participates in the ADME mechanisms for drugs. This is especially in the case of the cooccurrence of various polymorphisms for genes encoding proteins from the predicted PPI network. A connection has been shown between the occurrence of variants of the *ABCG2* and *NR1I2* genes and the pharmacokinetics of dolutegravir, used in HIV infection [68]. On the other hand, variants of the genes encoding SLCO1B1 and ABCG2 may affect the level of statins in the blood of patients treated with them [69,70]. Therefore, most of these interactions are associated with the potential development of drug resistance. For example, increased expressions of ABCC1 and ABCG2 reduced the therapeutic effect in an ovarian cancer cell line [71].

The *ABCG2* gene may also be involved in the process of carcinogenesis indirectly, by influencing such processes as apoptosis, autophagy, or ferroptosis. In a normal placenta, reduced or no expression of this gene results in increased sensitivity of placental trophoblast cells to apoptosis in response to cytokines or ceramides. Therefore, the presence of *ABCG2* gene expression protects the cell from apoptosis. However, in the case of cancer cells, this may have a negative effect, leading to an excessive proliferation of these cells and promoting carcinogenesis. Additionally, it has been shown that the overexpression of *ABCG2* in cancer cells enhances the process of autophagy induced by non-substrate stressors (such as radiation or nutrient starvation), contributing to increased cell survival and promoting cancer progression [72,73]. The ABCG2 as a potential heme exporter may be associated with the effect on ferroptosis, although the mechanism has not been fully elucidated, but it is believed that the amount of heme in the cell affects their sensitivity to this phenomenon. Reducing the amount of heme potentially lowers ferroptosis [74].

Although it has been shown in a mouse model that vascular endothelial progenitor cells with the overexpression of *ABCG2* have a higher potential for vessel formation in vivo compared to mature endothelial cells, no association has been demonstrated between *ABCG2* gene expression and *VEGF* gene expression and tumor vascularization in patients with retinoblastoma [75,76].

5. Conclusions

This study demonstrates the potential of *ABCG2* gene expression as well as its methylation evaluation as a biomarker in cancer through in silico and wet analyses. The low *ABCG2* mRNA level is a feature of NSCLC, with no correlation to clinical aggressiveness. This gene appears to have a particularly significant impact on the survival of patients because higher expression improved overall survival in LUAD patients. Additionally, the study highlighted CpG sites influencing the prognosis and drug resistance. The effect of immunotherapy related to immune cell infiltration also significantly depends on the *ABCG2* expression. To the best of our knowledge, this study is the first to present the most comprehensive analysis of the expression of this gene in NSCLC. Despite the fact that there were no differences of *ABCG2* gene expression in blood between subgroups of investigated lung cancer patients (before surgery and 100 days and one year after the surgical removal of the tumor), it is the first such investigation; hence, it was not possible to confront/discuss obtained results and draw unequivocal conclusions. Therefore, these findings require confirmation on a larger group of participants.

Supplementary Materials: The following supporting information can be downloaded at: https://www.mdpi.com/article/10.3390/biomedicines12102394/s1. Figure S1: Association between *ABCG2* expression and clinicopathological characteristics, including (**A**) cancer stage, (**B**) nodal metastasis status, (**C**) smoking status, and (**D**) *TP53* mutation status, in LUAD and LUSC (* $p < 0.05$; UALCAN); Figure S2: Association of *ABCG2* expression (**A**) with clinicopathological and demographic features, (**B**) and analysis of promoter region methylation in LUAD from TCGA datasets ($n = 861$) (*** $p < 0.001$; MEXPRESS); Figure S3: Association of *ABCG2* expression (**A**) with clinicopathological and demographic features, (**B**) and analysis of promoter region methylation in LUSC from TCGA datasets ($n = 758$) (* $p < 0.05$; ** $p < 0.01$; *** $p < 0.001$; MEXPRESS); Figure S4: The correlation of *ABCG2* gene expression (low vs. high expression level) with overall survival (OS) in subgroups of patients with LUAD. The analysis included subgroups formed according to the cancer stage ((**A**) stage 1; (**B**) stage 2; (**C**) stage 3), tumor grade ((**D**) G1; (**E**) G2; (**F**) G3), receiving chemotherapy ((**G**) yes; (**H**) no), gender ((**I**) male; (**J**) female), and tobacco smoking ((**K**) those who never smoked; (**L**) those who smoke or have smoked in the past). HR, hazard ratio; red: high expression; black: low expression ($p < 0.05$; Kaplan–Meier plotter); Figure S5: *ABCG2* gene expression levels in the blood of lung cancer patients depending on the (**A**) age at diagnosis ($p = 0.1995$), (**B**) histological type of the cancer ($p = 0.2638$), (**C**) grade of histological malignancy ($p = 0.6334$), (**D**) cancer stage ($p = 0.8486$), (**E**) gender ($p = 0.8433$), and (**F**) cigarette smoking ($p = 0.3604$); (**G**) The comparison of relative *ABCG2* expression in blood taken from patients at three points during the diagnostic–therapeutic procedure ($p = 0.8187$).

Author Contributions: Conceptualization, A.J.; methodology, A.J., M.Ż.-N. and D.S.-K.; formal analysis, A.J.; investigation, A.J., M.Ż.-N. and M.Ł.; resources, M.Ł.; writing—original draft preparation, A.J., M.Ż.-N. and D.S.-K.; writing—review and editing, A.J., M.Ż.-N., D.S.-K. and E.B.; supervision, E.B.; funding acquisition, E.B. All authors have read and agreed to the published version of the manuscript.

Funding: The present study was supported by statutory funds of the Department of Pharmaceutical Biochemistry and Molecular Diagnostics, Medical University of Lodz (No. 503/3-015-02/503-31-001).

Institutional Review Board Statement: The study was conducted in accordance with the Declaration of Helsinki and approved by the Ethical Committee of the Medical University of Lodz (no. RNN/85/20/KE and no. KE/649/23).

Informed Consent Statement: Informed consent was obtained from all subjects involved in the study.

Data Availability Statement: In the case of the in silico analysis, data are derived from publicly available datasets (TIMER 2.0, UALCAN, TNMplot, MEXPRESS, cBioPortal, MethSurv, KM Plotter, STRING, ShinyGO 0.80). In the case of the wet lab, data are available on request from the Corresponding Author.

Conflicts of Interest: The authors declare no conflicts of interest.

References

1. World Cancer Research Fund International. Lung Cancer Statistics. Available online: https://www.wcrf.org/cancer-trends/lung-cancer-statistics/ (accessed on 4 February 2024).
2. Sharma, R. Mapping of global, regional and national incidence, mortality and mortality-to-incidence ratio of lung cancer in 2020 and 2050. *Int. J. Clin. Oncol.* **2022**, *27*, 665–675. [CrossRef] [PubMed]
3. LoPiccolo, J.; Gusev, A.; Christiani, D.C.; Jänne, P.A. Lung cancer in patients who have never smoked—An emerging disease. *Nat. Rev. Clin. Oncol.* **2024**, *21*, 121–146. [CrossRef] [PubMed]
4. Zhang, Z.; Zhang, X.; Gao, Y.; Chen, Y.; Qin, L.; Wu, I.X. Risk factors for the development of lung cancer among never smokers: A systematic review. *Cancer Epidemiol.* **2022**, *81*, 102274. [CrossRef]
5. Kuśnierczyk, P. Genetic differences between smokers and never-smokers with lung cancer. *Front. Immunol.* **2023**, *2*, 1063716. [CrossRef]
6. Corrales, L.; Rosell, R.; Cardona, A.F.; Martín, C.; Zatarain-Barrón, Z.L.; Arrieta, O. Lung cancer in never smokers: The role of different risk factors other than tobacco smoking. *Crit. Rev. Oncol. Hematol.* **2020**, *148*, 102895. [CrossRef] [PubMed]
7. Dias, M.; Linhas, R.; Campainha, S.; Conde, S.; Barroso, A. Lung cancer in never-smokers—What are the differences? *Acta Oncol.* **2017**, *56*, 931–935. [CrossRef]
8. Jeleń, A.M.; Strehl, B.; Szmajda-Krygier, D.; Pązik, M.; Balcerczak, E. Bioinformatics-Based Characterization of ATP-Binding Cassette Subfamily B Member 1 (ABCB1) Gene Expression in Non-Small-Cell Lung Cancer (NSCLC). *Appl. Sci.* **2023**, *13*, 6576. [CrossRef]

9. Yu, Z.Z.; Xu, B.Q.; Wang, Y.Y.; Zhang, P.W.; Shu, Y.B.; Shi, Z. GSK2606414 Sensitizes ABCG2-Overexpressing Multidrug-Resistant Colorectal Cancer Cells to Chemotherapeutic Drugs. *Biomedicines* **2023**, *11*, 3103. [CrossRef]
10. Zhang, Y.S.; Yang, C.; Han, L.; Liu, L.; Liu, Y.J. Expression of BCRP/ABCG2 Protein in Invasive Breast Cancer and Response to Neoadjuvant Chemotherapy. *Oncol. Res. Treat.* **2022**, *45*, 94–101. [CrossRef]
11. Damiani, D.; Tiribelli, M. ATP-Binding Cassette Subfamily G Member 2 in Acute Myeloid Leukemia: A New Molecular Target? *Biomedicines* **2024**, *12*, 111. [CrossRef]
12. Majam, T.; Sukasem, C.; Reungwetwattana, T.; Chansriwong, P.; Atasilp, C.; Trachu, N.; Thamrongjirapat, T.; Sukprasong, R.; Meanwatthana, J. CYP450 and drug efflux transporters polymorphism influence clinical outcomes of Thai osimertinib-treated non-small cell lung cancer patients. *Front. Pharmacol.* **2023**, *14*, 1222435. [CrossRef] [PubMed]
13. Sito, H.; Sharzehan, M.A.K.; Islam, M.A.; Tan, S.C. Genetic Variants Associated With Response to Platinum-Based Chemotherapy in Non-Small Cell Lung Cancer Patients: A Field Synopsis and Meta-Analysis. *Br. J. Biomed. Sci.* **2024**, *81*, 11835. [CrossRef]
14. Loos, N.H.C.; Retmana, I.A.; Rijmers, J.; Wang, Y.; Gan, C.; Lebre, M.C.; Sparidans, R.W.; Beijnen, J.H.; Schinkel, A.H. Pharmacokinetics of the KRASG12C inhibitor adagrasib is limited by CYP3A and ABCB1, and influenced by binding to mouse plasma carboxylesterase 1c. *Biomed. Pharmacother.* **2023**, *166*, 115304. [CrossRef]
15. Budagaga, Y.; Sabet, Z.; Zhang, Y.; Novotná, E.; Hanke, I.; Rozkoš, T.; Hofman, J. Tazemetostat synergistically combats multidrug resistance by the unique triple inhibition of ABCB1, ABCC1, and ABCG2 efflux transporters in vitro and ex vivo. *Biochem. Pharmacol.* **2023**, *216*, 115769. [CrossRef] [PubMed]
16. Strachowska, M.; Gronkowska, K.; Sobczak, M.; Grodzicka, M.; Michlewska, S.; Kołacz, K.; Sarkar, T.; Korszun, J.; Ionov, M.; Robaszkiewicz, A. I-CBP112 declines overexpression of ATP-binding cassette transporters and sensitized drug-resistant MDA-MB-231 and A549 cell lines to chemotherapy drugs. *Biomed. Pharmacother.* **2023**, *168*, 115798. [CrossRef]
17. Zhang, Y.; Vagiannis, D.; Budagaga, Y.; Sabet, Z.; Hanke, I.; Rozkoš, T.; Hofman, J. Sonidegib potentiates the cancer cells' sensitivity to cytostatic agents by functional inhibition of ABCB1 and ABCG2 in vitro and ex vivo. *Biochem. Pharmacol.* **2022**, *199*, 115009. [CrossRef] [PubMed]
18. Cervenak, J.; Andrikovics, H.; Ozvegy-Laczka, C.; Tordai, A.; Német, K.; Váradi, A.; Sarkadi, B. The role of the human ABCG2 multidrug transporter and its variants in cancer therapy and toxicology. *Cancer Lett.* **2006**, *234*, 62–72. [CrossRef]
19. Duvivier, L.; Gerard, L.; Diaz, A.; Gillet, J.P. Linking ABC transporters to the hallmarks of cancer. *Trends Cancer* **2024**, *10*, 124–134. [CrossRef]
20. Jonker, J.W.; Buitelaar, M.; Wagenaar, E.; Van Der Valk, M.A.; Scheffer, G.L.; Scheper, R.J.; Plosch, T.; Kuipers, F.; Elferink, R.P.; Rosing, H.; et al. The breast cancer resistance protein protects against a major chlorophyll-derived dietary phototoxin and protoporphyria. *Proc. Natl. Acad. Sci. USA* **2002**, *99*, 15649–15654. [CrossRef]
21. Vlaming, M.L.; Teunissen, S.F.; van de Steeg, E.; van Esch, A.; Wagenaar, E.; Brunsveld, L.; de Greef, T.F.; Rosing, H.; Schellens, J.H.; Beijnen, J.H.; et al. Bcrp1;Mdr1a/b;Mrp2 combination knockout mice: Altered disposition of the dietary carcinogen PhIP (2-amino-1-methyl-6-phenylimidazo[4,5-b]pyridine) and its genotoxic metabolites. *Mol. Pharmacol.* **2014**, *85*, 520–530. [CrossRef]
22. Ajenu, E.O.; Seideneck, A.M.; Pandellapalli, E.; Shinsky, E.M.; Humphries, C.L.; Aparicio, N.L.; Sharma, M.; Marden, J.H.; Krasilnikova, M.M. ABCG2 transporter reduces protein aggregation in cigarette smoke condensate-exposed A549 lung cancer cells. *PLoS ONE* **2024**, *19*, e0297661. [CrossRef] [PubMed]
23. Nie, S.; Huang, Y.; Shi, M.; Qian, X.; Li, H.; Peng, C.; Kong, B.; Zou, X.; Shen, S. Protective role of ABCG2 against oxidative stress in colorectal cancer and its potential underlying mechanism. *Oncol. Rep.* **2018**, *40*, 2137–2146. [CrossRef] [PubMed]
24. Andersen, V.; Svenningsen, K.; Knudsen, L.A.; Hansen, A.K.; Holmskov, U.; Stensballe, A.; Vogel, U. Novel understanding of ABC transporters ABCB1/MDR/P-glycoprotein, ABCC2/MRP2, and ABCG2/BCRP in colorectal pathophysiology. *World J. Gastroenterol.* **2015**, *21*, 11862–11876. [CrossRef] [PubMed]
25. Sun, Y.; Wen, M.; Liu, Y.; Wang, Y.; Jing, P.; Gu, Z.; Jiang, T.; Wang, W. The human microbiome: A promising target for lung cancer treatment. *Front. Immunol.* **2023**, *14*, 1091165. [CrossRef]
26. Zheng, J.; Shi, W.; Yang, Q.; Huang, J.; Shen, J.; Yin, L.; Zhang, P.; Zhang, S.; Yang, M.; Qian, A.; et al. Hospital-treated infectious diseases, infection burden and risk of Parkinson disease: An observational and Mendelian randomization study. *Brain Behav. Immun.* **2024**, *120*, 352–359. [CrossRef]
27. Mounika, P. Helicobacter pylori Infection and Risk of Lung Cancer: A Meta-Analysis. *Lung Cancer Int.* **2013**, *2013*, 131869. [CrossRef]
28. Yang, Y.; Fan, Y.; Qi, Y.; Liu, D.; Wu, K.; Wen, F.; Zhao, S. Side population cells separated from A549 lung cancer cell line possess cancer stem cell-like properties and inhibition of autophagy potentiates the cytotoxic effect of cisplatin. *Oncol. Rep.* **2015**, *34*, 929–935. [CrossRef]
29. Zhang, L.; Shen, L.; Wu, D. Clinical significance of cancer stem cell markers in lung carcinoma. *Acta Biochim. Pol.* **2021**, *68*, 187–191. [CrossRef] [PubMed]
30. Yang, B.; Wang, Y.; Chen, Z.; Feng, Y.M.; Shi, L.L. Effects of Apatinib on the "Stemness" of Non-Small-Cell Lung Cancer Cells In Vivo and Its Related Mechanisms. *Can. Respir. J.* **2020**, *2020*, 2479369. [CrossRef]
31. Thirusangu, P.; Ray, U.; Sarkar Bhattacharya, S.; Oien, D.B.; Jin, L.; Staub, J.; Kannan, N.; Molina, J.R.; Shridhar, V. PFKFB3 regulates cancer stemness through the hippo pathway in small cell lung carcinoma. *Oncogene* **2022**, *41*, 4003–4017. [CrossRef]
32. Chen, Q.; Sun, Z.; Li, J.; Zhang, D.; Guo, B.; Zhang, T. SET Domain-Containing Protein 5 Enhances the Cell Stemness of Non-Small Cell Lung Cancer via the PI3K/Akt/mTOR Pathway. *J. Environ. Pathol. Toxicol. Oncol.* **2021**, *40*, 55–63. [CrossRef] [PubMed]

33. Nelakurthi, V.M.; Paul, P.; Reche, A. Bioinformatics in Early Cancer Detection. *Cureus* **2023**, *15*, e46931. [CrossRef] [PubMed]
34. Jiang, P.; Sinha, S.; Aldape, K.; Hannenhalli, S.; Sahinalp, C.; Ruppin, E. Big data in basic and translational cancer research. *Nat. Rev. Cancer* **2022**, *22*, 625–639. [CrossRef]
35. Li, T.; Fu, J.; Zeng, Z.; Cohen, D.; Li, J.; Chen, Q.; Li, B.; Liu, X.S. TIMER2.0 for analysis of tumor-infiltrating immune cells. *Nucleic Acids Res.* **2020**, *48*, W509–W514. [CrossRef]
36. Li, T.; Fan, J.; Wang, B.; Traugh, N.; Chen, Q.; Liu, J.S.; Li, B.; Liu, X.S. TIMER: A Web Server for Comprehensive Analysis of Tumor-Infiltrating Immune Cells. *Cancer Res.* **2017**, *77*, e108–e110. [CrossRef]
37. Bartha, Á.; Győrffy, B. TNMplot.com: A Web Tool for the Comparison of Gene Expression in Normal, Tumor and Metastatic Tissues. *Int. J. Mol. Sci.* **2021**, *22*, 2622. [CrossRef]
38. Chandrashekar, D.S.; Karthikeyan, S.K.; Korla, P.K.; Patel, H.; Shovon, A.R.; Athar, M.; Netto, G.J.; Qin, Z.S.; Kumar, S.; Manne, U.; et al. UALCAN: An update to the integrated cancer data analysis platform. *Neoplasia* **2022**, *25*, 18–27. [CrossRef]
39. Chandrashekar, D.S.; Bashel, B.; Balasubramanya, S.A.H.; Creighton, C.J.; Ponce-Rodriguez, I.; Chakravarthi, B.V.S.K.; Varambally, S. UALCAN: A Portal for Facilitating Tumor Subgroup Gene Expression and Survival Analyses. *Neoplasia* **2017**, *19*, 649–658. [CrossRef] [PubMed]
40. Koch, A.; De Meyer, T.; Jeschke, J.; Van Criekinge, W. MEXPRESS: Visualizing expression, DNA methylation and clinical TCGA data. *BMC Genomics* **2015**, *16*, 636. [CrossRef]
41. Koch, A.; Jeschke, J.; Van Criekinge, W.; van Engeland, M.; De Meyer, T. MEXPRESS update 2019. *Nucleic Acids Res* **2019**, *47*, W561–W565. [CrossRef]
42. Cerami, E.; Gao, J.; Dogrusoz, U.; Gross, B.E.; Sumer, S.O.; Aksoy, B.A.; Jacobsen, A.; Byrne, C.J.; Heuer, M.L.; Larsson, E.; et al. The cBio cancer genomics portal: An open platform for exploring multidimensional cancer genomics data. *Cancer Discov.* **2012**, *2*, 401–404. [CrossRef] [PubMed]
43. Modhukur, V.; Iljasenko, T.; Metsalu, T.; Lokk, K.; Laisk-Podar, T.; Vilo, J. MethSurv: A web tool to perform multivariable survival analysis using DNA methylation data. *Epigenomics* **2018**, *10*, 277–288. [CrossRef]
44. Győrffy, B. Transcriptome-level discovery of survival-associated biomarkers and therapy targets in non-small-cell lung cancer. *Br. J. Pharmacol.* **2024**, *181*, 362–374. [CrossRef]
45. Gao, J.; Aksoy, B.A.; Dogrusoz, U.; Dresdner, G.; Gross, B.; Sumer, S.O.; Sun, Y.; Jacobsen, A.; Sinha, R.; Larsson, E.; et al. Integrative analysis of complex cancer genomics and clinical profiles using the cBioPortal. *Sci. Signal* **2013**, *6*, pl1. [CrossRef]
46. de Bruijn, I.; Kundra, R.; Mastrogiacomo, B.; Tran, T.N.; Sikina, L.; Mazor, T.; Li, X.; Ochoa, A.; Zhao, G.; Lai, B.; et al. Analysis and Visualization of Longitudinal Genomic and Clinical Data from the AACR Project GENIE Biopharma Collaborative in cBioPortal. *Cancer Res.* **2023**, *83*, 3861–3867. [CrossRef] [PubMed]
47. Szklarczyk, D.; Kirsch, R.; Koutrouli, M.; Nastou, K.; Mehryary, F.; Hachilif, R.; Gable, A.L.; Fang, T.; Doncheva, N.T.; Pyysalo, S.; et al. The STRING database in 2023: Protein-protein association networks and functional enrichment analyses for any sequenced genome of interest. *Nucleic Acids Res* **2023**, *51*, D638–D646. [CrossRef] [PubMed]
48. Ge, S.X.; Jung, D.; Yao, R. ShinyGO: A graphical gene-set enrichment tool for animals and plants. *Bioinformatics* **2020**, *36*, 2628–2629. [CrossRef]
49. Lu, X.; Chen, M.; Shen, J.; Xu, Y.; Wu, H. IL-1β functionally attenuates ABCG2 and PDZK1 expression in HK-2 cells partially through NF-κB activation. *Cell Biol. Int.* **2019**, *43*, 279–289. [CrossRef]
50. Mosaffa, F.; Kalalinia, F.; Lage, H.; Afshari, J.T.; Behravan, J. Pro-inflammatory cytokines interleukin-1 beta, interleukin 6, and tumor necrosis factor-alpha alter the expression and function of ABCG2 in cervix and gastric cancer cells. *Mol. Cell Biochem.* **2012**, *363*, 385–393. [CrossRef]
51. Eckenstaler, R.; Benndorf, R.A. 3D structure of the transporter ABCG2-What's new? *Br. J. Pharmacol.* **2020**, *177*, 1485–1496. [CrossRef]
52. Nickel, S.; Selo, M.A.; Fallack, J.; Clerkin, C.G.; Huwer, H.; Schneider-Daum, N.; Lehr, C.M.; Ehrhardt, C. Expression and Activity of Breast Cancer Resistance Protein (BCRP/ABCG2) in Human Distal Lung Epithelial Cells In Vitro. *Pharm. Res.* **2017**, *34*, 2477–2487. [CrossRef] [PubMed]
53. Yoh, K.; Ishii, G.; Yokose, T.; Minegishi, Y.; Tsuta, K.; Goto, K.; Nishiwaki, Y.; Kodama, T.; Suga, M.; Ochiai, A. Breast cancer resistance protein impacts clinical outcome in platinum-based chemotherapy for advanced non-small cell lung cancer. *Clin. Cancer Res.* **2004**, *10*, 1691–1697. [CrossRef] [PubMed]
54. Lyu, C.; Wang, L.; Stadlbauer, B.; Buchner, A.; Pohla, H. A Pan-Cancer Landscape of ABCG2 across Human Cancers: Friend or Foe? *Int. J. Mol. Sci.* **2022**, *23*, 15955. [CrossRef] [PubMed]
55. Jaromi, L.; Csongei, V.; Vesel, M.; Abdelwahab, E.M.M.; Soltani, A.; Torok, Z.; Smuk, G.; Sarosi, V.; Pongracz, J.E. KRAS and EGFR Mutations Differentially Alter ABC Drug Transporter Expression in Cisplatin-Resistant Non-Small Cell Lung Cancer. *Int. J. Mol. Sci.* **2021**, *22*, 5384. [CrossRef] [PubMed]
56. Tada, H.; Gonda, K.; Kitamura, N.; Ishida, T. Clinical Significance of ABCG2/BCRP Quantified by Fluorescent Nanoparticles in Breast Cancer Patients Undergoing Neoadjuvant Chemotherapy. *Cancers* **2023**, *15*, 2365. [CrossRef]
57. Ma, R.; Luo, F.; Zhao, J.; He, H.; Wang, H.; Huang, X.; Sun, F.; Xu, Z.; Zhou, W.; Zhu, Y.; et al. Role of ABCG2 as a potentially prognostic factor during the follow-up of renal cell carcinoma. *J. Clin. Urol.* **2016**, *31*, 986–990. [CrossRef]
58. Emery, I.F.; Gopalan, A.; Wood, S.; Chow, K.H.; Battelli, C.; George, J.; Blaszyk, H.; Florman, J.; Yun, K. Expression and function of ABCG2 and XIAP in glioblastomas. *J. Neurooncol.* **2017**, *133*, 47–57. [CrossRef]

59. Bircsak, K.M.; Moscovitz, J.E.; Wen, X.; Archer, F.; Yuen, P.Y.S.; Mohammed, M.; Memon, N.; Weinberger, B.I.; Saba, L.M.; Vetrano, A.M.; et al. Interindividual Regulation of the Breast Cancer Resistance Protein/ABCG2 Transporter in Term Human Placentas. *Drug Metab. Dispos.* **2018**, *46*, 619–627. [CrossRef]
60. Liang, S.C.; Yang, C.Y.; Tseng, J.Y.; Wang, H.L.; Tung, C.Y.; Liu, H.W.; Chen, C.Y.; Yeh, Y.C.; Chou, T.Y.; Yang, M.H.; et al. ABCG2 localizes to the nucleus and modulates CDH1 expression in lung cancer cells. *Neoplasia* **2015**, *17*, 265–278. [CrossRef]
61. Nimisha; Saluja, S.S.; Sharma, A.K.; Nekarakanti, P.K.; Apurva; Kumar, A.; Sattar, R.S.A.; Anjum, H.; Batra, V.V.; Husain, S.A. Molecular aspects of ABCB1 and ABCG2 in Gallbladder cancer and its clinical relevance. *Mol. Cell Biochem.* **2023**, *478*, 2379–2394. [CrossRef]
62. Ahmed Aglan, S.; Mohamad Zaki, A.; Sobhy El Sedfy, A.; Gaber El-Sheredy, H.; Hussein Elgaddar, O. O6-Methylguanine-DNA Methyltransferase and ATP-Binding Cassette Membrane Transporter G2 Promotor Methylation: Can Predict the Response to Chemotherapy in Advanced Breast Cancer? *Rep. Biochem. Mol. Biol.* **2022**, *11*, 20–29. [CrossRef] [PubMed]
63. Erdogan, B.; Webb, D.J. Cancer-associated fibroblasts modulate growth factor signaling and extracellular matrix remodeling to regulate tumor metastasis. *Biochem. Soc. Trans.* **2017**, *45*, 229–236. [CrossRef] [PubMed]
64. Zhai, Y.; Zhai, X. ABCG2 predicts the prognosis and is associated with immune infiltration in lung cancer: A bioinformatics study. *Discov. Oncol.* 2024; *preprint is under review*. [CrossRef]
65. Liu, W.; Yu, C.; Li, J.; Fang, J. The Roles of EphB2 in Cancer. *Front. Cell Dev. Biol.* **2022**, *10*, 788587. [CrossRef]
66. Ullah, A.; Razzaq, A.; Zhou, C.; Ullah, N.; Shehzadi, S.; Aziz, T.; Alfaifi, M.Y.; Elbehairi, S.E.I.; Iqbal, H. Biological Significance of EphB4 Expression in Cancer. *Curr. Protein Pept. Sci.* **2024**, *25*, 244–255. [CrossRef]
67. Wang, H.; Luo, F.; Zhu, Z.; Xu, Z.; Huang, X.; Ma, R.; He, H.; Zhu, Y.; Shao, K.; Zhao, J. ABCG2 is a potential prognostic marker of overall survival in patients with clear cell renal cell carcinoma. *BMC Cancer* **2017**, *17*, 222. [CrossRef]
68. Elliot, E.R.; Neary, M.; Else, L.; Khoo, S.; Moyle, G.; Carr, D.F.; Wang, X.; Mcclure, M.; Boffito, M.; Owen, A. Genetic influence of ABCG2, UGT1A1 and NR1I2 on dolutegravir plasma pharmacokinetics. *J. Antimicrob. Chemother.* **2020**, *75*, 1259–1266. [CrossRef]
69. Liu, M.; Wu, X.J.; Zhao, G.L.; Zhang, T.; Xu, S.S.; Sun, Y.X.; Qiu, F.; Zhao, L.M. Effects of Polymorphisms in NR1H4, NR1I2, SLCO1B1, and ABCG2 on the Pharmacokinetics of Rosuvastatin in Healthy Chinese Volunteers. *J. Cardiovasc. Pharmacol.* **2016**, *68*, 383–390. [CrossRef]
70. Rattanacheeworn, P.; Chamnanphon, M.; Thongthip, S.; Kittanamongkolchai, W.; Townamchai, N.; Avihingsanon, Y.; Udomnilobol, U.; Prueksaritanont, T.; Jianmongkol, S.; Chariyavilaskul, P. *SLCO1B1* and *ABCG2* Gene Polymorphisms in a Thai Population. *Pharmgenomics Pers. Med.* **2020**, *13*, 521–530. [CrossRef]
71. Teng, Q.X.; Lei, Z.N.; Wang, J.Q.; Yang, Y.; Wu, Z.X.; Acharekar, N.D.; Zhang, W.; Yoganathan, S.; Pan, Y.; Wurpel, J.; et al. Overexpression of ABCC1 and ABCG2 confers resistance to talazoparib, a poly (ADP-Ribose) polymerase inhibitor. *Drug Resist. Updat.* **2024**, *73*, 101028. [CrossRef]
72. Evseenko, D.A.; Murthi, P.; Paxton, J.W.; Reid, G.; Emerald, B.S.; Mohankumar, K.M.; Lobie, P.E.; Brennecke, S.P.; Kalionis, B.; Keelan, J.A. The ABC transporter BCRP/ABCG2 is a placental survival factor, and its expression is reduced in idiopathic human fetal growth restriction. *FASEB J.* **2007**, *21*, 3592–3605. [CrossRef] [PubMed]
73. Ding, R.; Jin, S.; Pabon, K.; Scotto, K.W. A role for ABCG2 beyond drug transport: Regulation of autophagy. *Autophagy* **2016**, *12*, 737–751. [CrossRef] [PubMed]
74. Wang, Y.; Zhang, Z.; Jiao, W.; Wang, Y.; Wang, X.; Zhao, Y.; Fan, X.; Tian, L.; Li, X.; Mi, J. Ferroptosis and its role in skeletal muscle diseases. *Front. Mol. Biosci.* **2022**, *9*, 1051866. [CrossRef]
75. Kim, M.; Kim, J.H.; Kim, J.H.; Kim, D.H.; Yu, Y.S. Differential expression of stem cell markers and vascular endothelial growth factor in human retinoblastoma tissue. *Korean J. Ophthalmol.* **2010**, *24*, 35–39. [CrossRef]
76. Lin, Y.; Gil, C.H.; Banno, K.; Yokoyama, M.; Wingo, M.; Go, E.; Prasain, N.; Liu, Y.; Hato, T.; Naito, H.; et al. ABCG2-Expressing Clonal Repopulating Endothelial Cells Serve to Form and Maintain Blood Vessels. *Circulation* **2024**, *150*, 451–465. [CrossRef]

biomedicines

MDPI

Article

Interplay of RNA m^{6}A Modification-Related Geneset in Pan-Cancer

Boyu Zhang [1,†], Yajuan Hao [2,3,†], Haiyan Liu [1], Jiarun Wu [1], Lu Lu [4], Xinfeng Wang [1], Akhilesh K. Bajpai [4,*] and Xi Yang [1,*]

[1] Department of Hematology, Affiliated Hospital of Nantong University, Nantong 226007, China; 2031110059@stmail.ntu.edu.cn (B.Z.); haiyan1223@126.com (H.L.); 2331110594@stmail.ntu.edu.cn (J.W.); wxf5204079@126.com (X.W.)

[2] Department of Urology, Shanghai Tenth People's Hospital, Tongji University, Shanghai 200072, China; haoyajuan1989@126.com

[3] Urologic Cancer Institute, School of Medicine, Tongji University, Shanghai 200072, China

[4] Department of Genetics, Genomics, and Informatics, University of Tennessee Health Science Center, Memphis, UT 38163, USA; llu@uthsc.edu

* Correspondence: abajpai3@uthsc.edu (A.K.B.); yangxi209@163.com (X.Y.)

† These authors contributed equally to this work.

Abstract: Background: N^6-methyladenosine (m^{6}A), is the most common modification found in mRNA and lncRNA in higher organisms and plays an important role in physiology and pathology. However, its role in pan-cancer has not been explored. **Results**: A total of 31 m^{6}A modification regulators, including 12 writers, 2 erasers, and 17 readers are identified in the current study. The functional analysis of the regulators results in the enrichment of processes, primarily related to RNA modification and metabolism, and the PPI network reveals multiple interactions among the regulators. The mRNA expression analysis reveals a high expression for most of the regulators in pan-cancer. Most of the m^{6}A regulators are found to be mutated across the cancers, with *ZC3H13*, *VIRMA*, and *PRRC2A* having a higher frequency rate. Significant correlations of the regulators with clinicopathological parameters, such as age, gender, tumor stage, and grade are identified in pan-cancer. The m^{6}A regulators' expression is found to have significant positive correlations with the miRNAs in pan-cancer. The expression pattern of the m^{6}A regulators is able to classify the tumors into different subclusters as well as into high- and low-risk groups. These tumor groups show differential patterns in terms of their immune cell infiltration, tumor stemness score, genomic heterogeneity score, expression of immune regulatory/checkpoint genes, and correlations between the regulators and the drugs. **Conclusions**: Our study provide a comprehensive overview of the functional roles, genetic and epigenetic alterations, and prognostic value of the RNA m^{6}A regulators in pan-cancer.

Keywords: m^{6}A; pan-cancer; prognosis; immune cell infiltration; tumor stemness; genomic heterogeneity

1. Introduction

N^6-methyladenosine (m^{6}A) is the most common modification found in mRNA and other kinds of RNA in higher organisms, accounting for 0.1% to 0.4% of all adenine residues [1–3]. It typically occurs in the 3′ untranslated region (UTR) and near stop codons in mRNA [4,5]. The m^{6}A modification primarily includes m^{6}A methylation and m^{6}A demethylation.

The m^{6}A methylation is defined as the transfer of a methyl group to the N^6 position of RNA adenosine residues through the action of the methyltransferase complex, using S-adenosylmethionine (SAM) as the methyl donor [6]. The m^{6}A demethylation is defined as the removal of m^{6}A by the demethylating enzyme transforming it into A, thereby completing the removal of m^{6}A [7]. Due to the actions of methyltransferases and demethylases,

RNA methylation becomes a dynamic and reversible process. The m^{6}A modification could influence the stability and translation efficiency of RNA, which is controlled by three homologous factors, including 12 methyltransferases (defined as "writers", e.g., *METTL3* [8], *METTL14* [8], *WTAP* [8], *METTL16* [9], *VIRMA* [2], *ZC3H13* [10], *CBLL1* [11], *RBM15* [12], *RBM15B* [12], *METTL5* [13], *TRMT112* [13], and *ZCCHC4* [13]), 2 demethylation enzymes (named "erasers", e.g., *FTO* [14] and *ALKBH5* [15]), and 17 methylation-binding proteins (also known as "readers", e.g., *YTHDC1* [16], *YTHDC2* [17], *YTHDF1* [18], *YTHDF2* [19], *YTHDF3* [20], *HNRNPC* [21], *RBMX* [22], *FMR1* [23], *HNRNPA2B1* [24], *IGF2BP1* [25], *IGF2BP2* [25], *IGF2BP3* [25], *PRRC2A* [26], *RBM33* [27], *RBFOX2* [28], *LRPPRC* [29], and *FXR1* [30]). The m^{6}A modification reduces mRNA stability [31], increases mRNA translation [18], mediates cytoplasmic liquid–liquid phase separation [32], affectes mRNA splicing [33], and promotes mRNA export from the nucleus [34]. The presence of m^{6}A modifications on genes helps to promote/suppress multiple fundamental cellular functions, indicative of its association with many human diseases.

There have been multiple reports about the key role of m^{6}A modification in biological processes underlying cancer. The expression of *METTL3* has been shown to be increased in acute myeloid leukemia (AML) patients, suppressing cell differentiation and apoptosis, and promoting cell proliferation through increased translation of *c-MYC*, *BCL2*, and *PTEN*. Further, *METTL3* activates the PI3K/AKT signaling pathway to control cell differentiation and self-renewal in AML [35]. Another study shows that miR-33a inhibits proliferation and promotes differentiation of non-small cell lung cancer cells (NSCLCs) by binding to the 3′UTR of *METTL3* [36], which suggests that *METTL3* may be a novel therapeutic target for NSCLC. Similarly, an increased expression of *METTL3* has been reported in hepatocellular carcinoma (HCC) patients, as well as in in vivo experiments. Furthermore, *METTL3* is found to promote cell growth and migration of HCC, both in vivo and in vitro, and enhances the tumorigenicity, growth, and lung metastasis of liver cancer [37]. The *WTAP* deficiency has been shown to inhibit cell migration, invasion, and tumorigenicity of cholangiocarcinoma (CCA). cDNA microarray and real-time PCR results of CCA have demonstrated that *WTAP* enhances the expression of metastasis-related genes, such as *MMP7*, *MMP28*, and *MUC1* [38].

Other m^{6}A regulators also play vital roles in various kinds of cancers, and the same regulator may act contrariwise in different cancers [39]. The eraser *ALKBH5* is downregulated and acts as a tumor suppressor in esophageal squamous cell carcinoma by inhibiting m^{6}A/DGCR8-dependent miR-194-2 biogenesis and releasing RAI1 expression, as well as through positive feedback between miR-193a-3p and *ALKBH5*. *ALKBH5* increases in gastric cancer and demethylates lncRNA NEAT1, thus upregulating its expression, and also promotes FAD7 translation in an m^{6}A-dependent manner. *ALKBH5* demethylates lncRNA KCNK15-AS1, is decreased in pancreatic cancer, resulting in reduced tumor migration, invasion, and EMT. *ALKBH5* is decreased in non-small cell lung cancer and reduces m^{6}A levels on YAP pre-mRNA, leading to suppressed tumor proliferation, migration, invasion, and EMT. However, *ALKBH5* is increased in lung adenocarcinoma and reduces the m^{6}A level of FOXM1 mRNA, contributing to an oncogenic role in tumor proliferation and invasion. Another eraser, *FTO*, is elevated, reduces the USP7 mRNA m^{6}A level, and promotes the proliferation of non-small cell lung cancer. *FTO* is also elevated, and promotes proliferation and invasion, but inhibits apoptosis by reducing the MZF1 mRNA m^{6}A level in lung squamous cell carcinoma. In cervical cancer, *FTO* is upregulated, and promotes proliferation and migration by controlling the m^{6}A modification of E2F1 and MYC, also promoting drug resistance by reducing the β-catenin m^{6}A level, thereby positively regulating β-catenin expression. *FTO* is increased in acute myeloid leukemia, and regulates the ASB2 and RARA levels by demethylating the m^{6}A modification on their RNA, leading to elevated tumor proliferation and reduced apoptosis. *FTO* is also upregulated in breast cancer and mediates the m^{6}A demethylation of BNIP3 mRNA, inducing its degradation, leading to an oncogene role in proliferation and metastasis.

The methytransferase *METTL14* is reduced in hepatocellular carcinoma, and promotes pri-miR-126 processing through an m^{6}A/DGCR8-dependent manner, thus acting as a tumor suppressor. *METTL14* is also decreased in colorectal cancer and represses tumor progression by promoting SOX4 expression and reducing XIST in an m^{6}A-YTHDF2-dependent manner, and by promoting pri-miR-375 processing through an m^{6}A/DGCR8-dependent mechanism. *METTL14* also acts as a tumor suppressor in bladder cancer and renal cell carcinoma by inhibiting Notch1 and P2RX6 separately through m^{6}A modification. However, *METTL14* is elevated in acute myeloid leukemia by regulating its mRNA targets through m^{6}A modification, including MYB, MYC, and SPL1. *KIAA1429* induces GATA3 pre-mRNA methylation and promotes its degradation, leading to the progression of hepatocellular carcinoma.

The m^{6}A reader *HNRNPA2B1* upregulates the expression of ACLY and ACC1, leading to the tumor progression of esophageal squamous cell carcinoma. *YTHDF1* promotes FZD7 translation in an m^{6}A-dependent manner and is increased to promote the proliferation and metastasis in gastric cancer. *YTHDF1* is also increased and enhanced EIF3C translation using m^{6}A modification in ovarian cancer. *YTHDF1* also acts as an oncogene in melanoma by promoting the translation of methylated HINT2 mRNA. *YTHDF2* degrades IL11 and SERPINE2 mRNA, and inhibits tumor growth, vascular density and permeability, and inflammation in hepatocellular carcinoma. *YTHDF2* also increases and promotes 6PGD mRNA translation, leading to lung cancer proliferation. *YTHDF2* is also upregulated in prostate cancer and alters the tumor proliferation and migration using miR-493-3p. *YTHDF3* degrades GAS5 using m^{6}A modification and is elevated and enhanced the proliferation and invasion of colorectal cancer. *YTHDC2* increases HIF-1α translation and is increased and promotes the metastasis of colorectal cancer. *IGF2BP2* enhances HMGA2 stability in an m^{6}A-independent manner and plays an oncogenic role to promote colorectal cancer migration and invasion. *IGF2BP2* also regulates DANCR stability and enhances pancreatic cancer proliferation and stem cell like properties.

The m^{6}A modification has been considered as a key regulator of T cell homeostasis and immune response against bacterial and viral infections. Selectively altering m^{6}A levels and other types of immune therapies may be effective strategies for the management of various immune disorders [40,41]. The loss of *YTHDF1* inhibits tumor growth is due to increased infiltration of tumor-specific CD8$^+$ T cells in the cancer tissue. The m^{6}A modification affectes the turnover and translation of signaling molecules, including that of *MAVS*, *TRAF3*, and *TRAF6*, and thus regulating the production of interferon in antiviral innate immune response [41]. Therefore, m^{6}A modification plays important roles in the occurrence and development of cancer, and is thus considered for anti-tumor and anti-viral immune therapies.

In this study, we focuses on the association between m^{6}A modification genes and multiple cancers at the genomic, transcriptomic, and proteomic levels, exploring the pan-cancer regulatory mechanism of m^{6}A modification.

2. Materials and Methods

2.1. Geneset Collection, Protein-Protein Interaction (PPI), and Gene Annotation of m^{6}A Modifiers

The genes related to the writers, readers, and erasers of m^{6}A modification are collected from the literature and are shown in Supplementary Table S1. The protein–protein interaction network of the m^{6}A modification genes is analyzed and visualized using the STRING database (https://string-db.org/ accessed on 30 May 2024) [42,43]. Furthermore, the Metascape tool (https://metascape.org/ accessed on 30 May 2024) [44] is utilized to explore the Gene Ontology (GO) annotations associated with m^{6}A modification genes.

2.2. Data Collection and Processing

We download the gene expression data at TPM levels from the GTEx project (https://gtexportal.org/home/ accessed on 30 May 2024) and the Cancer Genome Atlas (TCGA) database (http://cancergenome.nih.gov accessed on 30 May 2024). We collect normal and tumor samples corresponding to 28 tissues, based on the information provided by the GTEx and TCGA databases. To eliminate batch effects, we use the combat algorithm from the sva (v 3.5) package [45]. To analyze the differential expression of genes between normal and tumor samples for each tissue, we employ the Wilcoxon rank sum and signed rank test [46]. In addition, we gather clinical information, mutation data, and miRNA expression data for these 28 types of cancer from the TCGA database [47,48].

2.3. Cox Regression Analysis

The univariate Cox regression model in the survival (v 3.2-7) package (https://cran.r-project.org/web/packages/survival/index.html, accessed on 1 March 2024) is used to assess the prognostic significance of each gene by considering their survival time, survival status, and gene expression levels.

2.4. Copy Number Variants (CNVs), Single Nucleotide Variations (SNVs), and Methylation Level Analysis

We obtain copy number variants (CNVs), single nucleotide variants (SNVs), and methylation data for multiple cancer types from the GDC (https://portal.gdc.cancer.gov/ accessed on 30 May 2024) database. For each cancer, we calculate the percentages of heterozygous amplifications, homozygous amplifications, heterozygous deletions, and homozygous deletions of m^6A modification genes. Additionally, we determine the correlation between CNV, methylation status, and RNA expression, as well as the SNV percentage and methylation differences for each cancer. Furthermore, we use the univariate Cox regression model to analyze the survival impact of CNVs and compare the differences between mutant and wild-type cases.

2.5. Consensus Cluster Analysis

The R package *ConsensusClusterPlus* (v 1.64.0) is utilized to identify distinct clusters based on the gene expression pattern of each cancer type, using a consensus-clustering approach [49]. The number of clusters is determined based on the area under the curve of the cumulative distribution function and the value of k. To enhance the reliability of the classification outcomes, the classification procedure is repeated 1000 times.

2.6. Risk Model Construction

The LASSO regression analysis is used to create a risk model for each cancer, considering factors, such as survival time, survival status, and gene expression levels. This is done using the *glmnet* (v 4.1-7) and *survival* (v 3.5-5) packages [50]. The best model is determined through a 10-fold cross-validation. The *maxstat* (v 0.7-25) package is utilized to calculate the optimal cutoff value for the Risk Score, with the requirement that the minimum group sample size be greater than 25% and the maximum group sample size be less than 75% [51]. Patients are then divided into high- and low-risk groups based on this optimal cutoff value, and further analysis is conducted to examine the prognostic differences between the two groups.

2.7. Immune Cell Infiltration, Stemness Features, and Tumor Heterogeneity Analysis

The *CIBERSORT* algorithm from the *IOBR* (v 0.99.9) package is used to elucidate immune cell infiltrations [52]. We collect various scores for tumor dryness, including DNAss (DNA methylation-based), EREG-METHss (epigenetically regulated DNA methylation-based), DMPss (differentially methylated probe-based), ENHss (enhancer element/DNA methylation-based), RNAss (RNA expression-based), and EREG.EXPss (epigenetically regulated RNA expression-based). These scores are calculated using the mRNA expression levels and methylation signatures for each tumor, based on the method outlined in Malta et al.'s research [53]. The tmb function from the maftools package (v 2.18) is used to calculate the tumor mutation burden (TMB) score for each tumor. The inferHeterogeneity function, also from the maftools package, is used to calculate the MATH score (mutant-allele tumor heterogeneity) [54]. The microsatellite instability (MSI) score is calculated based on the method described in Bonneville et al.'s study [55]. Additionally, the neoantigen (NEO) score, purity, ploidy, homologous recombination deficiency (HRD), and loss of heterozygosity (LOH) scores are calculated based on the method outlined in Thorsson et al.'s study [56]. We also calculate the correlation between immune cell infiltrations (or stemness features and tumor heterogeneity) and m^6A modification genes. Furthermore, we identify the different immune cells (or stemness features and tumor heterogeneity) among clusters, as well as between the high- and low-risk groups.

2.8. Immune Regulator and Immune Checkpoint Gene Analysis

The immune regulatory and checkpoint genes are gathered from the study conducted by Hu et al. in 2021 [57]. These genes encompass chemokine receptors, MHC genes, immunoinhibitors, immunestimulators, inhibitory, and stimulatory genes. We perform a calculation to ascertain the correlations between the immune regulator and immune checkpoint genes with m^6A modification genes. Additionally, we identify distinct immune regulator and immune checkpoint genes among clusters, as well as between the high- and low-risk groups.

2.9. Immune Score and miRNA Analysis

The ESTIMATE package (v 1.0.13) is utilized to compute the immune scores for each patient according to the gene expression profiles specific to their respective cancers [58]. Subsequently, we determine the correlations between immune scores and m^6A modification genes. The miRNA expression data of each tumor patient are acquired from the TCGA database. Then, we compute the correlation coefficient between the miRNAs and m^6A modification genes.

2.10. Drug Prediction

The oncoPredict (v 0.2) package is utilized to analyze the IC50 value of each drug from the Genomics of Drug Sensitivity in Cancer (GDSC) database (https://www.cancerrxgene.org/ accessed on 30 May 2024) [59,60] for each patient, based on their gene expression levels. We select the top 11 drugs with the lowest IC50 values for each cancer type. Subsequently, we compute the differences in the selected drugs between the high- and low-risk groups.

2.11. Statistical Analyses

The R (v 4.2.3) software packages are used for data processing, statistical analysis, and plotting. The Pearson's correlation coefficient is used to calculate the correlation between two continuous variables. The *chi-squared* test is conducted to compare the categorical variables, and the Wilcoxon rank-sum test or *t*-test is used to compare continuous variables.

2.12. Identifying m^6A-Related Biomarkers by Three Machine Learning Algorithms

Three machine-learning algorithms, including LASSO, support vector machine-recursive feature elimination (SVM–RFE) [61], and random forest (RF) [62] algorithms are used to identify the m^6A-related biomarkers in each cancer type based on the RNA expression and CNV. We introduce the LASSO algorithm above. We use the SVM algorithm to train a model based on the RNA or CNV data [63], and then the SVM–RFE algorithm is employed to iteratively refine the feature set by eliminating the least significant features and enhancing the model's predictive accuracy [61]. The RF algorithm is used to rank the importance of genes [62]. The genes with a relative importance score above 0.25 are considered significant. The biomarkers are identified by the intersection results of LASSO, SVM-RFE, and RF methods.

3. Results

3.1. Expression Pattern and Functional Analysis of RNA m^{6}A Modification Regulators in Pan-Cancer and Normal Tissues

In the current study, we screen a total of 31 RNA m^{6}A modification regulators including 12 writers, 2 erasers, and 17 readers from the published literatures (Supplementary Table S1). The m^{6}A modification regulators are studied across 28 cancer types from the TCGA database (Supplementary Table S2) and 45 normal tissue types from both the TCGA and GTEx databases (Supplementary Table S3). The PPI network analysis suggests multiple interactions among the regulators, except for PRRC2A, RBM33, LRPPRC, and RBFOX2 (Figure 1A). The GO analysis of the regulators reveals the enrichment of processes mainly associated with mRNA metabolism, RNA modification, and regulation of mRNA stability, and translational and stem cell population maintenance (Figure 1B). To investigate the expression level of m^{6}A modification regulators in normal tissues, we analyze the protein expression of the regulators in 45 types of normal tissues from TCGA and GTEx. Our results find that most of the regulators are highly expressed across all normal tissues except IGF2BP1, IGF2BP3, and RBM15B (Figure 1C). Furthermore, we analyze the mRNA expression of the 31 regulators across 28 cancer types in the TCGA database, as well as compare them with TCGA and GTEx normal cohorts. Our results reveal that the m^{6}A regulators are highly expressed in most of the cancer types, such as CHOL, ESCA, GBM, HNSC, LGG, LAML, PAAD, and STAD, while they are decreased in a few tumor types, including ACC, KICH, OV, THCA, and UCS; *METTL3, YTHDC1, YTHDC2, RBM33,* and *RBFOX2* are preferably lower expressed, while *CBLL1, RBM15, RBM15B, METTL5, TRMT112, YTHDF1, YTHDF2, YTHDF3, HNRNPC, HNRNPA2B1, IGF2BP1, IGF2BP2, IGF2BP3, PRRC2A, LRPPRC* and *FXR1* are highly expressed in most tumor types (Figure 1D). Supplementary Figure S1A,B represents the expression differences in *IGF2BP2* and *IGF2BP3* between their normal and tumor tissues, respectively.

3.2. Correlations among RNA m^{6}A Modification Regulators in Pan-Cancer

To explore the relationship among the RNA m^{6}A regulators in pan-cancer, we calculate the correlation coefficients among the 31 regulators across the 28 cancer types at the mRNA level (Supplementary Figure S2). Interestingly, our results revealed that overall-positive correlations are more common than negative correlations, particularly in ACC, KIRP, KIRC, KICH, PCPG, THCA, and UCEC. *METTL5* and *TRMT112* are negatively related to other genes in some cancer types, especially in OV, PRAD, BRCA, and GBM.

3.3. Overall Survival (OS) Status Based on the Expression of RNA m^{6}A Modification Regulators in Pan-Cancer

We analyze the overall survival (OS) status of 28 TCGA cancer types based on the expression of 31 RNA m^{6}A regulators and find the genes to have prognostic significance in different cancer types. Some are found to have a good OS advantage, such as *METTL3* in LIHC, LAML, ACC, and KICH; *METTL14* in LGG and LAML; *WTAP* in LGG, CESC, and LIHC; *VIRMA* in LGG, CESC, and LIHC; *ZC3H13* in LAML; *CBLL1* in LGG and KICH; *RBM15* in LGG, LUAD, LIHC, THCA, LAML, ACC, and KICH; *RBM15B* in LIHC and ACC; *METTL5* in LUAD, KIRP, HNSC, LIHC, PAAD, LAML, ACC, and KICH; *TRMT112* in LGG, KIRP, HNSC, LIHC, LAML, ACC, and KICH; *ZCCHC4* in LGG, LIHC, LAML, and KICH; *FTO* in STAD, BLCA, and LAML; *ALKBH5* in LGG, GBM, BLCA, LAML, and KICH; *YTHDC2* in LGG; and *YTHDF1* in LGG, LIHC, THCA, and LAML (Supplementary Figure S3). A few genes have a bad OS disadvantage, such as *METTL3* in PAAD; *METTL14* in KIRC, SKCM, and READ; *METTL16* in CESC and PAAD; *WTAP* in SKCM; *VIRMA* in SKCM; *ZC3H13* in KIRC; *CBLL1* in KIRC; *RBM15* in KIRC and READ; *RBM15B* in KIRC; *METTL5* in OV; *TRMT112* in OV; *ZCCHC4* in KIRC and SKCM; *FTO* in KIRC; *ALKBH5* in ESCA, OV, and PAAD; *YTHDC1* in KIRC; *YTHDC2* in COAD, KIRC, and READ; and *YTHDF1* in READ (Supplementary Figure S3).

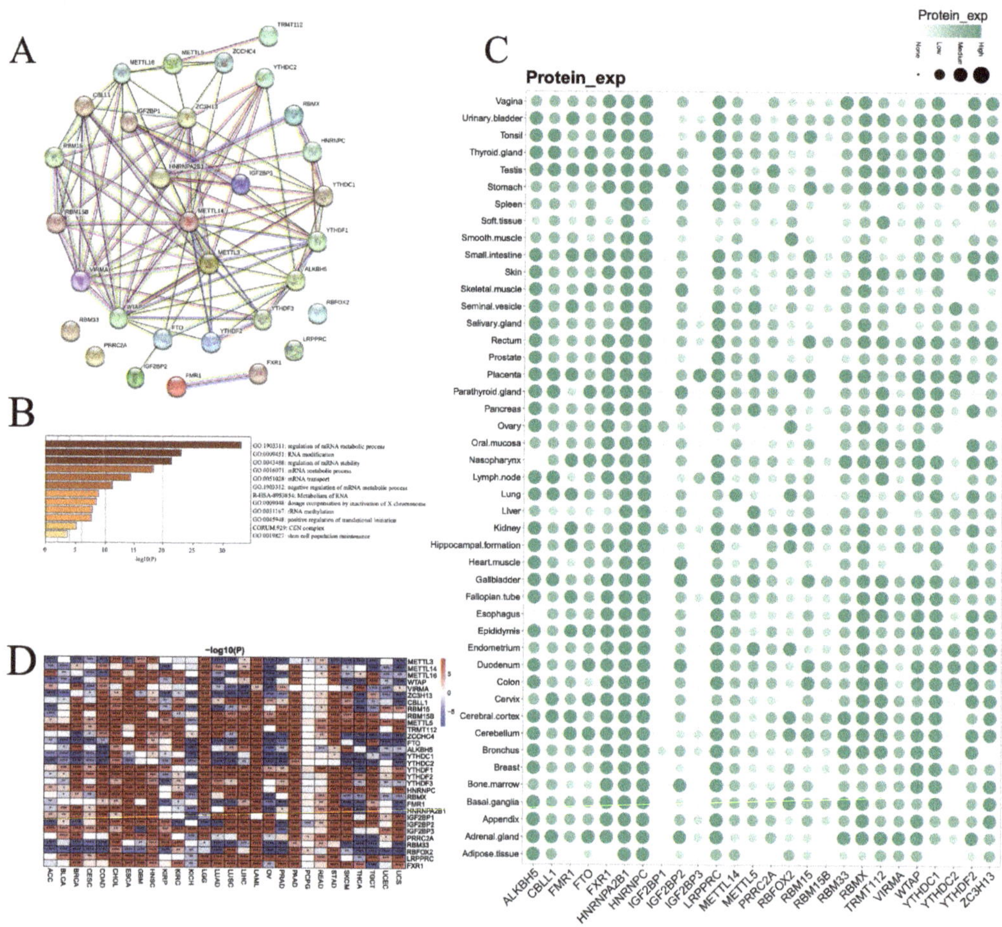

Figure 1. Expression levels of m^6A modification genes across cancer types. (**A**) Protein–protein interaction (PPI) analysis of genes. (**B**) GO annotation of genes. (**C**) Protein expression levels of genes in various tissues. (**D**) Expression differences in various normal and cancer tissues. (* $p < 0.05$, ** $p < 0.01$, *** $p < 0.001$, **** $p < 0.0001$).

3.4. Clinical Significance of RNA m^6A Modification Regulators in Pan-Cancer

To investigate the relationship between the expression levels of m^6A modification regulators and the clinicopathological features, such as age, gender, grade, stage, tumor T stage, lymph node metastasis, and distant metastasis in pan-cancer, we compare the mRNA expression of the 31 m^6A regulators in the TCGA pan-cancer cohort across different clinical features. We list the patients' number distribution of clinicopathological characteristics in each cancer cohort in Supplementary Table S4.

Most of the genes are found to be affected by age in KIRP, BRCA, ESCA, LUSC, PAAD, and THCA (Figure 2A). Furthermore, the expression of some genes varies significantly by the patients' gender in a few cancer types, such as HNSC, KIRP, KIRC, and LIHC (Figure 2B). Similarly, the expression of a few regulators is affected by the patients' tumor grade, in cancers such as HNSC, KIRC, LGG, LIHC, PAAD, and UCEC; *LRPPRC* and *TRMT112* are affected by tumor grade in most of the cancers (Figure 2C). As shown in Figure 2D, the expression of the regulators significantly varies based on tumor stage in a few cancers, including KIRP, KIRC, KICH, LIHC, OV, THCA, and TGCT; *IGF2BP2* in KIRC and THCA; *IGF2BP3* in KIRP, KIRC, and UCEC; and *LRPPRC* and *METTL14* in KIRC are the ones that are the most varied. Additionally, the expression of most of the regulators influences the tumor T feature of KIRC, LIHC, PRAD, STAD and THCA, especially *IGF2BP1* in BRCA; *IGF2BP2*, *IGF2BP3*, *LRPPRC*, and *METTL14* in KIRC; and *IGF2BP3* in KIRP (Figure 2E). The expression of some of the regulators is found to be affected by the tumor N feature in COAD, HNSC, KIRP, KICH, LUSC, PRAD and THCA, especially *ALKBH5* and *IGF2BP2* in THCA, and *FXR1* and *IGF2BP3* in KIRP (Figure 2F); and the tumor M feature in ACC, KIRC, and LUAD, especially *IGF2BP2* and *IGF2BP3* in KIRC, and *IGF2BP3* in KIRP (Figure 2G).

As shown in Supplementary Figure S4A, as a case study, the expression of *IGF2BP2* in some tumor types is positively correlated with the patients' age, i.e., the older the patient, the higher the expression, while its expression in a few tumor types is negatively correlated with age, i.e., the younger the patient, the higher the gene expression. Another gene, *YTHDF1*, has higher expression in males than in females in some cancers, while this trend is the opposite for a few other cancers (Supplementary Figure S4B). When we look at *IGF2BP2's* expression pattern, it is found to vary significantly among G1, G2, G3, and G4 grades in a few cancer types (Supplementary Figure S4C). The expression of *IGF2BP3* is found to be significantly different across stages I–IV in a few cancer types (Supplementary Figure S4D), and across T1–T4 groups (Supplementary Figure S4E). As shown in Supplementary Figures S4F,G, the expression pattern of a representative gene, *IGF2BP3*, varies significantly across N0–N3 groups and between M0 and M1 groups in some cancer types, respectively.

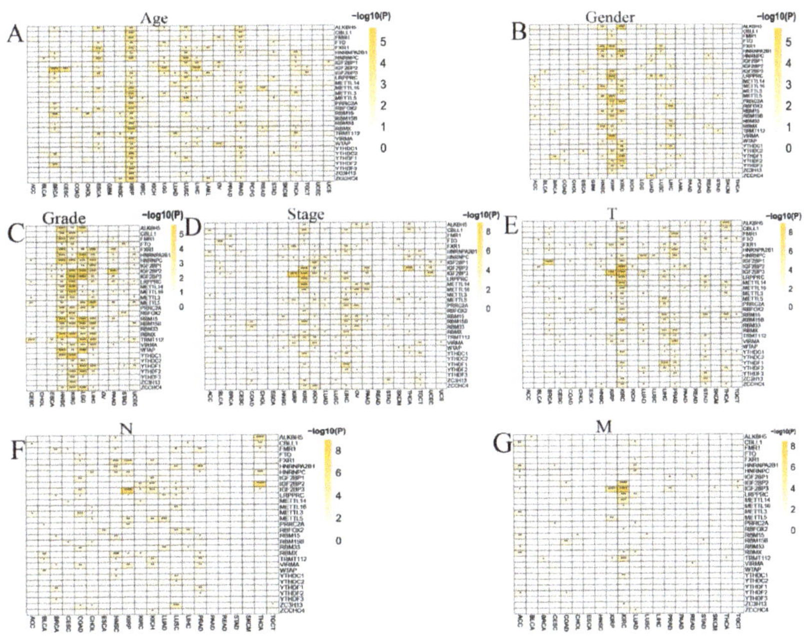

Figure 2. Clinicopathological characteristics of m^{6}A modification genes in each cancer. Expression of m^{6}A modification genes between (**A**) age groups, (**B**) gender, (**C**) grade, (**D**) stage, (**E**) T, (**F**) N, and (**G**) M groups. (* $p < 0.05$, ** $p < 0.01$, *** $p < 0.001$, **** $p < 0.0001$).

3.5. Correlation between Genetic or Epigenetic Alterations and Expression Levels of m^{6}A Regulators in Pan-Cancer

We analyze the correlations of copy number variation (CNV), single nucleotide variation (SNV), methylation levels or genomic variations, including missense mutation, nonsense mutation, frame-shift deletion, frame-shift insertion, in-frame deletion, and in-frame insertion, with the expression levels of the 31 RNA m^{6}A modification regulators and overall survival of the patients in pan-cancer.

The CNVs are mainly categorized into heterozygous and homologous amplifications and deletions. The deletions are found to be more common in *METTL16, ALKBH5, RBM15B, METTL14, ZC3H13, YTHDF2, WTAP, ZCCHC4, RBFOX2, YTHDC1, YTHDC2, RBM15, METTL3, HNRNPC, FTO, TRMT112*, and *RBMX*, whereas amplifications are more common in *FMR1, METTL5, PRRC2A, IGF2BP1, LRPPRC, IGF2BP2, FXR1, RBM33, CBLL1, YTHDF3, HNRNPA2B1, IGF2BP3, VIRMA*, and *YTHDF1* in most tumor types. However, a few cancer types, such as THCA, PRAD, LAML, and LGG have a lower percentage of CNVs than the others (Supplementary Figure S5A). Furthermore, we find a positive correlation between CNVs and mRNA expression levels for many of the regulators in most tumor types, especially in BRCA, LUSC, OV, LUAD, HNSC, BLCA, COAD, LIHC, CESC, STAD, SKCM, ESCA, and LGG, and *YTHDF1* in BRCA is the strongest among them (Figure 3A).

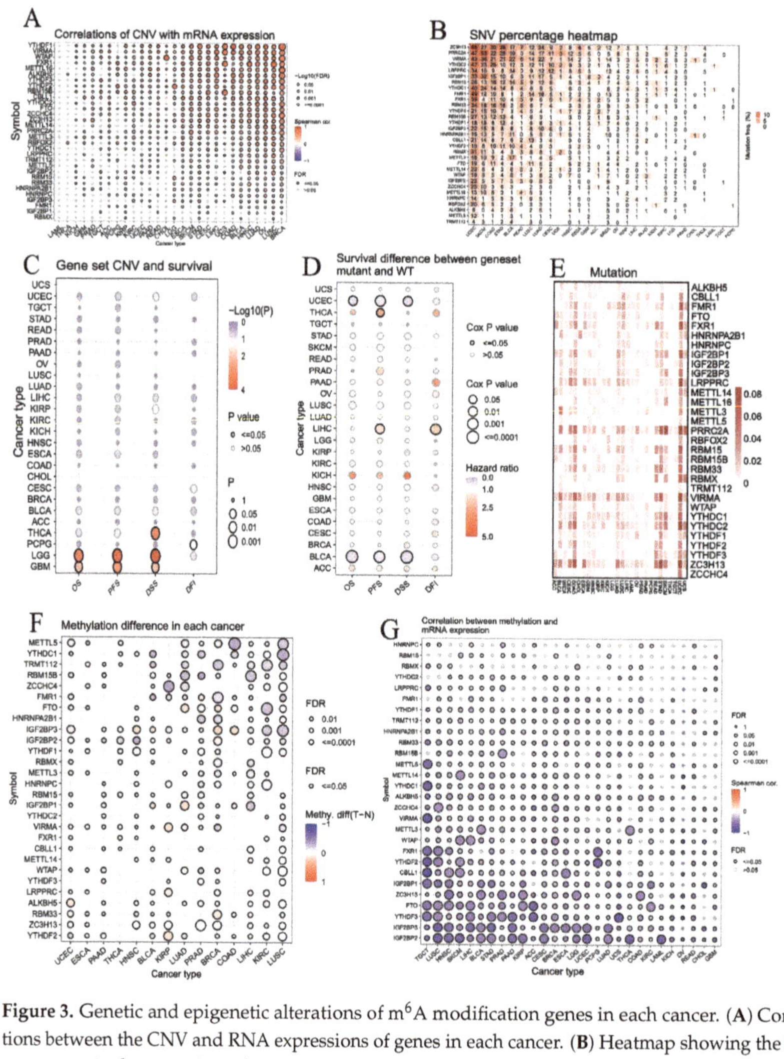

Figure 3. Genetic and epigenetic alterations of m^{6}A modification genes in each cancer. (**A**) Correlations between the CNV and RNA expressions of genes in each cancer. (**B**) Heatmap showing the SNV percentage in the genes in each cancer. (**C**) Association between geneset CNV and survival status

in each cancer. (**D**) Association between geneset SNV mutation and survival status in each cancer. (**E**) Heatmap showing the genomic variations, including missense mutation, nonsense mutation, frame-shift deletion, frame-shift insertion, in-frame deletion, and in-frame insertion of genes in different cancer types. (**F**) Methylation difference in each gene in each cancer. (**G**) Correlation between the methylation level and RNA expression of genes in each cancer.

Many of the m^{6}A regulators have a high SNV mutation frequency in most tumor types, especially in UCEC, SKCM, COAD, and STAD, furthermore, *ZC3H3* in UCEC and *PRRC2A* in SKCM are the top two whose mutation frequency is above 50% (Figure 3B).

Next, we analyze the correlation of patients' RNA m^{6}A regulators' geneset CNVs with four survival types, i.e., overall survival (OS), progression free survival (PFS), disease specific survival (DSS), and disease-free interval (DFI). Only a small proportion of tumors are found to be affected. For example, the CNVs of m^{6}A regulators are correlated with the OS, PFS, and DSS of LGG and GBM patients, while they are correlated with only the DSS of THCA patients. The CNVs of RNA m^{6}A regulators correlated with the DFI of PCPG patients (Figure 3C). Furthermore, we analyze the association between SNV mutations in m^{6}A regulators and patient survival. The SNV mutations in these regulators are significantly associated with the OS and DSS of UCEC and BLCA patients, the PFS of UCEC, THCA, LIHC, and BLCA patients, and the DFI of LIHC patients (Figure 3D).

We also analyze the genomic variations, including the missense mutation, nonsense mutation, frame-shift deletion, frame-shift insertion, in-frame deletion, and in-frame insertion of 31 RNA m^{6}A regulators across 28 types of TCGA pan-cancer cohorts. Most of them are found to be mutated in different cancers, especially in UCEC, COAD, STAD, BLCA, CESC, LUAD, LUSC, READ, and UCS (Figure 3E). *ZC3H13*, *VIRMA*, and *PRRC2A* almost have a higher mutation frequency rate in all cancer types (Figure 3E). Furthermore, we assess different genetic alteration types for *ZC3H13*. Our results reveal that *ZC3H13* has all the six types of alterations, while missense mutation is found to be the most frequent one (Supplementary Figure S5B).

The methylation levels of RNA m^{6}A regulators, such as *METTL5*, *YTHDC1*, *TRMT112*, *RBM15B*, *ZCCHC4*, *FMR1*, and *HNRNPA2B1* are found to be decreased in LUSC, KIRC, LIHC, COAD, BRCA, PRAD, LUAD, KIRP, and BLCA; however, the methylation levels of *FTO*, *IGF2BP3*, *IGF2BP2*, *IGF2BP1*, *WTAP*, and *RBM33* are increased in BRCA and LUAD, whereas the levels of *HNRNPC*, *VIRMA*, *LRPPRC*, *ZC3H13*, and *YTHDF2* increased in KIRP (Figure 3F). Interestingly, the methylation levels of most of the RNA m^{6}A regulators are negatively correlated with their mRNA expression in different cancer types, especially *METTL5*, *YTHDC1*, *VIRMA*, *FXR1*, *YTHDF2*, and *CBLL1* in TGCT; *IGF2BP3* and *IGF2BP2* in LUSC, HNSC, and PAAD; and *IGF2BP2* in THCA and LAML; and *YTHDF3* in UCS (Figure 3G).

3.6. Distinguishing Different Clusters of RNA m^{6}A Regulators in TCGA Pan-Cancer Cohort

The R package *ConsensusClusterPlus* is applied to classify patients by the similarity of the m^{6}A regulators' level into two to four different categories, that is, C1, C2, C3 and C4 in the TCGA pan-cancer cohort (Figure 4A). The discrepancy of the RNA m^{6}A regulators' level is found to be significant among C1–C4 groups in the TCGA pan-cancer cohort (Figure 4B). Figure 4C shows the comparison of the differential expression of a representative gene, *TRMT112* across the clusters in each tumor.

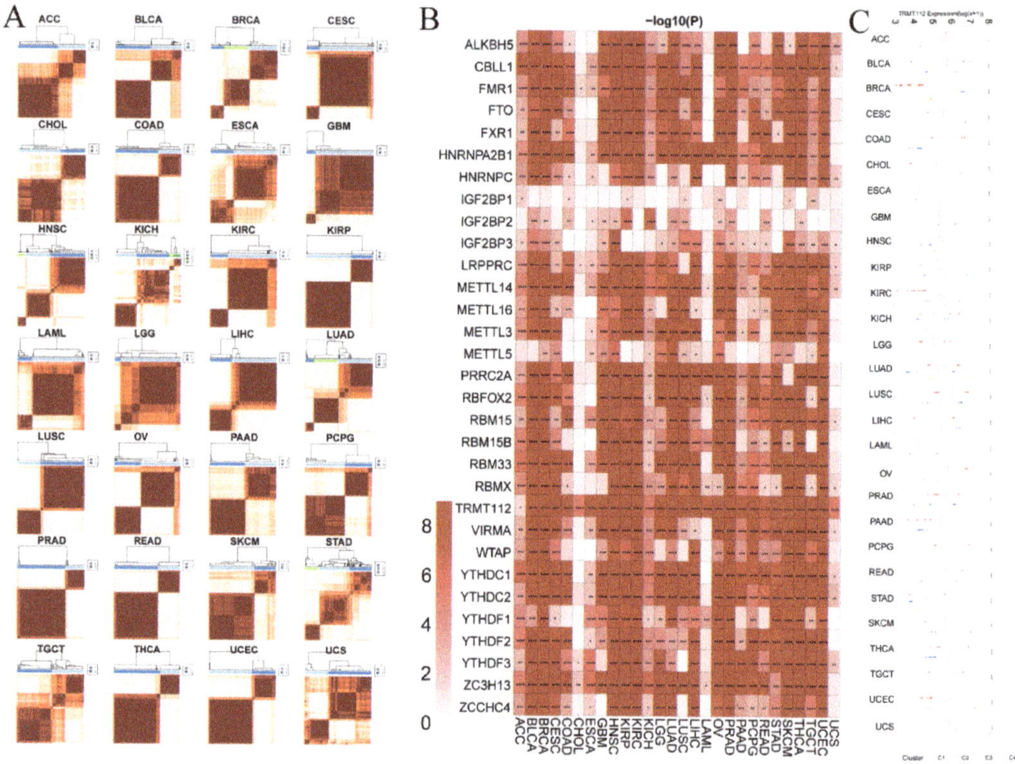

Figure 4. Consensus cluster analysis of m^{6}A modification genes in each cancer. (**A**) Consensus cluster analysis of different tumors. (**B**) Heatmap showing the differential expression of genes between the clusters in each tumor. (**C**) Differential expression of *TRMT112* between the clusters in each tumor. (* $p < 0.05$, ** $p < 0.01$, *** $p < 0.001$, **** $p < 0.0001$).

3.7. Evaluating the Prognostic Value of RNA m^{6}A Regulators in TCGA Pan-Cancer Cohort

The LASSO cox regression algorithm is applied to these RNA m^{6}A regulators in the TCGA pan-cancer cohort. A few candidate genes are screened out as they are considered to be prognosis-related in different cancers (Supplementary Table S5 and Figure 5A). We divide the patients into high- and low-risk groups according to the LASSO results. Patients in the high-risk group have a worse prognosis than the patients in the low-risk group in the TCGA pan-cancer cohort (Figure 5B). For example, *IGF2BP3* is found to be greater in high-risk than in low-risk group of ACC, BLCA, CESC, KIRP, KICH, LGG, LUAD, LIHC, LAML, and PAAD; however, the trend is the opposite for READ (Figure 5C). Figure 5D shows the differential expression of RNA m^{6}A regulators between the high- and low-risk groups in each tumor. Overall, the genes are found to be increased in the high-risk than in the low-risk group of ACC, BLCA, CESC, KIRP, KICH, LGG, LUAD, LIHC, and PAAD, while decreased in the high-risk compared to the low-risk group of KIRC and READ.

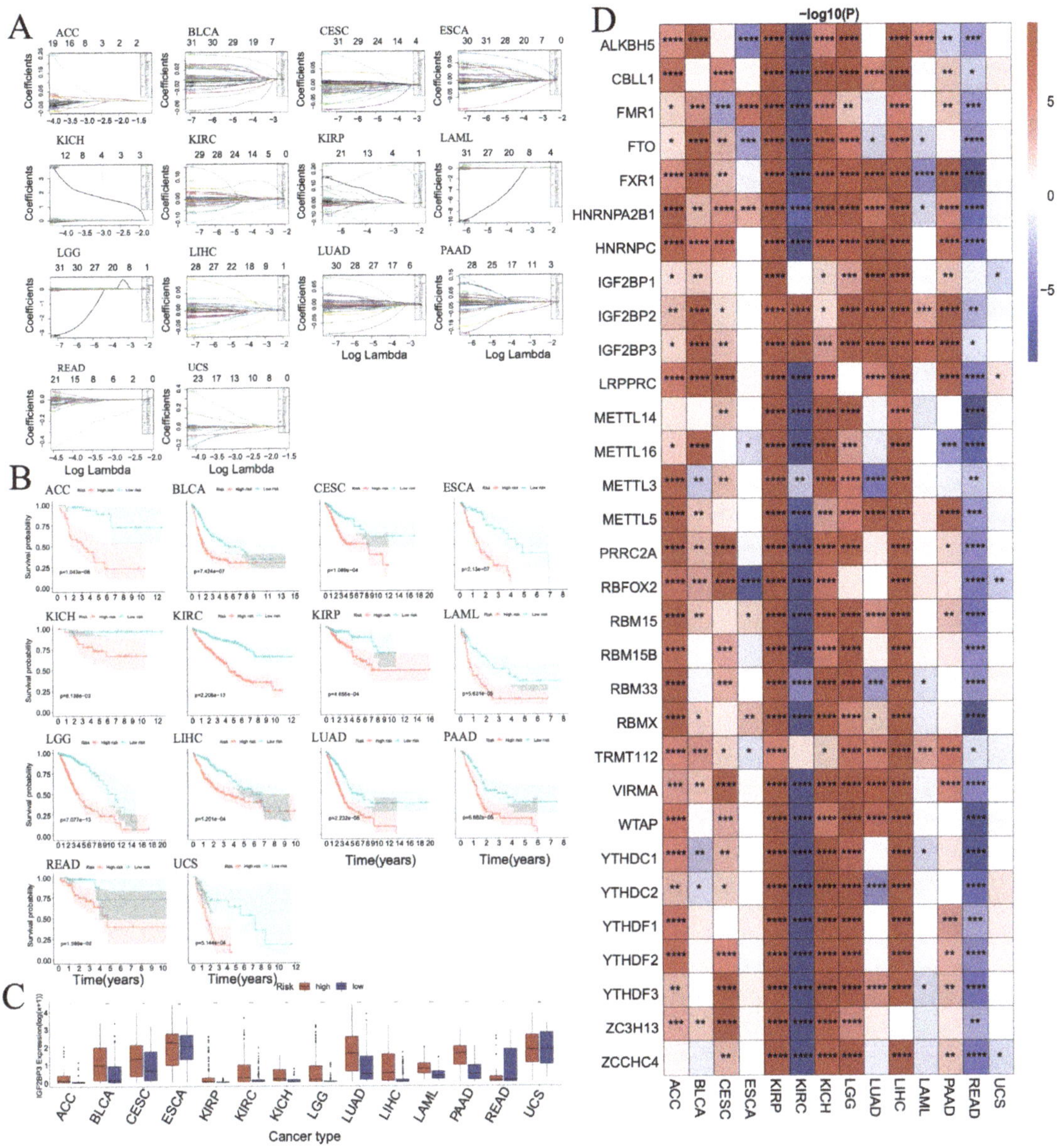

Figure 5. Prognostic model of m^6A modification genes in each cancer. (**A**) LASSO regression is used to screen for important genes in each tumor. (**B**) Survival curves of patients between high- and low-risk groups in each tumor. (**C**) Differential expression of *IGF2BP3* between high- and low-risk groups in each tumor. (**D**) Heatmap showing the differential expression of genes between high- and low-risk groups in each tumor. (* $p < 0.05$, ** $p < 0.01$, *** $p < 0.001$, **** $p < 0.0001$).

3.8. Correlation between Immune Infiltrating Score and RNA m^6A Regulators in TCGA Pan-Cancer Cohort

Next, we analyze the correlation between the immune infiltrating score with the expression of RNA m^6A regulators in the TCGA pan-cancer cohort. The genes are negatively related to the immune score in most cancer types except in COAD, KICH, LGG,

PAAD, and READ (Supplementary Figure S6A). *IGF2BP2*, *IGF2BP3*, *RBM15*, *WTAP*, and *YTHDC2* are positively correlated to the immune score in a few cancer types (Supplementary Figure S6A). Supplementary Figure S6B shows the most significant correlation of m^6A regulators with immune score in cancers. For instance, the genes negatively related to the immune score are *YTHDC2* in ACC; *METTL3* in BLCA and KIRP; *RBMX* in BRCA, GBM, LAML, OV, and TGCT; *LRPPRC* in CESC, ESCA, KIRC, LUAD, and SKCM; *METTL5* in HNSC and LUSC; *RBFOX2* in LGG; *ZCCHC4* in PCPG; *YTHDF1* in STAD; *ALKBH5* in THCA; *FXR1* in UCEC; and *PRRC2A* in UCS. The positively correlated genes with immune score include *ALKBH5* in COAD; *WTAP* in CHOL, LIHC, and PAAD; *IGF2BP1* in KICH; *IGF2BP2* in PRAD; and *RBFOX2* in READ (Supplementary Figure S6B).

3.9. *Association of Tumor Microenvironment (TME) Infiltrating Cells with RNA m^6A Regulators in Pan-Cancer by CIBERSORT*

To study the TME-infiltrating immune cells in TCGA pan-cancer, we use the CIBERSORT method to determine the cell types. Our results show that there are 22 types of tumor-infiltrated immune cells, including subtypes of B cells, T cells, NK cells, macrophages, dendritic cells, mast cells, monocytes, eosinophils, neutrophils, and plasma cells.

As shown in Supplementary Figure S7A, the m^6A regulators have a varying expression pattern in different immune cell types across the pan-cancer cohort. For instance, many RNA m^6A regulators have higher expression in resting CD4 memory T cells, resting NK cells, M0 macrophages, M1 macrophages, activated dendritic cells and activated mast cells, but lower expression in memory B cells, plasma cells, naïve CD4 T cells, and T regulatory cells in BLCA. In the case of BRCA, most RNA m^6A regulators are found to be increased in naïve B cells, resting CD4 memory T cells, M2 macrophages, resting mast cells, and neutrophils, while they are decreased in memory B cells, plasma cells, CD8 T cells, T follicular helper cells, T regulatory cells, and activated NK cells. However, in READ, most RNA m^6A regulators are found to be decreased in memory B cells and naïve CD4 T cells. Interestingly, most RNA m^6A regulators are found to be unaffected in UCS (Supplementary Figure S7A).

When we look at the differential immune cell infiltration between clusters in each TCGA pan-cancer cohort, most of the immune cells are found to be affected in BRCA, HNSC, KIRP, KIRC, PRAD, and STAD (Figure 6A). For instance, in the case of the BRCA cancer cohort, the cell percentage of naïve B cells, plasma cells, CD8 T cells, resting CD4 memory T cells, T follicular helper cells, T regulatory cells, gamma delta T cells, activated NK cells, resting dendritic cells, resting mast cells, and neutrophils is found to be significantly different among clusters C1, C2, and C3 (Supplementary Figure S7B). Furthermore, the differential immune cell infiltration analysis between high- and low-risk groups in each TCGA pan-cancer cohort reveals that most of the immune cells are affected in BLCA, KIRC, LGG, LUAD, LIHC, and PAAD (Figure 6B).

3.10. *Association of Tumor Stemness Score with RNA m^6A Regulators in TCGA Pan-Cancer Cohort*

We investigate the tumor stemness score in the TCGA pan-cancer cohort by analyzing DMPss, DNAss, ENHss, EREG.EXPss, EREG-METHss, and RNAss. The differential tumor stemness score analysis between clusters shows that a few cancer types, including KIRP, KICH, LUAD, LIHC, PAAD, and TGCT are significantly affected (Figure 6A). We also analyze the differential tumor stemness scores between the high- and low-risk groups in each cancer type (Figure 6B). Our results indicate that DMPss and DNAss are positively correlated with the high-risk group in LGG and LUAD. While ENHss is positively correlated with the high-risk group in LGG, it is negatively correlated with the high-risk group in KIRC. Furthermore, EREG.EXPss is positively correlated with the high-risk group in ACC, BLCA, LGG, LUAD, and PAAD, while negatively correlated with the high-risk group in KIRC. EREG-METHss is positively correlated with the high-risk group in LGG, LUAD, and PAAD. RNAss is positively correlated with the high-risk group in ACC, ESCA, LUAD, LIHC, and PAAD, while negatively correlated with the high-risk group in LGG and LAML.

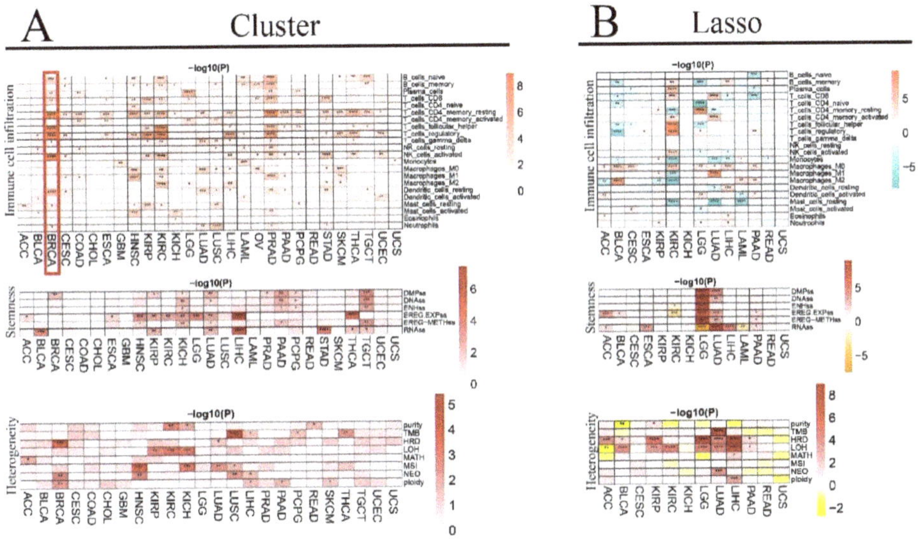

Figure 6. Association of immune cell infiltration, tumor stemness score, and genomic heterogeneity with RNA m^{6}A regulators in TCGA pan-cancer cohort. (**A**) Differential immune cell infiltration, tumor stemness score, and genomic heterogeneity between clusters in each tumor. (**B**) Differential immune cell infiltration, tumor stemness score, and genomic heterogeneity between high- and low-risk groups in each tumor. (* $p < 0.05$, ** $p < 0.01$, *** $p < 0.001$, **** $p < 0.0001$).

Next, we analyze the correlation between RNA m^{6}A modification genes and tumor stemness scores in each cancer type and find both positive and negative correlations between the genes and the stemness scores (Supplementary Figure S8). For example, the RNA m^{6}A regulators are positively correlated with RNAss in ACC, BLCA, BRCA, COAD, ESCA, GBM, HNSC, KIRC, LGG, LUAD, LUSC, LAML, PRAD, PCPG, STAD, TGCT, and UCEC, while they are negatively correlated with RNAss in KIRP and THCA. Additionally, the RNA m^{6}A regulators are positively correlated with EREG.EXPss in ACC, KIRC, LGG, LUAD, LAML, PRAD, PAAD, and STAD, whereas they are negatively correlated with EREG.EXPss in BLCA, BRCA, KIRP, LIHC, and THCA. Further, the analysis suggests that several RNA m^{6}A regulators are positively correlated with the DMPss, DNAss, ENHss, and EREG-METHss in HNSC, LGG, LUAD, LUSC, STAD, and TGCT, while negatively correlated with BRCA and LIHC. *CBLL1*, *HNRNPA2B1*, *HNRNPC*, *LRPPRC*, *METTL5*, *PRRC2A*, *RBFOX2*, *RBM15*, *TRMT112*, *WTAP*, and *YTHDF2* are usually positively related to EREG.EXPss in ACC, KIRC, LGG, and PRAD; they are also positively related to RNAss in BLCA, LUAD, LUSC, PRAD, PCPG, and STAD.

Some m^{6}A regulators are preferred to positively related to most of the stemness factors such as *YTHDF2* in CHOL, *RBM15* in ESCA, *YTHDC2* in GBM; *IGF2BP1*, *IGF2BP2*, *IGF2BP3*, *LRPPRC*, and *YTHDF1* in HNSC; *RBM15B* and *ZC3H13* in KIRC, *ALKBH5*, *HNRNPA2B1*, *IGF2BP1*, *IGF2BP2*, *IGF2BP3*, *RBM15*, and *YTHDF2* in LGG and LUSC; *HNRNPA2B1* and *TRMT112* in PRAD and PCPG; *CBLL1*, *FXR1*, *LRPPRC*, *METTL16*, *METTL5*, *RBM15*, *VIRMA*, *YTHDF2*, and *YTHDF3* in TGCT; and *METTL5* in UCEC (Supplementary Figure S8).

Some m^{6}A regulators are preferred to negatively related to most of the stemness factors such as *METTL14*, *RBM15*, and *WTAP* in BLCA; *METTL14*, *RBM33*, *YTHDC1*, *YTHDC2*, *ZC3H13*, and *ZCCHC4* in BRCA; *ALKBH5*, *FTO*, and *RBFOX2* in COAD; *YTHDC2* in LUAD;

CBLL1, *HNRNPC*, *IGF2BP2*, *METTL16*, and *YTHDC1* in LIHC; *FTO* in LAML; *METTL14* and *YTHDC2* in PAAD; *RBFOX2* in PCPG; *FTO* and *RBFOX2* in STAD; and *FMR1*, *FTO*, *IGF2BP2*, *IGF2BP3*, *METTL14*, *RBFOX2*, and *RBM15B* in TGCT (Supplementary Figure S8).

3.11. Association of Genomic Heterogeneity with RNA m^6A Regulators in TCGA Pan-Cancer Cohort

We investigate the genomic heterogeneity score in TCGA pan-cancer cohort by analyzing purity, tumor mutation burden (TMB), homologous recombination deficiency (HRD), heterozygosity (LOH), mutant-allele tumor heterogeneity (MATH), microsatellite instability (MSI), neoantigen (NEO), and ploidy. Our results show differential genomic heterogeneity scores between clusters in each cancer type. Some of the affected cancer types include BRCA, HNSC, KIRC, KICH, LUAD, LUSC, and LIHC, and TBM in LUSC has the highest genomic heterogeneity score among them (Figure 6A). Further, we analyze the differential genomic heterogeneity scores between the high- and low-risk groups in each tumor type (Figure 6B). Our results suggest that purity is negatively correlated with the high-risk group in BLCA, while positively correlated with the high-risk group in KIRP. TMB is positively correlated with the high-risk group in LUAD. HRD is positively correlated with the high-risk group in ACC, BLCA, KIRP, LGG, LUAD, LIHC, and PAAD. LOH is negatively correlated with the high-risk group in ACC, while positively correlated with the high-risk group in BLCA, KIRP, KIRC, LGG, LUAD, LIHC, and PAAD. MATH is positively correlated with the high-risk group in LIHC. NEO is positively correlated with the high-risk group in LUAD. Ploidy is positively correlated with the high-risk group in LIHC.

Further, we analyze the correlation between RNA m^6A modification genes and genomic heterogeneity scores in each cancer type, and identify both positive and negative correlations between the genes and the genomic heterogeneity scores across different cancer types (Supplementary Figure S9). For example, many RNA m^6A regulators are found to be positively correlated with purity in ACC, BLCA, BRCA, CESC, GBM, HNSC, KIRP, LGG, LUAD, LUSC, SKCM, TGCT, and UCEC, while negatively correlated to it in READ. A positive correlation is observed between several RNA m^6A regulators and TMB in LUAD and READ, whereas negative correlation is observed in KIRP and THCA. While HDR is positively correlated with many RNA m^6A regulators in ACC, BLCA, GBM, HNSC, KIRP, KICH, LGG, LUAD, LUSC, LIHC, and PRAD, and it is negatively correlated with the regulators in TGCT. Many RNA m^6A regulators are positively correlated with LOH in BLCA, COAD, HNSC, KIRP, LGG, LUAD, LUSC, and LIHC, whereas they are negatively correlated in KIRC and THCA. There is a positive correlation between RNA m^6A regulators and MATH in BLCA, BRCA, COAD, LUAD, and LUSC. The MSI is positively correlated with RNA m^6A regulators in KIRC and LUSC; however, it is negatively correlated with the regulators in PRAD. Lastly, a positive correlation is observed between RNA m^6A regulators and ploidy in BRCA, COAD, HNSC, LUAD, and LIHC, while a negative correlation is observed in KIRC.

The positive correlation between some genes and some kind of genomic heterogeneity types in some cancer types is more significant than others; for example, the relationships of *IGF2BP1*, *IGF2BP3*, and HRD in ACC; *METTL3* and purity in BLCA; *IGF2BP2* and HRD, LOH in BRCA; *METTL16* and TMB in CESC; *ALKBH5* and TMB, MSI, and NEO in COAD; *YTHDF1* and HRD, LOH, MATH, and ploidy in COAD; *IGF2BP3* and LOH in CHOL; *CBLL1*, *FMR1*, *HNRNPA2B1*, *HNRNPC*, *METTL3*, *PRRC2A*, *RBMX*, and *YTHDC1*, and purity in GBM; *RBFOX2* and NEO in GBM; *METTL5*, and *RBMX*, and purity in HNSC; *FXR1*, *IGF2BP1*, *LRPPRC*, and *METTL5*, and HRD and LOH in HNSC; *FXR1* and HRD in KIRP; *IGF2BP3* and LOH in KIRP; *FXR1*, *IGF2BP1*, and *IGF2BP2*, and MSI and NEO in KIRC; *IGF2BP1*, *TRMT112*, and *ZCCHC4*, and HRD in KICH; *CBLL1*, *METTL16*, and *RBMX*, and purity in LGG; *RBM15*, and *YTHDF2*, and HRD in LGG; *RBMX* and purity in LUAD; *IGF2BP3* and HRD and LOH in LUAD; *HNRNPC*, and *RBMX*, and purity in LUSC; *YTHDF1* and HRD and LOH in LIHC; *HNRNPA2B1*, *METTL3*, and *TRMT112*, and purity, HRD, and LOH in PRAD; *TRMT112* and LOH in PAAD; *ALKBH5*, and *RBM15*, and TMB in

READ; *CBLL1*, and *METTL3*, and purity in SKCM; *CBLL1*, and HRD and ploidy in THCA; *IGF2BP2*, *IGF2BP3*, *METTL14*, *RBFOX2*, *RBM15B*, and *RBMX*, and purity in TGCT; and *IGF2BP2* and HRD in UCEC (Supplementary Figure S9).

The negative correlation between some genes and some kinds of genomic heterogeneity types in some cancer types is more significant than others, such as *METTL5* and LOH in ACC; *IGF2BP2* and purity in BLCA; *METTL14*, *METTL16*, *METTL3*, *YTHDC2*, and *ZCCHC4*, and HRD and LOH in BRCA; *YTHDF1* and TMB, MSI, and NEO in COAD; *PRRC2A*, *RBFOX2*, *RBMX*, *WTAP*, *YTHDC1*, and *YTHDF2*, and LOH in KIRC; *IGF2BP3* and MATH in LGG; *WTAP* and purity in LIHC; *METTL14*, and *YTHDF3*, and MSI in PRAD; *HNRNPC*, and *RBFOX2* and LOH in THCA; and *ALKBH5* and HRD in TGCT (Supplementary Figure S9).

3.12. Association of Immune Regulatory or Checkpoint Genes with RNA m^6A Regulators in TCGA Pan-Cancer Cohort

We analyze the immune regulatory genes, including chemokines, immunoinhibitors, immunostimulators, MHCs, and receptors, among different clusters in each tumor type and between high- and low-risk groups. We also investigate the immune checkpoint genes in the TCGA pan-cancer cohort by analyzing the inhibitory and stimulatory genes.

Our results demonstrate that the chemokines affect various cancer types among different clusters, including BLCA, BRCA, ESCA, HNSC, KIRP, KICH, LUAD, LUSC, LIHC, PRAD, STAD, SKCM, THCA, TGCT, and UCEC; some chemokines affect some cancer types quite significantly, such as *CX3CL1*, *CXCL9*, *CXCL12*, *CXCL13* and *CXCL16* in HNSC; *CXCL12* in KIRC; *CXCL8* in LUSC, *CXCL8*, *CXCL9*, *CXCL10*, *CXCL11*, *CXCL12, and CXCL16* in PRAD; and *CXCL12* in THCA (Figure 7A). The effect of chemokines is also observed between high- and low-risk groups in each cancer type. While some chemokines are positively correlated, others are negatively correlated with the high-risk group in different cancer types; for example, *CXCL13*, *XCL1*, and *XCL2* in KIRC and *CCL5*, *CXCL9*, *CXCL10*, *CXCL11*, and *CXCL16* in LGG are elevated, while *CCL15* in BLCA, *CX3CL1* and *CXCL12* in KIRC, *CXCL17* in LUAD, *CCL14* and *CCL16* in LIHC, and *CCL14* in PAAD are reduced in the high-risk group (Figure 7B).

The immunoinhibitors affect some cancer types among different clusters, including BLCA, BRCA, CESC, ESCA, GBM, HNSC, KIRP, KIRC, LUAD, LUSC, LIHC, OV, PRAD, PCPG, READ, STAD, THCA, and UCEC; *IL10RB*, *KDR* and *TGFBR1* are significantly affected most tumor types (Figure 7A). Furthermore, a few immunoinhibitors are positively correlated, while some are negatively correlated with the high-risk group in various cancer types; *IL10RB*, *PVRL2*, and *TGFBR1* in most of the tumor types are increased while *ADORA2A* in KIRC and PAAD, and *KDR* and *TGFBR1* in KIRC are the most significantly decreased in the high-risk group (Figure 7B).

The immunostimulators affect various cancer types among different clusters, including BLCA, BRCA, CESC, ESCA, GBM, HNSC, KIRP, KIRC, KICH, LGG, LUAD, LUSC, LIHC, OV, PRAD, READ, STAD, THCA, TGCT, and UCEC; *CD28*, *ENTPD1*, *IL6R*, *NT5E*, *PVR*, *TMEM173*, *TNFSF15*, *TNFSF18* and *TNFSF4* are affected in most tumor types (Figure 7A). Some of the immunostimulators are positively correlated, while a few are negatively correlated with the high-risk group in various cancer types; *CD276*, *MICB*, *PVR*, *TNFSF4*, and *ULBP1* in most tumor types are elevated, while *C10orf54*, *CXCL12*, *ENTPD1*, *IL6R*, *NT5E*, *RAET1E*, *TNFSF13*, and *TNFSF15* in KIRC, and *IL6R*, *TMEM173*, *TNFRSF14*, and *TNFSF15* in LUAD are the most significantly reduced in the high-risk group (Figure 7B).

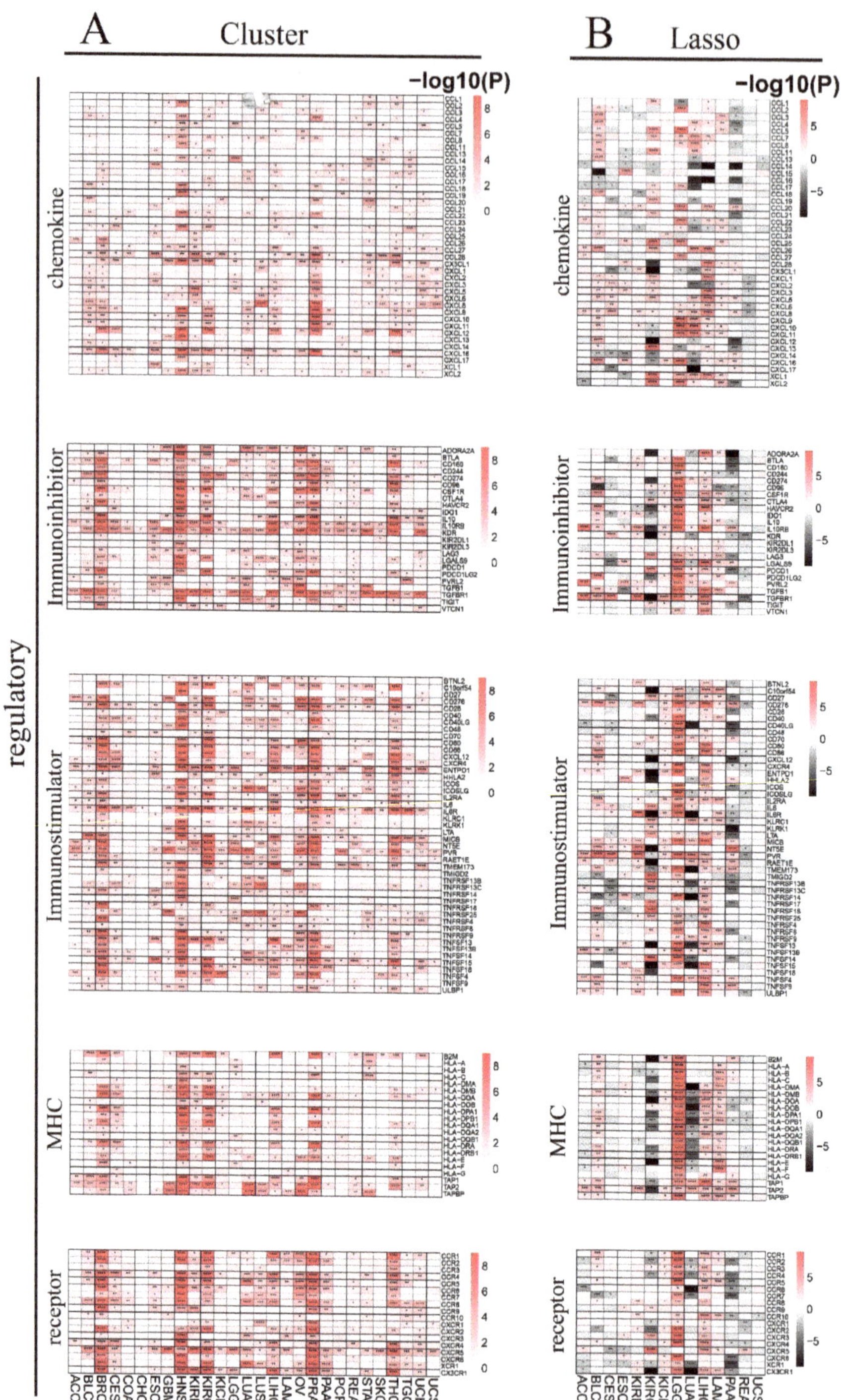

Figure 7. *Cont.*

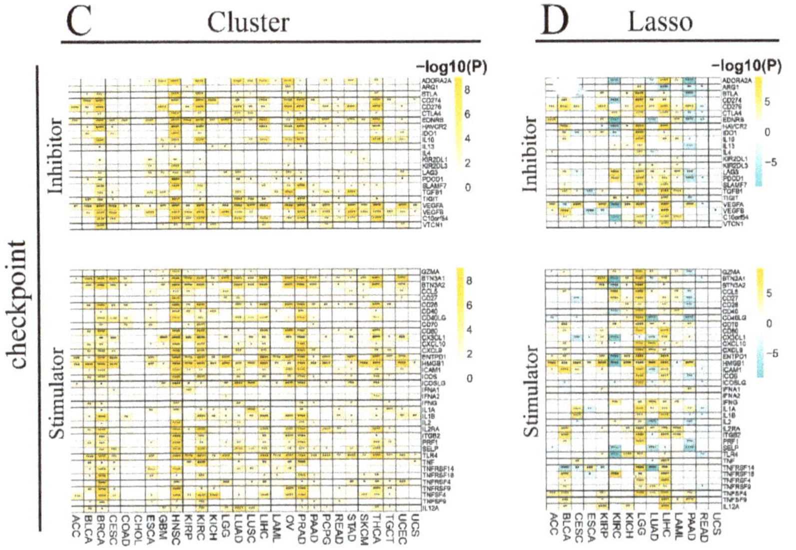

Figure 7. Association of immune regulatory and checkpoint genes with RNA m^6A regulators in multiple cancers. (**A**) Differential immune regulatory genes including chemokine, immunoinhibitor, immunostimulator, MHC, and receptor genes between clusters in each cancer type. (**B**) Differential immune regulatory genes including chemokine, immunoinhibitor, immunostimulator, MHC, and receptor genes between high- and low-risk groups in each cancer type. (**C**) Differential immune checkpoint inhibitory and stimulatory genes between clusters in each cancer type. (**D**) Differential immune checkpoint inhibitory and stimulatory genes between high- and low-risk groups in each cancer type. (* $p < 0.05$, ** $p < 0.01$, *** $p < 0.001$, **** $p < 0.0001$).

The MHCs affect cancer types among different clusters, including BLCA, BRCA, CESC, HNSC, KIRP, KIRC, LIHC, PRAD, STAD, and THCA; *B2M*, *HLA-DOA*, *TAP1*, *TAP2*, and *TAPBP* are affected in most tumor types (Figure 7A). As shown in Figure 7B, a few MHCs are positively correlated, while some are negatively correlated with the high-risk group in various cancer types; most of the MHCs in BLCA, LGG, LIHC, and LAML are increased; however, in KIRC and LUAD, they are decreased in the high-risk group.

The receptors affect a few cancer types among different clusters, including BLCA, BRCA, CESC, HNSC, KIRP, KIRC, LUAD, LUSC, LIHC, OV, PRAD, PAAD, THCA, TGCT, and UCEC; *CCR1*, *CCR2*, *CCR4*, *CCR5*, *CCR6*, *CCR8*, *CXCR5*, *XCR1* and *CX3CR1* are affected in most tumor types (Figure 7A). Furthermore, some receptors are positively correlated, while a few are negatively correlated with the high-risk group in various kinds of tumors; most of the receptors in LGG and LIHC are elevated while those in KIRC, LUAD, and PAAD are reduced, especially *CCR6* in LUAD, *CX3CR1* in KIRC, and LUAD in the high-risk group (Figure 7B).

The immune checkpoint inhibitory genes are found to affect various cancer types among different clusters, including BLCA, BRCA, CESC, ESCA, GBM, HNSC, KIRP, KIRC, KICH, LUAD, LUSC, LIHC, OV, PRAD, PCPG, STAD, SKCM, THCA, and UCEC; *CD274*, *CD276*, *EDNRB*, *VEGFA*, and *VEGFB* are the most affected tumor types (Figure 7C). Furthermore, the immune checkpoint inhibitory genes influence the high- and low-risk groups in each cancer type. While some immune checkpoint inhibitory genes are positively correlated, some are negatively correlated with the high-risk group in various cancer types; most immune checkpoint inhibitory genes in LGG and LIHC are increased while those in KIRC and PAAD are decreased, especially *VEGFA* and *C10orf54* in KIRC in the high-risk group (Figure 7D).

The immune checkpoint stimulatory genes affect various TCGA cancer types among different clusters, including BLCA, BRCA, CESC, ESCA, GBM, HNSC, KIRP, KIRC, LGG, LUAD, LUSC, LIHC, OV, PRAD, PAAD, PCPG, READ, STAD, SKCM, THCA, TGCT, and UCEC; *BTN3A1*, *BTN3A2*, *CD28*, *ENTPD1*, *HMGB1*, and *TLR4* are the most affected tumor types (Figure 7C). We also detect the influence of immune checkpoint stimulatory genes between high- and low-risk groups in each cancer type. Some immune checkpoint stimulatory genes are positively correlated, while some are negatively correlated with the high-risk group in various cancer types; most immune checkpoint stimulatory genes in LGG, LIHC, and BLCA are elevated; however, *BTN3A1*, *CX3CL1*, *ENTPD1*, *HMGB1*, and *TLR4* in KIRC; *CD40LG*, *IL2*, and *TNFRSF14* in LUAD; and *CD40LG* and *SELP* in PAAD are significantly reduced in the high-risk group (Figure 7D).

3.13. Correlation between microRNAs (miRNAs) and the RNA m^{6}A Regulators in TCGA Pan-Cancer

As shown in Supplementary Figure S10, we analyze the correlations between the miRNAs and RNA m^{6}A regulators in the TCGA pan-cancer cohort. Our results demonstrate that most of the genes are positively correlated with miRNAs in CESC, HNSC, LUAD, LIHC, TGCT, and UCEC. However, in the case of LAML, THCA, and UCS, most of the regulators show a negative correlation with miRNAs. We present the top 10 miRNAs, which have the most significant correlation with m^{6}A regulators in each cancer type.

3.14. Drug Prediction Based on m^{6}A Modification Genes in TCGA Pan-Cancer Cohort

To investigate the drug sensitivity in pan-cancer patients, we use *oncoPredict* to predict the relationships between RNA m^{6}A regulators and existing drugs in GDSC drug databases. The top 11 predicted drugs are vinorelbine, vinblastine, staurosporine, sepantronium.bromide, paclitaxel, eg5, docetaxel, dinaciclib, daporinad, dactinomycin, and bortezomib. Our results show that most of the genes are negatively correlated with these drugs (based on IC50 values) between high- and low-risk groups in each tumor except for *RBFOX2* in some tumors, *YTHDF1* in SKCM and LUAD, *FTO* in LUSC and TGCT, and *FMR1* in OV and UCS (Supplementary Figure S11).

3.15. Identified m^{6}A-Related Biomarkers by Three Machine Learning Algorithms

To investigate whether m^{6}A-related genes could serve as a biomarker for prognosis in each cancer type, we use LASSO, SVM-RFE, and RF algorithms to identify the important prognosis-related genes. The biomarkers are identified in 10 cancer types based on the RNA expression (Figure 8A). *IGF2BP1* is found to be a biomarker for BLCA, KICH, KIRP, and UCS; while *IGF2BP2* is found to be a biomarker for ACC, CESC, LAML, LGG, and PAAD; *HNRNPC* is a biomarker for LGG; and *RBMX* is the biomarker for ESCA (Figure 8A). We also identify prognostic biomarkers in each cancer type based on the CNV data with three machine-learning algorithms (Supplementary Table S6 and Figure 8B). *IGF2BP3* and *YTHDF3* are found to be the biomarkers for BLCA; *METTL14* for CHOL; *RBFOX2* for GBM and KIRP; *RBM15B*, *TRMT112*, and *YTHDF2* for KIRP; *FMR1* and *METTL3* for LGG; *YTHDC2* and *ZCCHC4* for LUAD; *ALKBH5*, *FMR1*, *HNRNPA2B1*, *YTHDC2*, *YTHDF2*, and *ZC3H13* for OV; and *YTHDF2* for PCPG (Figure 8B).

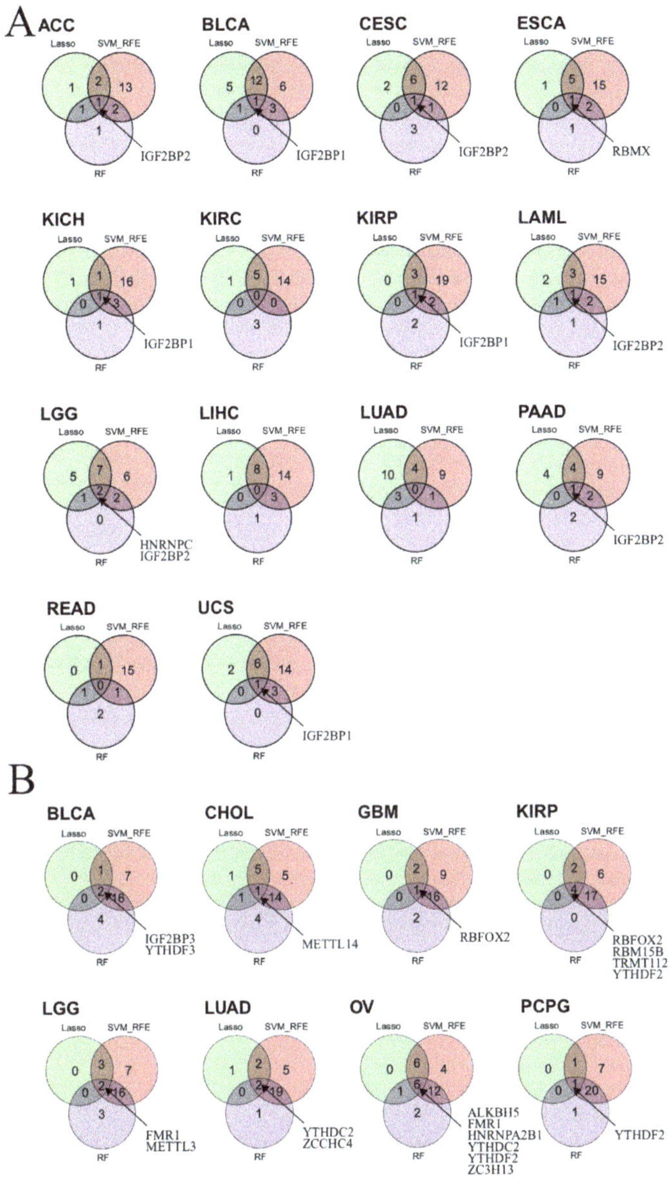

Figure 8. Identifying m^{6}A-related biomarkers using three machine-learning algorithms. (**A**) The Venn plot shows biomarkers obtained from the intersection of results from SVM-RFE, RF, and LASSO algorithms, based on the RNA expression levels in each cancer type. (**B**) The Venn plot shows biomarkers obtained from the intersection of results from SVM-RFE, RF, and LASSO algorithms based on the CNV data in each cancer type.

4. Discussion

In the current study, we collect a total of 31 m^{6}A modification regulators, including 12 writers, 2 erasers, and 17 readers. The mRNA expression, and the genetic and epigenetic alterations of the modifiers are explored by retrieving the expression and genomic data in pan-cancer from the TCGA database. The m^6A modification regulators are found to be highly expressed across various cancers and most of them harbored genetic aberrations, including SNVs and CNVs. Furthermore, the differential expression analysis between the cancer and normal tissues of the m^6A modifiers reveals significant differences for most regulators. Additionally, the m^6A regulators are found to be significantly correlated with the clinical parameters, such as age, gender, tumor stage, and grade in pan-cancer. Based on the expression of m^6A modifiers, we classify the tumors into different clusters or high- and low-risk groups. The m^6A modifiers are then evaluated among different clusters or between the high- and low-risk groups in the context of tumor microenvironment infiltrating immune cells, various tumor stemness, genomic heterogeneity properties, and immune regulatory or checkpoint genes. Lastly, the m^6A modifiers are correlated with miRNA expression and drug sensitivity in different pan-cancer clusters as well as high- and low-risk tumor groups. Finally, we identify some m^6A-related biomarkers using three machine-learning algorithms: LASSO, support vector machine-recursive feature elimination (SVM-RFE), and random forest (RF), according to their RNA expression or CNV data. For example, *IGF2BP1, IGF2BP2, HNRNPC,* and *RBMX* are found to be prognostic biomarkers based on their RNA levels. *IGF2BP3, YTHDF3, METTL14, RBFOX2, RBM15B, TRMT112, YTHDF2, FMR1, METTL3, YTHDC2, ZCCHC4, ALKBH5, HNRNPA2B1,* and *ZC3H13* are found to be prognostic biomarkers based on their CNV levels.

m^6A RNA modification is associated with multiple processes related to cancer, such as tumorigenesis, drug resistance, tumor epithelial-mesenchymal transition (EMT), and tumor metastasis. It also contributes to the self-renewal and differentiation of cancer stem cells, and resistance to radiotherapy and chemotherapy [64]. Some evidence agrees with the high/low expression of m^6A regulators across different cancers in our pan-cancer analysis. Accumulating evidence suggests that m^6A regulators act both as promoters and suppressors of oncogenesis. This is achieved by directly promoting/inhibiting the expression of m^6A regulators or indirectly influencing the downstream oncogenes or tumor suppressors during different stages or in different cancer types [65]. For instance, *METTL3* is highly expressed and promotes bladder cancer by promoting the expressions of *MYC* and *AFF4*; inhibition of *METTL3* reduces bladder tumor cell proliferation, migration, and invasion [66]. In endometrial tumors, reduced *METTL3* expression or *METTL14* mutation causes reduced levels of m^6A, leading to enhanced cell proliferation, colony formation, migration, and invasion of tumor cells [65,67].

When the genomic alterations are investigated, most of the m^6A regulators harbor SNVs across different cancers, with *ZC3H13, VIRMA,* and *PRRC2A* having higher mutation frequencies. Multiple studies have reported genomic variations in m^6A regulators in different cancers [68–70]. *ZC3H13* (zinc finger CCCH-type containing 13) is a canonical zinc finger protein, which harbors a somatic frame-shift mutation in colorectal cancer [68,71]. *VIRMA* (vir-like m^6A methyltransferase associated) is known to promote the progression of cancer and is associated with poor survival in multiple types of cancer [72]. *PRRC2A* (Proline-rich coiled-coil2A), also named *BAT2*, is localized near the genes coding for TNF alpha and TNF beta, and all these genes are within the human major histocompatibility complex class III region [73]. Furthermore, mutations in *PRRC2A* have been found to be associated with multiple cancers [74–76].

The survival analysis suggests involvement of the m^6A regulators with overall survival, both positively and negatively. For instance, *METTL3* is found to be positively associated with the prognosis of LIHC and LAML; it is negatively associated with PAAD. Similarly, another gene from the same family, *METTL14*, is positively associated with the prognosis of LGG and LAML, while negatively associated with KIRC, SKCM, and READ. There is accumulating biological evidence that these genes are associated with the prognosis of multiple cancers. A meta-analysis by Liu et al. [77] suggests that the upregulation of *METTL3* is significantly associated with poor prognosis. *METTL14* (Methyltransferase-like 14) is the central component of the m^6A methyltransferase complex and acts as both an oncogene and tumor suppressor gene. A review by Guan et al. [78] systematically summarizes the latest research on *METTL14*. The downregulated *METTL14* acts as a tumor suppressor in breast cancer and predicts poor prognosis [79].

Furthermore, we find a significant association between the clinicopathological parameters and the m^6A modification regulators in the current study. Such an association has been reported by multiple studies in literature. For instance, a meta-analysis by Su et al. [80] on human cancers identifies *METTL3* and *METTL14* to be the most important prognostic markers in cancer. A study by Zheng et al. [81] evaluates the relationship between m^6A modification and clinicopathological characteristics in breast cancer and identifies *CBLL1* as a promising prognostic biomarker.

Further, we classify the cancer patients based on the similarity of their m^6A regulators' levels into two to four clusters using the consensus-cluster method and evaluate the differential expression of the m^6A regulators across different clusters. The consensus-cluster method has been widely used to analyze m^6A regulators-related immune characteristics in various conditions, including spondylitis [82], prostate cancer [83], AML [84], and hepatitis B virus-related hepatocellular carcinoma [85].

The LASSO Cox regression method is suitable for constructing models when there are a large number of independent variables and in the case of restricted sample size [86]. Previously, LASSO regression has been used to construct the m^6A regulators-based risk signature in various conditions, including head and neck cancer [87], colorectal cancer [88,89], hepatocellular carcinoma [90], and AML [84]. We apply the LASSO Cox regression model to the pan-cancer cohort to identify high- and low-risk groups based on m^6A regulators-based prognostic signatures. Different sets of prognostic signatures are identified for different cancers by us, and *IGF2BP3*, a well-known m^6A regulator, is found to be highly expressed in a high-risk group of several cancers. The importance of this gene in cancer prognosis has been shown by other studies as well [91–93].

We further evaluate the differential immune cell infiltration between the high- and low-risk groups. Tumor–immune cell infiltration is closely related to clinical outcomes and the composition of tumor-infiltrating immune cells can serve as a diagnostic and prognostic biomarker [94–96]. Our results indicate a significant differential infiltration rate of multiple immune cell types between high- and low-risk KIRC along with a few other cancer types including LUAD, LGG, BLCA, and LIHC. A study by Zuo et al. [96] on immune cell infiltration patterns across 32 cancer types reveals that patients with high immune cell infiltration have worse OS, but PFS compared to those with low immune cell infiltration. Further, the authors suggest considerable heterogeneity in the prognostic value of these cells in different cancer types, which is in agreement with our results on pan-cancer analysis. Another pan-cancer study by Guo et al. [97] suggests that *METTL3* regulates the tumor immune microenvironment and epithelial–mesenchymal transition by modulating RNA modification and metabolism.

The correlation of the m^6A regulators with immune checkpoint genes and immune regulatory genes, including chemokines, immunoinhibitors, immunostimulators, and MHCs, results in significant correlations across different cancers.

We investigate the tumor stemness score in the TCGA pan-cancer cohort by analyzing DMPss, DNAss, ENHss, EREG.EXPss, EREG-METHss, and RNAss. The tumor stemness score of a few cancer types, including KIRP, KICH, LUAD, LIHC, PAAD, and TGCT, are significantly varied among different clusters. Also, there is an obvious discrepancy in tumor stemness between high- and low-risk groups in multiple cancer types.

Additionally, we investigate the genomic heterogeneity score in pan-cancer by analyzing different parameters, such as TMB, HRD, LOH, MSI, MATH, and NEO. Our analysis show significant differences in different parameters between the high- and low-risk groups across different tumor types. When the m^6A modification genes are correlated with the heterogeneity scores, we observe significant positive and negative correlations in different cancer types. The genomic heterogeneity properties have been shown to be useful as prognostic biomarkers and in therapy selection [98]. Recent studies have shed light on the key roles of m^6A modifiers in modulating DNA repair and genome integrity and stability [99].

A few m^6A regulators can regulate the RNA levels involved in DNA damage and repair, in turn affecting the genomic instability [100].

Next, we analyze the correlations between m^6A regulators and miRNAs in pan-cancer. Overall, our results show a positive correlation between the regulators and miRNAs in several cancer types. Recently, increasing evidence has suggested an interplay between miRNAs and m^6A modification. m^6A modification plays an important role in regulating miRNA biosynthesis, while miRNAs affect m^6A levels by targeting m^6A regulatory RNAs. A review by Han et al. [101] discusses, in detail, the interaction between m^6A modification and miRNAs.

Further, the drug sensitivity analysis predicts the relationship between the m^6A regulators and multiple drugs. Some of the top drugs that are identified to target these genes include vinorelbine, vinblastine, and staurosporine. Vinorelbine, an alkaloid, is an antineoplastic drug and is used as first-line chemotherapy for metastatic cancers [102]. Vinblastine, another alkaloid, is used to treat mainly blood cancers by inducing acute cell cycle phase-independent apoptosis [103,104]. Staurosporine, a highly successful anti-cancer drug, is produced by a soil-dwelling microbe. It acts by inhibiting protein kinases, particularly tyrosine kinases, and has a remarkably strong cytotoxic effect on cancer cells [105].

Although our study obtain several interesting findings, there are a few limitations. In this study, several important molecules are found to affect different cancers; however, further validations using other datasets as well as experiments are required to confirm their exact roles. Furthermore, additional external validations using other cohorts are needed to evaluate whether the m^6A molecular subtypes and risk-groups still perform well in various cancer types.

Supplementary Materials: The following supporting information can be downloaded at https://www.mdpi.com/article/10.3390/biomedicines12102211/s1, Figure S1: Differential expression of IGF2BP2 (A) and IGF2BP3 (B) in various normal and cancer tissues; Figure S2: Correlation between m^6A modification genes in 28 cancer types; Figure S3: Survival analysis of m^6A modification genes in 28 tumor types; Figure S4: Clinicopathological characteristics of representative m^6A modification genes in each cancer; Figure S5: Genetic and epigenetic alterations of m^6A modification genes in each cancer; Figure S6: The relationship between m^6A modification genes and ImmuneScore in multiple cancers; Figure S7: Association of immune cell infiltration with RNA m^6A regulators in TCGA pan-cancer cohort; Figure S8: Correlation between m^6A modification genes and tumor stemness scores in each cancer type; Figure S9: Correlation between m^6A modification genes and genomic heterogeneity scores in each cancer type; Figure S10: The relationship between m^6A modification genes and miRNAs in pan-cancer; Figure S11: Drug prediction based on m^6A modification genes; Table S1: Regulators of RNA m^6A modification; Table S2: 28 types of cancers in TCGA database; Table S3: 45 types of normal tissue in TCGA and GTEx database; Table S4: Patients' number distribution of clinicopathological characteristics in each cancer cohort; Table S5: Prognosis related genes in each tumor type based on LASSO cox regression; Table S6: Prognosis related genes in each tumor type based on CNV data with three machine learning algorithms.

Author Contributions: L.L. and X.W. conceive this project and supervise all the bioinformatics analyses. Y.H., A.K.B. and X.Y. write the manuscript. B.Z., H.L., J.W. and X.Y. perform the bioinformatics analyses and analyze the data. All authors have read and agreed to the published version of the manuscript.

Funding: This work is supported by the Postdoctoral Fund of Affiliated Hospital of Nantong University (BSH202307, BSH202309), and the Social Development Science and Technology Program of Nantong City (JC2020050).

Institutional Review Board Statement: Not applicable.

Informed Consent Statement: Not applicable.

Data Availability Statement: The datasets presented in this study can be found in online repositories.

Code Availability Statement: The full code used during this study is available at https://github.com/NTUWangLab/m6a_pancancer (accessed on 30 August 2024).

Conflicts of Interest: The authors declare no competing financial interests.

References

1. Linder, B.; Grozhik, A.V.; Olarerin-George, A.O.; Meydan, C.; Mason, C.E.; Jaffrey, S.R. Single-nucleotide-resolution mapping of m6A and m6Am throughout the transcriptome. *Nat. Methods* **2015**, *12*, 767–772. [CrossRef] [PubMed]
2. Schwartz, S.; Mumbach, M.R.; Jovanovic, M.; Wang, T.; Maciag, K.; Bushkin, G.G.; Mertins, P.; Ter-Ovanesyan, D.; Habib, N.; Cacchiarelli, D.; et al. Perturbation of m6A writers reveals two distinct classes of mRNA methylation at internal and 5′ sites. *Cell Rep.* **2014**, *8*, 284–296. [CrossRef] [PubMed]
3. Mattick, J.S.; Amaral, P.P.; Carninci, P.; Carpenter, S.; Chang, H.Y.; Chen, L.L.; Chen, R.; Dean, C.; Dinger, M.E.; Fitzgerald, K.A.; et al. Long non-coding RNAs: Definitions, functions, challenges and recommendations. *Nat. Rev. Mol. Cell Biol.* **2023**, *24*, 430–447. [CrossRef]
4. Meyer, K.D.; Saletore, Y.; Zumbo, P.; Elemento, O.; Mason, C.E.; Jaffrey, S.R. Comprehensive analysis of mRNA methylation reveals enrichment in 3′ UTRs and near stop codons. *Cell* **2012**, *149*, 1635–1646. [CrossRef]
5. Dominissini, D.; Moshitch-Moshkovitz, S.; Schwartz, S.; Salmon-Divon, M.; Ungar, L.; Osenberg, S.; Cesarkas, K.; Jacob-Hirsch, J.; Amariglio, N.; Kupiec, M.; et al. Topology of the human and mouse m^6A RNA methylomes revealed by m^6A-seq. *Nature* **2012**, *485*, 201–206. [CrossRef]
6. Xu, W.; He, C.; Kaye, E.G.; Li, J.; Mu, M.; Nelson, G.M.; Dong, L.; Wang, J.; Wu, F.; Shi, Y.G.; et al. Dynamic control of chromatin-associated m^6A methylation regulates nascent RNA synthesis. *Mol. Cell* **2022**, *82*, 1156–1168.e7. [CrossRef]
7. Li, Z.; Weng, H.; Su, R.; Weng, X.; Zuo, Z.; Li, C.; Huang, H.; Nachtergaele, S.; Dong, L.; Hu, C.; et al. FTO Plays an Oncogenic Role in Acute Myeloid Leukemia as a N^6-Methyladenosine RNA Demethylase. *Cancer Cell* **2017**, *31*, 127–141. [CrossRef] [PubMed]
8. Ping, X.L.; Sun, B.F.; Wang, L.; Xiao, W.; Yang, X.; Wang, W.J.; Adhikari, S.; Shi, Y.; Lv, Y.; Chen, Y.S.; et al. Mammalian WTAP is a regulatory subunit of the RNA N^6-methyladenosine methyltransferase. *Cell Res.* **2014**, *24*, 177–189. [CrossRef]
9. Mendel, M.; Chen, K.M.; Homolka, D.; Gos, P.; Pandey, R.R.; McCarthy, A.A.; Pillai, R.S. Methylation of structured RNA by the m^6A writer METTL16 is essential for mouse embryonic development. *Mol. Cell* **2018**, *71*, 986–1000.e11. [CrossRef]
10. Wen, J.; Lv, R.; Ma, H.; Shen, H.; He, C.; Wang, J.; Jiao, F.; Liu, H.; Yang, P.; Tan, L.; et al. ZC3H13 regulates nuclear RNA m^6A methylation and mouse embryonic stem cell self-renewal. *Mol. Cell* **2018**, *69*, 1028–1038.e6. [CrossRef]
11. Ruzicka, K.; Zhang, M.; Campilho, A.; Bodi, Z.; Kashif, M.; Saleh, M.; Eeckhout, D.; El-Showk, S.; Li, H.; Zhong, S.; et al. Identification of factors required for m^6A mRNA methylation in Arabidopsis reveals a role for the conserved E3 ubiquitin ligase HAKAI. *New Phytol.* **2017**, *215*, 157–172. [CrossRef] [PubMed]
12. Patil, D.P.; Chen, C.K.; Pickering, B.F.; Chow, A.; Jackson, C.; Guttman, M.; Jaffrey, S.R. m^6A RNA methylation promotes XIST-mediated transcriptional repression. *Nature* **2016**, *537*, 369–373. [CrossRef] [PubMed]
13. van Tran, N.; Ernst, F.G.M.; Hawley, B.R.; Zorbas, C.; Ulryck, N.; Hackert, P.; Bohnsack, K.E.; Bohnsack, M.T.; Jaffrey, S.R.; Graille, M.; et al. The human 18S rRNA m^6A methyltransferase METTL5 is stabilized by TRMT112. *Nucleic Acids Res.* **2019**, *47*, 7719–7733. [CrossRef] [PubMed]
14. Jia, G.; Fu, Y.; Zhao, X.; Dai, Q.; Zheng, G.; Yang, Y.; Yi, C.; Lindahl, T.; Pan, T.; Yang, Y.G.; et al. N^6-methyladenosine in nuclear RNA is a major substrate of the obesity-associated FTO. *Nat. Chem. Biol.* **2011**, *7*, 885–887. [CrossRef] [PubMed]
15. Zheng, G.; Dahl, J.A.; Niu, Y.; Fedorcsak, P.; Huang, C.M.; Li, C.J.; Vagbo, C.B.; Shi, Y.; Wang, W.L.; Song, S.H.; et al. ALKBH5 is a mammalian RNA demethylase that impacts RNA metabolism and mouse fertility. *Mol. Cell* **2013**, *49*, 18–29. [CrossRef]
16. Xiao, W.; Adhikari, S.; Dahal, U.; Chen, Y.S.; Hao, Y.J.; Sun, B.F.; Sun, H.Y.; Li, A.; Ping, X.L.; Lai, W.Y.; et al. Nuclear m^6A reader YTHDC1 regulates mRNA splicing. *Mol. Cell* **2016**, *61*, 507–519. [CrossRef]
17. Hsu, P.J.; Zhu, Y.; Ma, H.; Guo, Y.; Shi, X.; Liu, Y.; Qi, M.; Lu, Z.; Shi, H.; Wang, J.; et al. Ythdc2 is an N^6-methyladenosine binding protein that regulates mammalian spermatogenesis. *Cell Res.* **2017**, *27*, 1115–1127. [CrossRef]
18. Wang, X.; Zhao, B.S.; Roundtree, I.A.; Lu, Z.; Han, D.; Ma, H.; Weng, X.; Chen, K.; Shi, H.; He, C. N^6-methyladenosine Modulates Messenger RNA Translation Efficiency. *Cell* **2015**, *161*, 1388–1399. [CrossRef]
19. Wang, X.; Lu, Z.; Gomez, A.; Hon, G.C.; Yue, Y.; Han, D.; Fu, Y.; Parisien, M.; Dai, Q.; Jia, G.; et al. N^6-methyladenosine-dependent regulation of messenger RNA stability. *Nature* **2014**, *505*, 117–120. [CrossRef]
20. Li, A.; Chen, Y.S.; Ping, X.L.; Yang, X.; Xiao, W.; Yang, Y.; Sun, H.Y.; Zhu, Q.; Baidya, P.; Wang, X.; et al. Cytoplasmic m^6A reader YTHDF3 promotes mRNA translation. *Cell Res.* **2017**, *27*, 444–447. [CrossRef]
21. Liu, N.; Dai, Q.; Zheng, G.; He, C.; Parisien, M.; Pan, T. N^6-methyladenosine-dependent RNA structural switches regulate RNA-protein interactions. *Nature* **2015**, *518*, 560–564. [CrossRef] [PubMed]
22. Liu, N.; Zhou, K.I.; Parisien, M.; Dai, Q.; Diatchenko, L.; Pan, T. N^6-methyladenosine alters RNA structure to regulate binding of a low-complexity protein. *Nucleic Acids Res.* **2017**, *45*, 6051–6063. [CrossRef]
23. Edupuganti, R.R.; Geiger, S.; Lindeboom, R.G.H.; Shi, H.; Hsu, P.J.; Lu, Z.; Wang, S.Y.; Baltissen, M.P.A.; Jansen, P.; Rossa, M.; et al. N^6-methyladenosine (m^6A) recruits and repels proteins to regulate mRNA homeostasis. *Nat. Struct. Mol. Biol.* **2017**, *24*, 870–878. [CrossRef]
24. Alarcon, C.R.; Goodarzi, H.; Lee, H.; Liu, X.; Tavazoie, S.; Tavazoie, S.F. HNRNPA2B1 is a mediator of m^6A-dependent nuclear RNA processing events. *Cell* **2015**, *162*, 1299–1308. [CrossRef] [PubMed]

25. Huang, H.; Weng, H.; Sun, W.; Qin, X.; Shi, H.; Wu, H.; Zhao, B.S.; Mesquita, A.; Liu, C.; Yuan, C.L.; et al. Recognition of RNA N^6-methyladenosine by IGF2BP proteins enhances mRNA stability and translation. *Nat. Cell Biol.* **2018**, *20*, 285–295. [CrossRef] [PubMed]
26. Wu, R.; Li, A.; Sun, B.; Sun, J.G.; Zhang, J.; Zhang, T.; Chen, Y.; Xiao, Y.; Gao, Y.; Zhang, Q.; et al. A novel m^6A reader Prrc2a controls oligodendroglial specification and myelination. *Cell Res.* **2019**, *29*, 23–41. [CrossRef]
27. Yu, F.; Zhu, A.C.; Liu, S.; Gao, B.; Wang, Y.; Khudaverdyan, N.; Yu, C.; Wu, Q.; Jiang, Y.; Song, J.; et al. RBM33 is a unique m^6A RNA-binding protein that regulates ALKBH5 demethylase activity and substrate selectivity. *Mol. Cell* **2023**, *83*, 2003–2019.e6. [CrossRef]
28. Dou, X.; Xiao, Y.; Shen, C.; Wang, K.; Wu, T.; Liu, C.; Li, Y.; Yu, X.; Liu, J.; Dai, Q.; et al. RBFOX2 recognizes N^6-methyladenosine to suppress transcription and block myeloid leukaemia differentiation. *Nat. Cell Biol.* **2023**, *25*, 1359–1368. [CrossRef]
29. Arguello, A.E.; DeLiberto, A.N.; Kleiner, R.E. RNA chemical proteomics reveals the N^6-Methyladenosine (m^6A)-regulated protein-RNA interactome. *J. Am. Chem. Soc.* **2017**, *139*, 17249–17252. [CrossRef]
30. Deng, S.; Zhang, J.; Su, J.; Zuo, Z.; Zeng, L.; Liu, K.; Zheng, Y.; Huang, X.; Bai, R.; Zhuang, L.; et al. RNA m^6A regulates transcription via DNA demethylation and chromatin accessibility. *Nat. Genet.* **2022**, *54*, 1427–1437. [CrossRef]
31. Sommer, S.; Lavi, U.; Darnell, J.E., Jr. The absolute frequency of labeled N-6-methyladenosine in HeLa cell messenger RNA decreases with label time. *J. Mol. Biol.* **1978**, *124*, 487–499. [CrossRef] [PubMed]
32. Ries, R.J.; Zaccara, S.; Klein, P.; Olarerin-George, A.; Namkoong, S.; Pickering, B.F.; Patil, D.P.; Kwak, H.; Lee, J.H.; Jaffrey, S.R. m^6A enhances the phase separation potential of mRNA. *Nature* **2019**, *571*, 424–428. [CrossRef] [PubMed]
33. Wilkinson, F.L.; Holaska, J.M.; Zhang, Z.; Sharma, A.; Manilal, S.; Holt, I.; Stamm, S.; Wilson, K.L.; Morris, G.E. Emerin interacts in vitro with the splicing-associated factor, YT521-B. *Eur. J. Biochem.* **2003**, *270*, 2459–2466. [CrossRef] [PubMed]
34. Roundtree, I.A.; Luo, G.Z.; Zhang, Z.; Wang, X.; Zhou, T.; Cui, Y.; Sha, J.; Huang, X.; Guerrero, L.; Xie, P.; et al. YTHDC1 mediates nuclear export of N^6-methyladenosine methylated mRNAs. *Elife* **2017**, *6*, e31311. [CrossRef]
35. Vu, L.P.; Pickering, B.F.; Cheng, Y.; Zaccara, S.; Nguyen, D.; Minuesa, G.; Chou, T.; Chow, A.; Saletore, Y.; MacKay, M.; et al. The N^6-methyladenosine (m^6A)-forming enzyme METTL3 controls myeloid differentiation of normal hematopoietic and leukemia cells. *Nat. Med.* **2017**, *23*, 1369–1376. [CrossRef]
36. Du, M.; Zhang, Y.; Mao, Y.; Mou, J.; Zhao, J.; Xue, Q.; Wang, D.; Huang, J.; Gao, S.; Gao, Y. MiR-33a suppresses proliferation of NSCLC cells via targeting METTL3 mRNA. *Biochem. Biophys. Res. Commun.* **2017**, *482*, 582–589. [CrossRef]
37. Chen, M.; Wei, L.; Law, C.T.; Tsang, F.H.; Shen, J.; Cheng, C.L.; Tsang, L.H.; Ho, D.W.; Chiu, D.K.; Lee, J.M.; et al. RNA N6-methyladenosine methyltransferase-like 3 promotes liver cancer progression through YTHDF2-dependent posttranscriptional silencing of SOCS2. *Hepatology* **2018**, *67*, 2254–2270. [CrossRef]
38. Kennedy, L.; Hargrove, L.; Demieville, J.; Francis, N.; Seils, R.; Villamaria, S.; Francis, H. Recent Advances in Understanding Cholangiocarcinoma. *F1000Research* **2017**, *6*, 1818. [CrossRef]
39. Xue, C.; Chu, Q.; Zheng, Q.; Jiang, S.; Bao, Z.; Su, Y.; Lu, J.; Li, L. Role of main RNA modifications in cancer: N^6-methyladenosine, 5-methylcytosine, and pseudouridine. *Signal Transduct. Target. Ther.* **2022**, *7*, 142. [CrossRef]
40. Benci, J.L.; Xu, B.; Qiu, Y.; Wu, T.J.; Dada, H.; Twyman-Saint Victor, C.; Cucolo, L.; Lee, D.S.M.; Pauken, K.E.; Huang, A.C.; et al. Tumor Interferon Signaling Regulates a Multigenic Resistance Program to Immune Checkpoint Blockade. *Cell* **2016**, *167*, 1540–1554.e12. [CrossRef]
41. Zheng, Q.; Hou, J.; Zhou, Y.; Li, Z.; Cao, X. The RNA helicase DDX46 inhibits innate immunity by entrapping m^6A-demethylated antiviral transcripts in the nucleus. *Nat. Immunol.* **2017**, *18*, 1094–1103. [CrossRef] [PubMed]
42. Szklarczyk, D.; Gable, A.L.; Nastou, K.C.; Lyon, D.; Kirsch, R.; Pyysalo, S.; Doncheva, N.T.; Legeay, M.; Fang, T.; Bork, P.; et al. The STRING database in 2021: Customizable protein-protein networks, and functional characterization of user-uploaded gene/measurement sets. *Nucleic Acids Res.* **2021**, *49*, D605–D612. [CrossRef]
43. Bajpai, A.K.; Davuluri, S.; Tiwary, K.; Narayanan, S.; Oguru, S.; Basavaraju, K.; Dayalan, D.; Thirumurugan, K.; Acharya, K.K. Systematic comparison of the protein-protein interaction databases from a user's perspective. *J. Biomed. Inform.* **2020**, *103*, 103380. [CrossRef] [PubMed]
44. Zhou, Y.; Zhou, B.; Pache, L.; Chang, M.; Khodabakhshi, A.H.; Tanaseichuk, O.; Benner, C.; Chanda, S.K. Metascape provides a biologist-oriented resource for the analysis of systems-level datasets. *Nat. Commun.* **2019**, *10*, 1523. [CrossRef] [PubMed]
45. Leek, J.T.; Johnson, W.E.; Parker, H.S.; Jaffe, A.E.; Storey, J.D. The sva package for removing batch effects and other unwanted variation in high-throughput experiments. *Bioinformatics* **2012**, *28*, 882–883. [CrossRef]
46. Wang, Y.; Zhang, B.; Zhang, Z.; Ge, J.; Xu, L.; Mao, J.; Zhou, X.; Mao, L.; Xu, Q.; Sang, M. Predicting Prognosis and Immunotherapy Response in Multiple Cancers Based on the Association of PANoptosis-Related Genes with Tumor Heterogeneity. *Genes* **2023**, *14*, 1994. [CrossRef]
47. Tomczak, K.; Czerwinska, P.; Wiznerowicz, M. The Cancer Genome Atlas (TCGA): An immeasurable source of knowledge. *Contemp. Oncol.* **2015**, *19*, A68–A77. [CrossRef]
48. Schaschl, H.; Wallner, B. Population-specific, recent positive directional selection suggests adaptation of human male reproductive genes to different environmental conditions. *BMC Evol. Biol.* **2020**, *20*, 27. [CrossRef]
49. Wilkerson, M.D.; Hayes, D.N. ConsensusClusterPlus: A class discovery tool with confidence assessments and item tracking. *Bioinformatics* **2010**, *26*, 1572–1573. [CrossRef]

50. Friedman, J.; Hastie, T.; Tibshirani, R. Regularization Paths for Generalized Linear Models via Coordinate Descent. *J. Stat. Softw.* **2010**, *33*, 1–22. [CrossRef]
51. Hothorn, T.; Lausen, B. On the exact distribution of maximally selected rank statistics. *Comput. Stat. Data Anal.* **2003**, *43*, 121–137. [CrossRef]
52. Zeng, D.; Ye, Z.; Shen, R.; Yu, G.; Wu, J.; Xiong, Y.; Zhou, R.; Qiu, W.; Huang, N.; Sun, L.; et al. IOBR: Multi-Omics Immuno-Oncology Biological Research to Decode Tumor Microenvironment and Signatures. *Front. Immunol.* **2021**, *12*, 687975. [CrossRef] [PubMed]
53. Malta, T.M.; Sokolov, A.; Gentles, A.J.; Burzykowski, T.; Poisson, L.; Weinstein, J.N.; Kaminska, B.; Huelsken, J.; Omberg, L.; Gevaert, O.; et al. Machine Learning Identifies Stemness Features Associated with Oncogenic Dedifferentiation. *Cell* **2018**, *173*, 338–354.e15. [CrossRef]
54. Mayakonda, A.; Lin, D.C.; Assenov, Y.; Plass, C.; Koeffler, H.P. Maftools: Efficient and comprehensive analysis of somatic variants in cancer. *Genome Res.* **2018**, *28*, 1747–1756. [CrossRef]
55. Bonneville, R.; Krook, M.A.; Kautto, E.A.; Miya, J.; Wing, M.R.; Chen, H.Z.; Reeser, J.W.; Yu, L.; Roychowdhury, S. Landscape of Microsatellite Instability across 39 Cancer Types. *JCO Precis. Oncol.* **2017**, *2017*, PO.17.00073. [CrossRef] [PubMed]
56. Thorsson, V.; Gibbs, D.L.; Brown, S.D.; Wolf, D.; Bortone, D.S.; Ou Yang, T.H.; Porta-Pardo, E.; Gao, G.F.; Plaisier, C.L.; Eddy, J.A.; et al. The Immune Landscape of Cancer. *Immunity* **2018**, *48*, 812–830.e14. [CrossRef]
57. Hu, J.; Yu, A.; Othmane, B.; Qiu, D.; Li, H.; Li, C.; Liu, P.; Ren, W.; Chen, M.; Gong, G.; et al. Siglec15 shapes a non-inflamed tumor microenvironment and predicts the molecular subtype in bladder cancer. *Theranostics* **2021**, *11*, 3089–3108. [CrossRef]
58. Yoshihara, K.; Shahmoradgoli, M.; Martinez, E.; Vegesna, R.; Kim, H.; Torres-Garcia, W.; Trevino, V.; Shen, H.; Laird, P.W.; Levine, D.A.; et al. Inferring tumour purity and stromal and immune cell admixture from expression data. *Nat. Commun.* **2013**, *4*, 2612. [CrossRef]
59. Yang, W.; Soares, J.; Greninger, P.; Edelman, E.J.; Lightfoot, H.; Forbes, S.; Bindal, N.; Beare, D.; Smith, J.A.; Thompson, I.R.; et al. Genomics of Drug Sensitivity in Cancer (GDSC): A resource for therapeutic biomarker discovery in cancer cells. *Nucleic Acids Res.* **2013**, *41*, D955–D961. [CrossRef]
60. Maeser, D.; Gruener, R.F.; Huang, R.S. oncoPredict: An R package for predicting in vivo or cancer patient drug response and biomarkers from cell line screening data. *Brief Bioinform.* **2021**, *22*, bbab260. [CrossRef]
61. Huang, M.L.; Hung, Y.H.; Lee, W.M.; Li, R.K.; Jiang, B.R. SVM-RFE based feature selection and Taguchi parameters optimization for multiclass SVM classifier. *Sci. World J.* **2014**, *2014*, 795624. [CrossRef] [PubMed]
62. Rigatti, S.J. Random forest. *J. Insur. Med.* **2017**, *47*, 31–39. [CrossRef] [PubMed]
63. Zhang, J.; Xu, J.; Hu, X.; Chen, Q.; Tu, L.; Huang, J.; Cui, J. Diagnostic method of diabetes based on support vector machine and tongue images. *BioMed Res. Int.* **2017**, *2017*, 7961494. [CrossRef] [PubMed]
64. Wang, C.; Danli, M.; Yu, H.; Zhuo, Z.; Ye, Z. N6-methyladenosine (m6A) as a regulator of carcinogenesis and drug resistance by targeting epithelial-mesenchymal transition and cancer stem cells. *Heliyon* **2023**, *9*, e14001. [CrossRef]
65. He, L.; Li, H.; Wu, A.; Peng, Y.; Shu, G.; Yin, G. Functions of N6-methyladenosine and its role in cancer. *Mol. Cancer* **2019**, *18*, 176. [CrossRef]
66. Cheng, M.; Sheng, L.; Gao, Q.; Xiong, Q.; Zhang, H.; Wu, M.; Liang, Y.; Zhu, F.; Zhang, Y.; Zhang, X.; et al. The m^6A methyltransferase METTL3 promotes bladder cancer progression via AFF4/NF-kappaB/MYC signaling network. *Oncogene* **2019**, *38*, 3667–3680. [CrossRef]
67. Liu, J.; Eckert, M.A.; Harada, B.T.; Liu, S.M.; Lu, Z.; Yu, K.; Tienda, S.M.; Chryplewicz, A.; Zhu, A.C.; Yang, Y.; et al. m^6A mRNA methylation regulates AKT activity to promote the proliferation and tumorigenicity of endometrial cancer. *Nat. Cell Biol.* **2018**, *20*, 1074–1083. [CrossRef]
68. Li, W.; Gao, Y.; Jin, X.; Wang, H.; Lan, T.; Wei, M.; Yan, W.; Wang, G.; Li, Z.; Zhao, Z.; et al. Comprehensive analysis of N6-methylandenosine regulators and m6A-related RNAs as prognosis factors in colorectal cancer. *Mol. Ther. Nucleic Acids* **2022**, *27*, 598–610. [CrossRef]
69. Zhao, H.; Xu, Y.; Xie, Y.; Zhang, L.; Gao, M.; Li, S.; Wang, F. m6A Regulators Is Differently Expressed and Correlated with Immune Response of Esophageal Cancer. *Front. Cell Dev. Biol.* **2021**, *9*, 650023. [CrossRef]
70. Luo, Y.; Sun, X.; Xiong, J. Characterization of m6A Regulator-Mediated Methylation Modification Patterns and Tumor Microenvironment Infiltration in Ovarian Cancer. *Front. Cell Dev. Biol.* **2021**, *9*, 794801. [CrossRef]
71. Zhu, D.; Zhou, J.; Zhao, J.; Jiang, G.; Zhang, X.; Zhang, Y.; Dong, M. ZC3H13 suppresses colorectal cancer proliferation and invasion via inactivating Ras-ERK signaling. *J. Cell. Physiol.* **2019**, *234*, 8899–8907. [CrossRef] [PubMed]
72. Zhu, W.; Wang, J.Z.; Wei, J.F.; Lu, C. Role of m6A methyltransferase component VIRMA in multiple human cancers (Review). *Cancer Cell Int.* **2021**, *21*, 172. [CrossRef]
73. Banerji, J.; Sands, J.; Strominger, J.L.; Spies, T. A gene pair from the human major histocompatibility complex encodes large proline-rich proteins with multiple repeated motifs and a single ubiquitin-like domain. *Proc. Natl. Acad. Sci. USA* **1990**, *87*, 2374–2378. [CrossRef]
74. Pan, Q.; Ning, Y.; Chen, L.Z.; Zhang, S.; Liu, Z.Z.; Yang, X.X.; Wei, W.; Wei, H.; Li, Q.G.; Yue, H.N.; et al. Association of MHC class-III gene polymorphisms with ER-positive breast cancer in Chinese Han population. *Genet. Mol. Res.* **2012**, *11*, 4299–4306. [CrossRef]

75. Walsh, K.M.; Gorlov, I.P.; Hansen, H.M.; Wu, X.; Spitz, M.R.; Zhang, H.; Lu, E.Y.; Wenzlaff, A.S.; Sison, J.D.; Wei, C.; et al. Fine-mapping of the 5p15.33, 6p22.1-p21.31, and 15q25.1 regions identifies functional and histology-specific lung cancer susceptibility loci in African-Americans. *Cancer Epidemiol. Biomark. Prev.* **2013**, *22*, 251–260. [CrossRef] [PubMed]
76. Nieters, A.; Conde, L.; Slager, S.L.; Brooks-Wilson, A.; Morton, L.; Skibola, D.R.; Novak, A.J.; Riby, J.; Ansell, S.M.; Halperin, E.; et al. PRRC2A and BCL2L11 gene variants influence risk of non-Hodgkin lymphoma: Results from the InterLymph consortium. *Blood* **2012**, *120*, 4645–4648. [CrossRef]
77. Liu, K.; Gao, Y.; Gan, K.; Wu, Y.; Xu, B.; Zhang, L.; Chen, M. Prognostic Roles of N6-Methyladenosine METTL3 in Different Cancers: A System Review and Meta-Analysis. *Cancer Control* **2021**, *28*, 1073274821997455. [CrossRef]
78. Guan, Q.; Lin, H.; Miao, L.; Guo, H.; Chen, Y.; Zhuo, Z.; He, J. Functions, mechanisms, and therapeutic implications of METTL14 in human cancer. *J. Hematol. Oncol.* **2022**, *15*, 13. [CrossRef] [PubMed]
79. Gong, P.J.; Shao, Y.C.; Yang, Y.; Song, W.J.; He, X.; Zeng, Y.F.; Huang, S.R.; Wei, L.; Zhang, J.W. Analysis of N6-Methyladenosine Methyltransferase Reveals METTL14 and ZC3H13 as Tumor Suppressor Genes in Breast Cancer. *Front. Oncol.* **2020**, *10*, 578963. [CrossRef]
80. Su, Z.; Xu, L.; Dai, X.; Zhu, M.; Chen, X.; Li, Y.; Li, J.; Ge, R.; Cheng, B.; Wang, Y. Prognostic and clinicopathological value of m6A regulators in human cancers: A meta-analysis. *Aging* **2022**, *14*, 8818–8838. [CrossRef]
81. Zheng, F.; Du, F.; Qian, H.; Zhao, J.; Wang, X.; Yue, J.; Hu, N.; Si, Y.; Xu, B.; Yuan, P. Expression and clinical prognostic value of m6A RNA methylation modification in breast cancer. *Biomark. Res.* **2021**, *9*, 28. [CrossRef] [PubMed]
82. Guo, D.; Liu, J.; Li, S.; Xu, P. Analysis of m6A regulators related immune characteristics in ankylosing spondylitis by integrated bioinformatics and computational strategies. *Sci. Rep.* **2024**, *14*, 2724. [CrossRef]
83. Quan, Y.; Zhang, X.; Ping, H. Construction of a risk prediction model using m6A RNA methylation regulators in prostate cancer: Comprehensive bioinformatic analysis and histological validation. *Cancer Cell Int.* **2022**, *22*, 33. [CrossRef]
84. Ding, Y.; Bajpai, A.K.; Wu, F.; Lu, W.; Xu, L.; Mao, J.; Li, Q.; Pan, Q.; Lu, L.; Wang, X. 5-methylcytosine RNA modification regulators-based patterns and features of immune microenvironment in acute myeloid leukemia. *Aging* **2024**, *16*, 2340–2361. [CrossRef] [PubMed]
85. Zhang, Z.; Gao, W.; Liu, Z.; Yu, S.; Jian, H.; Hou, Z.; Zeng, P. Comprehensive analysis of m6A regulators associated with immune infiltration in Hepatitis B virus-related hepatocellular carcinoma. *BMC Gastroenterol.* **2023**, *23*, 259. [CrossRef]
86. Lee, S.; Seo, M.H.; Shin, Y. The lasso for high dimensional regression with a possible change point. *J. R. Stat. Soc. Ser. B Stat. Methodol.* **2016**, *78*, 193–210. [CrossRef] [PubMed]
87. Chen, Y.; Jiang, X.; Li, X.; Yan, D.; Liu, J.; Yang, J.; Yan, S. The methylation modification of m6A regulators contributes to the prognosis of head and neck squamous cell carcinoma. *Ann. Transl. Med.* **2021**, *9*, 1346. [CrossRef] [PubMed]
88. Zhang, D.; Wu, G.; Yang, L.; Wu, Q.; Yuan, L. The predictive significance of a 5-m6A RNA methylation regulator signature in colorectal cancer. *Heliyon* **2023**, *9*, e20172. [CrossRef]
89. Ji, L.; Chen, S.; Gu, L.; Zhang, X. Exploration of Potential Roles of m6A Regulators in Colorectal Cancer Prognosis. *Front. Oncol.* **2020**, *10*, 768. [CrossRef]
90. Li, W.; Liu, J.; Ma, Z.; Zhai, X.; Cheng, B.; Zhao, H. m^{6}A RNA Methylation Regulators Elicit Malignant Progression and Predict Clinical Outcome in Hepatocellular Carcinoma. *Dis. Markers* **2021**, *2021*, 8859590. [CrossRef]
91. Klingbeil, K.D.; Tang, J.P.; Graham, D.S.; Lofftus, S.Y.; Jaiswal, A.K.; Lin, T.L.; Frias, C.; Chen, L.Y.; Nakasaki, M.; Dry, S.M.; et al. IGF2BP3 as a Prognostic Biomarker in Well-Differentiated/Dedifferentiated Liposarcoma. *Cancers* **2023**, *15*, 4489. [CrossRef] [PubMed]
92. Sun, C.; Zheng, X.; Sun, Y.; Yu, J.; Sheng, M.; Yan, S.; Zhu, Q.; Lan, Q. Identification of IGF2BP3 as an Adverse Prognostic Biomarker of Gliomas. *Front. Genet.* **2021**, *12*, 743738. [CrossRef]
93. Huang, W.; Zhu, L.; Huang, H.; Li, Y.; Wang, G.; Zhang, C. IGF2BP3 overexpression predicts poor prognosis and correlates with immune infiltration in bladder cancer. *BMC Cancer* **2023**, *23*, 116. [CrossRef]
94. Bense, R.D.; Sotiriou, C.; Piccart-Gebhart, M.J.; Haanen, J.; van Vugt, M.; de Vries, E.G.E.; Schroder, C.P.; Fehrmann, R.S.N. Relevance of Tumor-Infiltrating Immune Cell Composition and Functionality for Disease Outcome in Breast Cancer. *J. Natl. Cancer Inst.* **2017**, *109*, djw192. [CrossRef] [PubMed]
95. Zhou, R.; Zhang, J.; Zeng, D.; Sun, H.; Rong, X.; Shi, M.; Bin, J.; Liao, Y.; Liao, W. Immune cell infiltration as a biomarker for the diagnosis and prognosis of stage I-III colon cancer. *Cancer Immunol. Immunother.* **2019**, *68*, 433–442. [CrossRef]
96. Zuo, S.; Wei, M.; Wang, S.; Dong, J.; Wei, J. Pan-Cancer Analysis of Immune Cell Infiltration Identifies a Prognostic Immune-Cell Characteristic Score (ICCS) in Lung Adenocarcinoma. *Front. Immunol.* **2020**, *11*, 1218. [CrossRef]
97. Guo, Y.; Heng, Y.; Chen, H.; Huang, Q.; Wu, C.; Tao, L.; Zhou, L. Prognostic Values of METTL3 and Its Roles in Tumor Immune Microenvironment in Pan-Cancer. *J. Clin. Med.* **2022**, *12*, 155. [CrossRef] [PubMed]
98. Lee, D.W.; Han, S.W.; Bae, J.M.; Jang, H.; Han, H.; Kim, H.; Bang, D.; Jeong, S.Y.; Park, K.J.; Kang, G.H.; et al. Tumor Mutation Burden and Prognosis in Patients with Colorectal Cancer Treated with Adjuvant Fluoropyrimidine and Oxaliplatin. *Clin. Cancer Res.* **2019**, *25*, 6141–6147. [CrossRef]
99. Qu, F.; Tsegay, P.S.; Liu, Y. N^6-Methyladenosine, DNA Repair, and Genome Stability. *Front. Mol. Biosci.* **2021**, *8*, 645823. [CrossRef]
100. Huang, W.; Chen, T.Q.; Fang, K.; Zeng, Z.C.; Ye, H.; Chen, Y.Q. N6-methyladenosine methyltransferases: Functions, regulation, and clinical potential. *J. Hematol. Oncol.* **2021**, *14*, 117. [CrossRef]

101. Han, X.; Guo, J.; Fan, Z. Interactions between m6A modification and miRNAs in malignant tumors. *Cell Death Dis.* **2021**, *12*, 598. [CrossRef] [PubMed]
102. Goa, K.L.; Faulds, D. Vinorelbine. A review of its pharmacological properties and clinical use in cancer chemotherapy. *Drugs Aging* **1994**, *5*, 200–234. [CrossRef] [PubMed]
103. Salerni, B.L.; Bates, D.J.; Albershardt, T.C.; Lowrey, C.H.; Eastman, A. Vinblastine induces acute, cell cycle phase-independent apoptosis in some leukemias and lymphomas and can induce acute apoptosis in others when Mcl-1 is suppressed. *Mol. Cancer Ther.* **2010**, *9*, 791–802. [CrossRef] [PubMed]
104. Dhyani, P.; Quispe, C.; Sharma, E.; Bahukhandi, A.; Sati, P.; Attri, D.C.; Szopa, A.; Sharifi-Rad, J.; Docea, A.O.; Mardare, I.; et al. Anticancer potential of alkaloids: A key emphasis to colchicine, vinblastine, vincristine, vindesine, vinorelbine and vincamine. *Cancer Cell Int.* **2022**, *22*, 206. [CrossRef]
105. Omura, S.; Asami, Y.; Crump, A. Staurosporine: New lease of life for parent compound of today's novel and highly successful anti-cancer drugs. *J. Antibiot.* **2018**, *71*, 688–701. [CrossRef]

biomedicines

Article

Prognostic Significance of *VAV3* Gene Variants and Expression in Renal Cell Carcinoma

Chi-Fen Chang [1,†], Bo-Ying Bao [2,†], Yu-Mei Hsueh [3,4], Pei-Ling Chen [5], Li-Hsin Chang [6], Chia-Yang Li [7,8], Jiun-Hung Geng [9,10], Te-Ling Lu [2], Chao-Yuan Huang [5,*] and Shu-Pin Huang [6,9,11,*]

1 Department of Anatomy, School of Medicine, China Medical University, Taichung 406, Taiwan; cfchang@mail.cmu.edu.tw
2 Department of Pharmacy, China Medical University, Taichung 406, Taiwan; bao@mail.cmu.edu.tw (B.-Y.B.); lutl@mail.cmu.edu.tw (T.-L.L.)
3 Department of Family Medicine, Wan Fang Hospital, Taipei Medical University, Taipei 110, Taiwan; ymhsueh@tmu.edu.tw
4 Department of Public Health, School of Medicine, College of Medicine, Taipei Medical University, Taipei 110, Taiwan
5 Department of Urology, National Taiwan University Hospital, College of Medicine, National Taiwan University, Taipei 100, Taiwan; 100117@ntuh.gov.tw
6 Graduate Institute of Clinical Medicine, College of Medicine, Kaohsiung Medical University, Kaohsiung 807, Taiwan; r120002@kmu.edu.tw
7 Graduate Institute of Medicine, College of Medicine, Kaohsiung Medical University, Kaohsiung 807, Taiwan; chiayangli@kmu.edu.tw
8 Department of Medical Research, Kaohsiung Medical University Hospital, Kaohsiung 807, Taiwan
9 Department of Urology, Kaohsiung Medical University Hospital, Kaohsiung 807, Taiwan; 1000596@kmuh.org.tw
10 Department of Urology, Kaohsiung Municipal Hsiao-Kang Hospital, Kaohsiung 812, Taiwan
11 Institute of Medical Science and Technology, College of Medicine, National Sun Yat-Sen University, Kaohsiung 804, Taiwan
* Correspondence: cyh0909@ntu.edu.tw (C.-Y.H.); shpihu@kmu.edu.tw (S.-P.H.)
† These authors contributed equally to this work.

Abstract: Renal cell carcinoma (RCC) is characterized by high mortality and morbidity rates. Vav guanine nucleotide exchange factors (VAVs), crucial for signal transduction between cell membrane receptors and intracellular mediators, have been implicated in carcinogenesis. However, their potential prognostic value in RCC remains unclear. The impact of 150 common *VAV* polymorphisms on RCC risk and survival was investigated in a cohort of 630 individuals. Publicly available gene expression datasets were utilized to analyze *VAV* gene expression in relation to patient outcomes. The *VAV3* rs17019888 polymorphism was significantly associated with RCC risk and overall survival after adjusting for false discovery rates. Expression quantitative trait loci analysis revealed that the risk allele of rs17019888 is linked to reduced *VAV3* expression. Analysis of 19 kidney cancer gene expression datasets revealed lower *VAV3* expression in RCC tissues compared to normal tissues, with higher expression correlating with better prognosis. Gene set enrichment analysis demonstrated that *VAV3* negatively regulates the ubiquitin–proteasome system, extracellular matrix and membrane receptors, inflammatory responses, matrix metalloproteinases, and cell cycle pathways. Furthermore, elevated *VAV3* expression was associated with increased infiltration of B cells, macrophages, and neutrophils into the RCC tumor microenvironment. Our findings suggest that *VAV3* gene variants influence RCC risk and survival, contributing to a favorable prognosis in RCC.

Keywords: renal cell carcinoma; vav guanine nucleotide exchange factor; genetic variants; gene set enrichment analysis; prognosis

1. Introduction

Renal cell carcinoma (RCC) is among the most prevalent forms of genitourinary cancer, with global incidence rates rising by approximately 2–3% annually [1]. From 1990 to 2019, the number of RCC cases worldwide has increased by 154.78% [2]. The mortality rate of RCC ranges from 30 to 40%, with a higher prevalence in males and in developed countries. The age of onset has shifted to younger populations, likely due to widespread health screening [3]. Despite this, the 5-year survival rate remained significantly lower in metastatic cases (13%) than in regional cases (70%) [4]. Current treatments for advanced unresectable RCC are inadequate, underscoring the urgent need for novel therapeutic strategies. Genetic factors and single-nucleotide polymorphisms (SNPs) such as *VHL* rs7629500 and *IRF5* rs3807306 play significant roles in RCC susceptibility [5]. Therefore, elucidating the genetic and molecular mechanisms underlying RCC may lead to the development of early diagnostic markers and effective treatments.

VAV genes function as guanine nucleotide exchange factors (GEFs) that activate Rho family GTPases [6]. In mammals, the *VAV* family comprises *VAV1*, *VAV2*, and *VAV3*, which have similar but not identical functions. *VAV1* is primarily expressed in hematopoietic cells, whereas *VAV2* and *VAV3* exhibit more widespread expression patterns [7]. VAVs play a crucial role in the intracellular signaling pathways downstream of receptors with tyrosine kinase activity [8]. Upon receptor stimulation, VAV proteins undergo tyrosine phosphorylation, activating Rho GTPases such as RhoA, Rac1, and Cdc42 [6], which, in turn, regulate various cellular processes, including phagocytosis, vesicular transport, cell growth, chemotaxis, migration, and adhesion [9].

Recent studies suggest that VAV proteins are essential for maintaining the homeostasis of cardiovascular, central nervous, and immune systems [6]. They are also implicated in numerous aspects of cancer biology, such as epithelial–mesenchymal transition, tumorigenesis, chemosensitivity, and metastasis [10,11]. *VAV1*, initially identified for its oncogenic activity [12], has been associated with poor survival rates in pancreatic [13], ovarian [14], and medulloblastoma tumors [15]. Conversely, *VAV1* may function as a tumor suppressor in immature T cells, with its loss leading to acute lymphoblastic leukemia in T cells [16,17]. Recent studies have investigated the relationship between genetic variants of *VAV* family genes and cancer susceptibility. For example, *VAV3* rs7521681 and rs4915076 have been linked to thyroid cancer risk [18], whereas rs12410676 has been associated with prostate cancer in Chinese males [19]. Additionally, *VAV2* rs12002767 may influence the overall survival of patients with non-small cell lung cancer by regulating *VAV2* expression [20]. However, the clinical significance of the genetic variants of *VAV* family genes in RCC remains unclear.

Given the critical role of *VAV* GEF family genes in signal transduction and cellular behavior, we hypothesized that genetic variants in *VAV* family genes are associated with RCC risk and survival. To test this hypothesis, we examined the relationship between 150 SNPs in *VAV* family genes and RCC risk and survival outcomes in a cohort of 630 participants. Additionally, we explored the functional significance of the implicated gene, *VAV3*, through gene ontology (GO) enrichment and pathway analyses to elucidate the potential biological mechanisms influencing RCC development.

2. Materials and Methods

2.1. Study Population and Data Collection

This study involved 630 participants recruited from Taipei Medical University Hospital, Taipei Municipal Wan Fang Hospital, and National Taiwan University Hospital. The cohort comprised 312 patients with pathologically confirmed RCC and 318 cancer-free controls matched for age (±1 year) and sex [21,22]. Demographic information was gathered through structured interviews, and clinical data were extracted from medical records. Our patient cohort consisted of 75.3% clear cell RCC (KIRC), 8.7% papillary RCC (KIRP), and 8% chromophobe RCC (KICH), closely mirroring the general cancer statistics where these subtypes represent approximately 75%, 10%, and 5% of all kidney cancers, respectively.

As shown in Table S1, the control group and patients with RCC were similar regarding sex, age, body mass index (BMI), and smoking status, but showed significant differences in alcohol intake, hypertension, and diabetes prevalence ($p < 0.001$). Most RCC cases were at stages I–II (81.4%) or grade I–II (75.2%). During the median follow-up period of 90 months, 34 (10.9%) patients died. All participants provided written informed consent prior to the interviews and specimen collection. This study was conducted in compliance with the Declaration of Helsinki and received approval from the Research Ethics Committee of the National Taiwan University Hospital (approval no. 9100201527, 2 July 2012).

2.2. SNP Selection and Genotyping

We selected haplotype-tagged SNPs for the *VAV* genes (*VAV1*, *VAV2*, and *VAV3*) using Han Chinese data from the 1000 Genomes Project and Haploview version 4.2, applying the criteria of minor allele frequency >0.03 and pairwise linkage disequilibrium $r^2 > 0.8$ [23,24]. A total of 150 SNPs was identified and genotyped. Genomic DNA was extracted from peripheral blood using the QIAamp DNA Blood Mini Kit (Qiagen, Valencia, CA, USA). Genotyping was performed using the Affymetrix Axiom Genotyping Arrays at the National Centre for Genome Medicine, Taiwan, in accordance with established protocols [25]. All SNPs were in Hardy–Weinberg equilibrium ($p > 0.001$), with genotyping rates between 97.9 and 100.0%.

2.3. Bioinformatic Analyses

Expression quantitative trait loci (eQTL) associations between SNPs and gene expression were evaluated using the Genotype-Tissue Expression (GTEx) portal [26]. Functional predictions of the SNPs were performed using HaploReg [27]. We analyzed 19 kidney cancer gene expression datasets from Gene Expression Omnibus [28–41], ArrayExpress [42,43], and The Cancer Genome Atlas (TCGA) [44] to explore correlations between gene expression and patient prognosis. For a deeper insight into the molecular mechanisms and pathways involving *VAV3*, we analyzed the genes correlated with *VAV3* in TCGA-KIRC kidney renal clear cell carcinoma samples using Pearson's correlation via LinkedOmics [45]. Enrichment analysis of GO terms and WikiPathways was conducted using gene set enrichment analysis (GSEA), with thresholds set at a false discovery rate (FDR) <0.05 and 1000 simulations. Tumor-infiltrating immune cell infiltration levels in TCGA-KIRC in relation to *VAV3* somatic copy number alterations and expression were compared using the TIMER database [46].

2.4. Statistical Analyses

Logistic regression was used to assess SNP associations with RCC risk by calculating odds ratios (ORs) and 95% confidence intervals (CIs) using the Statistical Package for the Social Sciences (version 19.0.0; IBM, Armonk, NY, USA). Statistical significance was defined as $p < 0.05$, and multiple testing corrections were applied using the FDR (q-value) [47]. *VAV3* expression levels in cancer and adjacent normal tissues were compared using standardized mean difference (SMD) and 95% CI with a random-effects model in Review Manager (RevMan version 5.4.1; Cochrane, London, UK). Associations between *VAV3* mRNA expression and RCC patient survival were evaluated by pooling hazard ratios (HRs) and 95% CIs using a random-effects model with RevMan.

3. Results

Logistic regression analysis was conducted to examine the association between genetic variants in *VAV* genes and the risk of RCC (Table S2). Of the 150 SNPs analyzed, seven SNPs within the *VAV* genes demonstrated a significant association with the risk of RCC ($p < 0.05$). Notably, the most significant association was observed for SNP rs17019888 in the *VAV3* gene, which had a q-value of 0.320, suggesting that 32.0% of these associations may be false positives (less than one false discovery). Specifically, each additional minor allele C of *VAV3* rs17019888 was associated with a 33% reduction in RCC risk (OR = 0.67, 95% CI = 0.50–0.88, $p = 0.005$; Table 1). This association remained significant after adjusting for confounding factors including sex, age, BMI, smoking status, alcohol intake, and history of diabetes and hypertension (adjusted OR = 0.59, 95% CI = 0.43–0.81, p = 0.001; Table 1).

Table 1. Association of *VAV3* rs17019888 with the risk of renal cell carcinoma.

Genotype	Controls, *n* (%)	Patients, *n* (%)	OR (95% CI)	*p*	*q*	OR (95% CI) [a]	*p* [a]
TT	191 (60.8)	214 (70.9)	1.00			1.00	
TC	104 (33.1)	79 (26.2)	0.68 (0.48–0.96)	0.030		0.56 (0.38–0.82)	0.003
CC	19 (6.1)	9 (3.0)	0.42 (0.19–0.96)	0.039		0.42 (0.17–1.05)	0.064
TC/CC			0.64 (0.46–0.89)	0.009		0.54 (0.37–0.78)	0.001
Trend			0.67 (0.50–0.88)	0.005	0.320	0.59 (0.43–0.81)	0.001

Abbreviations: OR, odds ratio; CI, confidence interval. [a] ORs were adjusted for sex, age, body mass index, smoking status, alcohol intake, and history of diabetes and hypertension.

The minor C allele of *VAV3* rs17019888 was also linked to overall survival among patients with RCC. Individuals carrying the minor allele C had a 68% reduction in the risk of all-cause mortality compared to those with the major allele homozygous genotype (TT) (HR = 0.32, 95% CI = 0.11–0.90, p = 0.032; Table 2 and Figure 1A). This association persisted after adjusting for sex, age, BMI, smoking status, alcohol intake, history of diabetes and hypertension, and disease stage and grade (adjusted HR = 0.12, 95% CI = 0.02–0.89, p = 0.038; Table 2).

Table 2. Association of *VAV3* rs17019888 with overall survival in patients with renal cell carcinoma.

Genotype	*n* of Patients	*n* of Events	5-y Survival Rate (%)	HR (95% CI)	*p*	HR (95% CI) [a]	*p* [a]
TT	214	30	89.6	1.00		1.00	
TC	79	3	95.9	0.27 (0.08–0.88)	0.029		
CC	9	1	100.0	0.74 (0.10–5.43)	0.767		
TC/CC	88	4	96.3	0.32 (0.11–0.90)	0.032	0.12 (0.02–0.89)	0.038
Trend				0.42 (0.17–1.03)	0.057	0.28 (0.07–1.08)	0.064

Abbreviations: HR, hazard ratio; CI, confidence interval. [a] HRs were adjusted for sex, age, body mass index, smoking status, alcohol intake, history of diabetes and hypertension, and disease stage and grade.

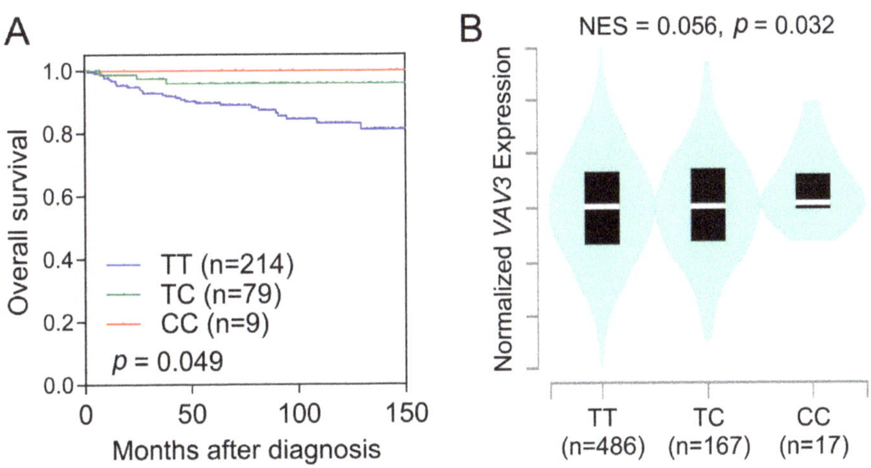

Figure 1. Survival and expression quantitative trait loci analyses for *VAV3* rs17019888. (**A**) Kaplan–Meier estimation displays overall survival of patients with renal cell carcinoma (RCC) categorized based on the rs17019888 genotype of *VAV3*. (**B**) Association between the genotypes of rs17019888 and the expression of *VAV3* in whole blood based on the Genotype-Tissue Expression dataset. NES, normalized effect size.

Subsequent eQTL analyses of 670 whole-blood samples from the GTEx project revealed that the minor C allele of rs17019888 was associated with increased *VAV3* mRNA expression ($p = 0.032$; Figure 1B). Despite rs17019888 being located within an intron of *VAV3*, functional prediction using HaploReg indicated that several SNPs in high linkage disequilibrium with rs17019888 coincided with potential promoter or enhancer regions (Table S3).

To better understand *VAV3*'s role in RCC, public kidney cancer datasets were analyzed. A pooled analysis of 1418 kidney cancer and 400 adjacent normal tissues across 17 studies revealed significant downregulation of *VAV3* in kidney cancer (SMD = −1.49, 95% CI = −1.81 to −1.18, $p < 0.001$; Figure 2A). Moreover, higher *VAV3* expression was significantly linked to improved patient survival (HR = 0.76, 95% CI = 0.59–0.97, $p = 0.03$; Figure 2B). Interestingly, *VAV3* exhibited downregulation (SMD from −0.63 to −1.70; Figure 2A) across all three TCGA datasets for the main RCC subtypes: KIRC, KIRP, and KICH. High *VAV3* expression was significantly associated with improved survival in the TCGA KIRC and KICH datasets, while it tended to be linked to poor survival in the KIRP dataset (Figure 2B).

A

Study or Subgroup	Cancer Mean	Cancer SD	Cancer Total	Normal Mean	Normal SD	Normal Total	Weight	Std. Mean Difference IV, Random, 95% CI
E-TABM-282	11.4605	0.6582	15	11.5486	0.4547	12	5.8%	-0.15 [-0.91, 0.61]
E-TABM-53	7.1951	1.0267	64	10.2285	0.391	9	5.3%	-3.08 [-3.94, -2.21]
GSE11024	9.2776	1.3598	67	10.6478	0.3901	12	6.4%	-1.07 [-1.71, -0.43]
GSE11151	9.3218	1.5466	61	10.5473	0.5626	6	5.3%	-0.81 [-1.66, 0.04]
GSE12606	10.0595	1.0166	7	10.7136	0.4813	3	3.2%	-0.65 [-2.05, 0.75]
GSE14762	9.4346	1.0907	10	10.6498	0.3849	12	4.8%	-1.49 [-2.46, -0.52]
GSE15641	8.9416	0.8498	69	10.3256	0.3247	23	6.9%	-1.82 [-2.36, -1.27]
GSE36895	9.7797	1.1348	29	11.0943	0.4467	23	6.5%	-1.44 [-2.06, -0.82]
GSE46699	9.6106	0.786	67	10.7086	0.4627	63	7.7%	-1.68 [-2.08, -1.28]
GSE53757	9.877	0.5347	72	10.9842	0.4003	72	7.5%	-2.33 [-2.76, -1.91]
GSE6280	7.7837	1.9048	14	10.2332	0.3271	6	4.3%	-1.44 [-2.52, -0.36]
GSE6344	9.1747	0.2992	10	10.1357	0.1747	10	2.8%	-3.76 [-5.32, -2.19]
GSE7023	9.9328	0.6516	35	10.7225	0.2578	12	6.0%	-1.34 [-2.05, -0.62]
GSE781	8.8969	0.6109	9	9.6094	0.2011	8	4.2%	-1.45 [-2.55, -0.35]
TCGA KICH	11.2801	0.9929	66	11.8402	0.5008	25	7.3%	-0.63 [-1.10, -0.16]
TCGA KIRC	10.4173	0.9359	533	11.9428	0.5449	72	8.2%	-1.70 [-1.96, -1.43]
TCGA KIRP	10.7937	0.7259	290	11.7108	0.3557	32	7.8%	-1.31 [-1.69, -0.93]
Total (95% CI)			**1418**			**400**	**100.0%**	**-1.49 [-1.81, -1.18]**

Heterogeneity: Tau² = 0.29; Chi² = 71.63, df = 16 ($p < 0.00001$); I² = 78%
Test for overall effect: Z = 9.31 ($p < 0.00001$)

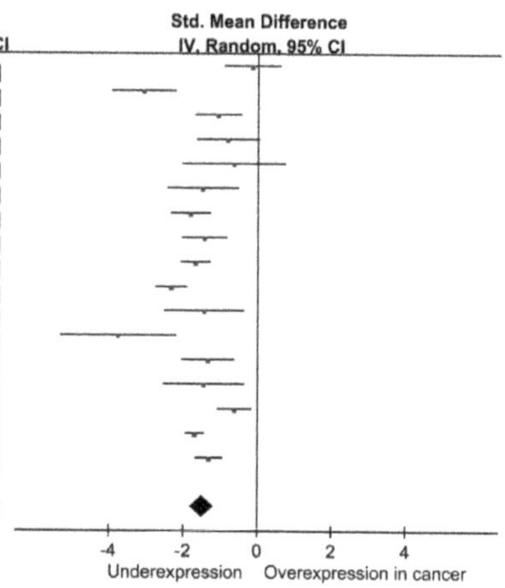

B

Study or Subgroup	log[Hazard Ratio]	SE	Weight	Hazard Ratio IV, Random, 95% CI
GSE22541	-0.1914	0.1798	18.8%	0.83 [0.58, 1.17]
GSE3538	-0.2281	0.0909	25.9%	0.80 [0.67, 0.95]
TCGA KICH	-0.8307	0.3019	11.3%	0.44 [0.24, 0.79]
TCGA KIRC	-0.4908	0.0763	26.9%	0.61 [0.53, 0.71]
TCGA KIRP	0.242	0.2038	17.0%	1.27 [0.85, 1.90]
Total (95% CI)			**100.0%**	**0.76 [0.59, 0.97]**

Heterogeneity: Tau² = 0.06; Chi² = 16.90, df = 4 ($p = 0.002$); I² = 76%
Test for overall effect: Z = 2.17 ($p = 0.03$)

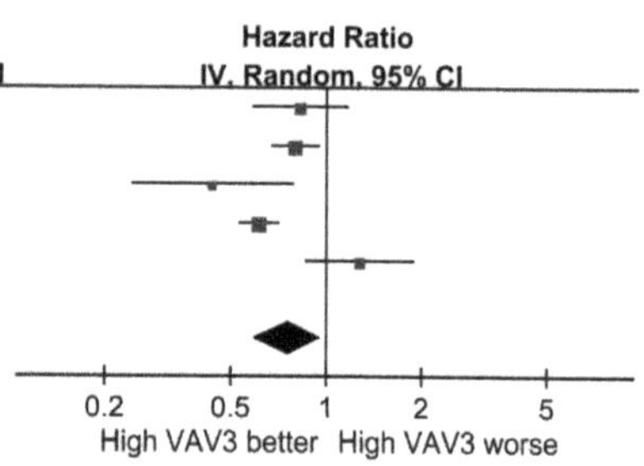

Figure 2. The mRNA expression of *VAV3* in kidney cancer. (**A**) Forest plot of differential expression of *VAV3* in kidney cancer and normal tissues. (**B**) Forest plot showing the association between *VAV3* expression and kidney cancer prognosis. SD, standard deviation; SE, standard error; IV, inverse variance; CI, confidence interval; Std, standardized; TCGA, The Cancer Genome Atlas; KICH, kidney chromophobe; KIRC, kidney renal clear cell carcinoma; KIRP, kidney renal papillary cell carcinoma; df, degrees of freedom [28–44].

To understand the biological significance of *VAV3* in RCC, we investigated *VAV3*-correlated genes in the TCGA-KIRC cohort. We identified 3298 positively correlated and 5606 negatively correlated genes based on FDR < 0.01 for Pearson's correlation. GO term annotation indicated that *VAV3*-correlated genes were involved in cellular components such as the collagen trimer, condensed chromatin, and extracellular matrix (Figure 3A).

These genes were primarily involved in biological processes such as collagen metabolic processes, chromosome segregation, and extracellular structure organization (Figure 3B). Molecular functions, such as extracellular matrix structural constituents, collagen binding, and nucleosome binding, were negatively regulated by *VAV3* (Figure 3C). WikiPathway enrichment analysis suggested that *VAV3* negatively regulates pathways related to the ubiquitin–proteasome system, extracellular matrix and membrane receptors, inflammatory response, matrix metalloproteinases, and cell cycle (Figure 3D), which indicate a protective role of *VAV3* against RCC.

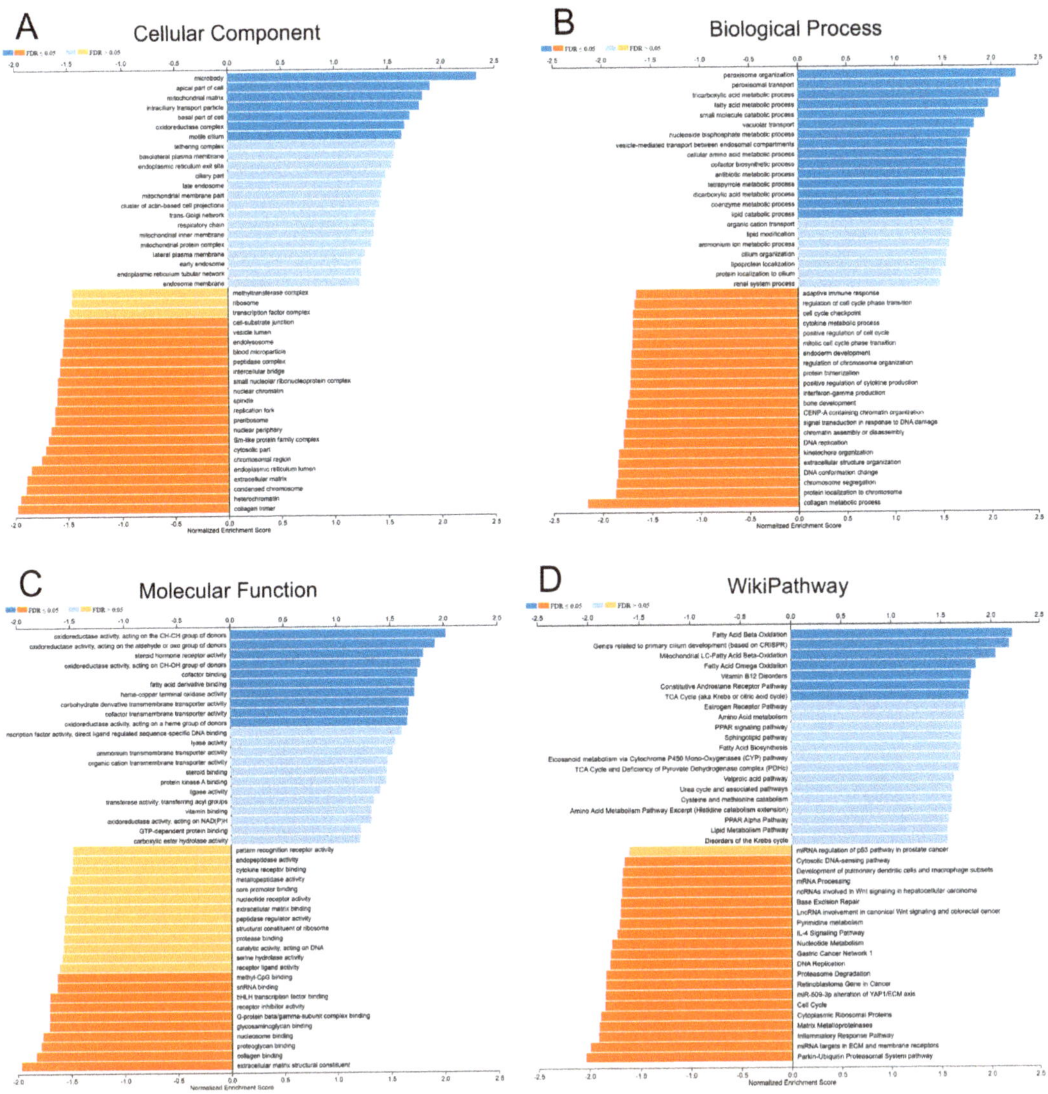

Figure 3. Potential biological functions of *VAV3* in kidney cancer. Gene ontology annotations of (**A**) cellular components, (**B**) biological processes, (**C**) molecular functions, and (**D**) WikiPathway enrichment analysis of *VAV3* correlated genes.

Given the association between the inflammatory response and cancer development, we examined the correlation between *VAV3* expression and immune cell infiltration in RCC. Arm-level deletion of *VAV3* was associated with the infiltration of various immune cells, including B cells, $CD8^+$ T cells, $CD4^+$ T cells, macrophages, neutrophils, and dendritic cells (Figure 4A). Furthermore, the infiltration levels of B cells, macrophages, and neutrophils positively correlated with *VAV3* expression in RCC (Figure 4B). These findings suggest that *VAV3* plays a crucial role in modulating immune cell infiltration, particularly in B cells, macrophages, and neutrophils, in RCC.

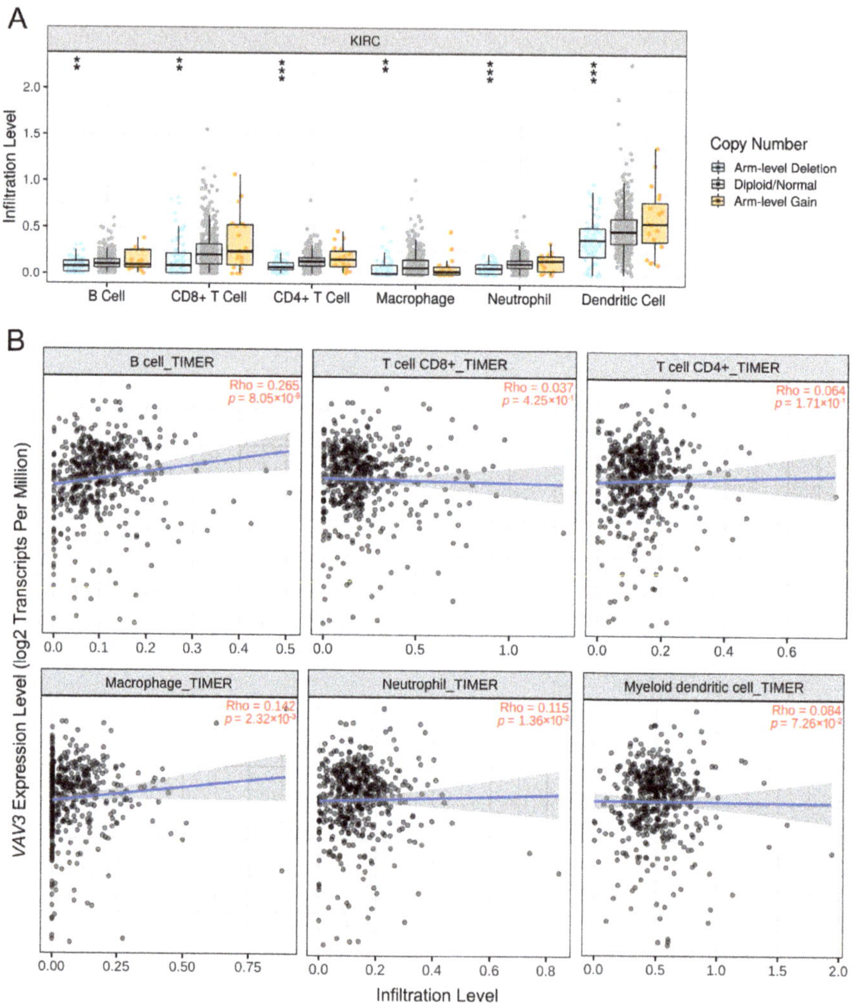

Figure 4. Correlation between *VAV3* expression and immune cell infiltration levels in the tumor microenvironment. (**A**) *VAV3* copy number variations affect the infiltration levels of multiple immune cell types in The Cancer Genome Atlas kidney renal clear cell carcinoma dataset. ** $p < 0.01$; *** $p < 0.001$. (**B**) Correlation between *VAV3* expression and the infiltrating levels of B cells, $CD8^+$ T cells, $CD4^+$ T cells, macrophages, neutrophils, and dendritic cells.

4. Discussion

In this study, we employed a combination of genetic and bioinformatics analyses to investigate the associations between genetic variants in *VAV* family genes and the risk and survival of RCC thoroughly. We identified a significant association between the *VAV3* rs17019888 T > C polymorphism and the risk and overall survival of patients with RCC, which remained robust after multivariate analysis and multiple testing correction. Carriers of the rs17019888 C allele exhibited a reduced risk of developing RCC and lower rates of all-cause mortality. Additionally, the rs17019888 C allele was significantly correlated with increased *VAV3* mRNA expression. Our pooled analysis of 19 studies indicated that *VAV3* may have tumor-suppressive properties, as it is downregulated in kidney cancers, and that higher *VAV3* mRNA expression levels were associated with better survival outcomes in patients with RCC. GSEA further suggested that *VAV3* may negatively regulate pathways related to the ubiquitin–proteasome system, extracellular matrix and membrane receptors, inflammatory response, matrix metalloproteinases, and cell cycle. Higher *VAV3* expression was also correlated with increased infiltration of anticancer immune cells, which is consistent with our genetic findings.

The VAV family of proteins, known as signal transducers, was initially identified for their protumorigenic activities. Various studies have reported that *VAV3* enhances cell proliferation in cancers such as breast cancer [11], gastric cancer [48], endometrial cancer [49], osteosarcoma [50], and acute lymphoblastic leukemia [51]. In addition, *VAV3* promotes cell migration and invasion in breast cancer [52], pancreatic cancer [53], gastric cancer [48], and osteosarcoma [50]. These findings highlight *VAV3* as the pivotal player in cancer progression. However, despite its oncogenic effects and upregulation in several tumors, *VAV3* expression is downregulated in certain cancers, including colon adenocarcinoma, head and neck squamous cell carcinoma, kidney cancer, lung adenocarcinoma, and prostate adenocarcinoma, as indicated by TCGA datasets. These data suggest that *VAV3* expression levels and their prognostic significance are highly cancer-dependent, necessitating further investigations to confirm *VAV3*'s specific role in different cancer types.

Furthermore, recent studies have shown that *VAV1*-deficient mice develop T-cell tumors at high frequencies upon aging or carcinogen treatment [17,54]. *VAV1* silences NOTCH1 signaling and suppresses T cell acute lymphoblastic leukemia by promoting the degradation of the intracellular domain of NOTCH1 (ICN1) through ubiquitination and proteasomal degradation [17]. Given the structural similarity and overlapping functions of VAV proteins, it is plausible that *VAV3* may also play tumor suppressor roles akin to *VAV1*. Studies have reported that *VAV3*-deficient mice develop certain tumors more frequently than their wild-type counterparts [55].

This study is the first to explore the clinical significance and role of *VAV3* in RCC using bioinformatic and functional analyses. Our pooled analysis of multiple datasets demonstrated that *VAV3* expression was reduced in RCC tumors and that patients with higher *VAV3* expression had longer survival times. GSEA revealed that genes co-expressed with *VAV3* were enriched in pathways related to the ubiquitin–proteasomal system, extracellular matrix and membrane receptors, inflammatory response, matrix metalloproteinases, and cell cycle. Additionally, high *VAV3* expression was correlated with increased infiltration of anticancer immune cells. These findings suggested that *VAV3* plays a suppressive role in RCC, possibly through ubiquitin-mediated proteasomal degradation, thereby influencing cancer-associated pathways. However, further research is required to elucidate the precise molecular mechanisms underlying *VAV3*'s involvement in RCC.

Despite these significant findings, this study has several limitations. First, the small sample size may have reduced the statistical power of detecting significant associations. Second, all study participants were Taiwanese, which may limit the generalizability of our findings to other ethnicities. Third, the lack of detailed clinical information from public datasets precluded adjustments to our analyses. Finally, the exact molecular mechanisms underlying the associations between the identified SNP and RCC survival remain unclear and require further investigation.

5. Conclusions

Our findings suggest that *VAV3* rs17019888 T > C polymorphism may serve as a novel prognostic biomarker for RCC. The rs17019888 variant may influence RCC progression by modulating *VAV3* expression and affecting cancer-related pathways and immune cell infiltration. However, it is essential to validate these results in larger studies and to conduct further mechanistic investigations to gain a comprehensive understanding of the underlying mechanisms.

Supplementary Materials: The following supporting information can be downloaded at https://www.mdpi.com/article/10.3390/biomedicines12081694/s1, Table S1. Clinical and demographic characteristics of healthy controls and patients with renal cell carcinoma. Table S2. Association between vav guanine nucleotide exchange factor gene polymorphisms and the risk of renal cell carcinoma. Table S3. Regulatory annotation of *VAV3* rs17019888.

Author Contributions: Conceptualization and methodology, C.-F.C., B.-Y.B., Y.-M.H., C.-Y.H. and S.-P.H.; resources and funding acquisition, B.-Y.B., C.-Y.H. and S.-P.H.; formal analysis and investigation, B.-Y.B., P.-L.C., L.-H.C. and C.-Y.L.; data curation and visualization, C.-F.C., J.-H.G. and T.-L.L. All authors have read and agreed to the published version of the manuscript.

Funding: This work was supported by the National Science and Technology Council of Taiwan (grant nos: 110-2314-B-002-113, 111-2314-B-002-240-MY3, 111-2320-B-039-021-MY3, 111-2218-E-037-001, and 112-2314-B-037-127), the Kaohsiung Medical University (grant no: KMUH109-9R63, KMUH109-9R64, KMUH112-2R59 and NHRIKMU-111-I002), and the China Medical University (grant nos: CMU110-MF-59, CMU111-MF-09, and CMU112-MF-10). The funders had no role in study design, data collection and analysis, decision to publish, or preparation of the manuscript.

Institutional Review Board Statement: This study was conducted in accordance with the Declaration of Helsinki and approved by the Research Ethics Committee of the National Taiwan University Hospital (approval no. 9100201527, 2 July 2012).

Informed Consent Statement: Written informed consent was obtained from all participants prior to the interviews and specimen collection.

Data Availability Statement: Data will be available on reasonable request.

Acknowledgments: The authors thank Chao-Shih Chen for data analysis, and the National Centre for Genome Medicine, Taiwan, for technical support. The results published here are based, in part, on data generated by the HaploReg, 1000 Genomes, GTEx, and TCGA projects.

Conflicts of Interest: The authors declare no conflicts of interest.

References

1. Capitanio, U.; Bensalah, K.; Bex, A.; Boorjian, S.A.; Bray, F.; Coleman, J.; Gore, J.L.; Sun, M.; Wood, C.; Russo, P. Epidemiology of Renal Cell Carcinoma. *Eur. Urol.* **2019**, *75*, 74–84. [CrossRef]
2. Zi, H.; He, S.H.; Leng, X.Y.; Xu, X.F.; Huang, Q.; Weng, H.; Zhu, C.; Li, L.Y.; Gu, J.M.; Li, X.H.; et al. Global, regional, and national burden of kidney, bladder, and prostate cancers and their attributable risk factors, 1990–2019. *Mil. Med. Res.* **2021**, *8*, 60. [CrossRef]
3. Pang, C.; Guan, Y.; Li, H.; Chen, W.; Zhu, G. Urologic cancer in China. *Jpn. J. Clin. Oncol.* **2016**, *46*, 497–501. [CrossRef]
4. Kase, A.M.; George, D.J.; Ramalingam, S. Clear Cell Renal Cell Carcinoma: From Biology to Treatment. *Cancers* **2023**, *15*, 665. [CrossRef]
5. Purdue, M.P.; Dutta, D.; Machiela, M.J.; Gorman, B.R.; Winter, T.; Okuhara, D.; Cleland, S.; Ferreiro-Iglesias, A.; Scheet, P.; Liu, A.; et al. Multi-ancestry genome-wide association study of kidney cancer identifies 63 susceptibility regions. *Nat. Genet.* **2024**, *56*, 809–818. [CrossRef]
6. Bustelo, X.R. Vav family exchange factors: An integrated regulatory and functional view. *Small GTPases* **2014**, *5*, 9. [CrossRef]
7. Movilla, N.; Bustelo, X.R. Biological and regulatory properties of Vav-3, a new member of the Vav family of oncoproteins. *Mol. Cell Biol.* **1999**, *19*, 7870–7885. [CrossRef]
8. Rodriguez-Fdez, S.; Bustelo, X.R. The Vav GEF Family: An Evolutionary and Functional Perspective. *Cells* **2019**, *8*, 465. [CrossRef]
9. Katoh, H.; Hiramoto, K.; Negishi, M. Activation of Rac1 by RhoG regulates cell migration. *J. Cell Sci.* **2006**, *119*, 56–65. [CrossRef] [PubMed]

10. Citterio, C.; Menacho-Marquez, M.; Garcia-Escudero, R.; Larive, R.M.; Barreiro, O.; Sanchez-Madrid, F.; Paramio, J.M.; Bustelo, X.R. The rho exchange factors vav2 and vav3 control a lung metastasis-specific transcriptional program in breast cancer cells. *Sci. Signal.* **2012**, *5*, ra71. [CrossRef] [PubMed]
11. Lee, K.; Liu, Y.; Mo, J.Q.; Zhang, J.; Dong, Z.; Lu, S. Vav3 oncogene activates estrogen receptor and its overexpression may be involved in human breast cancer. *BMC Cancer* **2008**, *8*, 158. [CrossRef]
12. Hornstein, I.; Pikarsky, E.; Groysman, M.; Amir, G.; Peylan-Ramu, N.; Katzav, S. The haematopoietic specific signal transducer Vav1 is expressed in a subset of human neuroblastomas. *J. Pathol.* **2003**, *199*, 526–533. [CrossRef]
13. Fernandez-Zapico, M.E.; Gonzalez-Paz, N.C.; Weiss, E.; Savoy, D.N.; Molina, J.R.; Fonseca, R.; Smyrk, T.C.; Chari, S.T.; Urrutia, R.; Billadeau, D.D. Ectopic expression of VAV1 reveals an unexpected role in pancreatic cancer tumorigenesis. *Cancer Cell* **2005**, *7*, 39–49. [CrossRef]
14. Wakahashi, S.; Sudo, T.; Oka, N.; Ueno, S.; Yamaguchi, S.; Fujiwara, K.; Ohbayashi, C.; Nishimura, R. VAV1 represses E-cadherin expression through the transactivation of Snail and Slug: A potential mechanism for aberrant epithelial to mesenchymal transition in human epithelial ovarian cancer. *Transl. Res.* **2013**, *162*, 181–190. [CrossRef]
15. Lindsey, J.C.; Kawauchi, D.; Schwalbe, E.C.; Solecki, D.J.; Selby, M.P.; McKinnon, P.J.; Olson, J.M.; Hayden, J.T.; Grundy, R.G.; Ellison, D.W.; et al. Cross-species epigenetics identifies a critical role for VAV1 in SHH subgroup medulloblastoma maintenance. *Oncogene* **2015**, *34*, 4746–4757. [CrossRef]
16. Abate, F.; da Silva-Almeida, A.C.; Zairis, S.; Robles-Valero, J.; Couronne, L.; Khiabanian, H.; Quinn, S.A.; Kim, M.Y.; Laginestra, M.A.; Kim, C.; et al. Activating mutations and translocations in the guanine exchange factor VAV1 in peripheral T-cell lymphomas. *Proc. Natl. Acad. Sci. USA* **2017**, *114*, 764–769. [CrossRef]
17. Robles-Valero, J.; Lorenzo-Martin, L.F.; Menacho-Marquez, M.; Fernandez-Pisonero, I.; Abad, A.; Camos, M.; Toribio, M.L.; Espinosa, L.; Bigas, A.; Bustelo, X.R. A Paradoxical Tumor-Suppressor Role for the Rac1 Exchange Factor Vav1 in T Cell Acute Lymphoblastic Leukemia. *Cancer Cell* **2017**, *32*, 608–623.E9. [CrossRef]
18. Ren, W.; Xu, C.; Wang, S.; Li, H.; Dai, H.; Yang, F.; Shao, Y.; Bai, Y. The effect of VAV3 polymorphisms on thyroid cancer. *Endocrine* **2022**, *75*, 178–184. [CrossRef]
19. Liu, M.; Miao, N.; Zhu, Y.; Gu, C.Y.; Shi, X.L.; Cui, W.L.; Zhang, W.; Li, Q.X. Association between polymorphism in Vav3 genes and risk of primary prostatic cancer in Chinese Han population. *Chin. J. Pathol.* **2016**, *45*, 451–456. [CrossRef]
20. Bai, Y.; Zheng, J.; Cheng, L.; Liu, Q.; Zhao, G.; Li, J.; Gu, Y.; Xu, W.; Wang, M.; Wei, Q.; et al. Potentially functional genetic variants of VAV2 and PSMA4 in the immune-activation pathway and non-small cell lung cancer survival. *J. Gene Med.* **2022**, *24*, e3447. [CrossRef]
21. Huang, C.Y.; Hsueh, Y.M.; Chen, L.C.; Cheng, W.C.; Yu, C.C.; Chen, W.J.; Lu, T.L.; Lan, K.J.; Lee, C.H.; Huang, S.P.; et al. Clinical significance of glutamate metabotropic receptors in renal cell carcinoma risk and survival. *Cancer Med.* **2018**, *7*, 6104–6111. [CrossRef]
22. Huang, C.Y.; Su, C.T.; Chu, J.S.; Huang, S.P.; Pu, Y.S.; Yang, H.Y.; Chung, C.J.; Wu, C.C.; Hsueh, Y.M. The polymorphisms of P53 codon 72 and MDM2 SNP309 and renal cell carcinoma risk in a low arsenic exposure area. *Toxicol. Appl. Pharmacol.* **2011**, *257*, 349–355. [CrossRef]
23. Genomes Project, C.; Abecasis, G.R.; Auton, A.; Brooks, L.D.; DePristo, M.A.; Durbin, R.M.; Handsaker, R.E.; Kang, H.M.; Marth, G.T.; McVean, G.A. An integrated map of genetic variation from 1,092 human genomes. *Nature* **2012**, *491*, 56–65. [CrossRef]
24. Li, C.Y.; Huang, S.P.; Chen, Y.T.; Wu, H.E.; Cheng, W.C.; Huang, C.Y.; Yu, C.C.; Lin, V.C.; Geng, J.H.; Lu, T.L.; et al. TNFRSF13B is a potential contributor to prostate cancer. *Cancer Cell Int.* **2022**, *22*, 180. [CrossRef]
25. Chang, H.H.; Lee, C.H.; Chen, Y.T.; Huang, C.Y.; Yu, C.C.; Lin, V.C.; Geng, J.H.; Lu, T.L.; Huang, S.P.; Bao, B.Y. Genetic Analysis Reveals the Prognostic Significance of the DNA Mismatch Repair Gene MSH2 in Advanced Prostate Cancer. *Cancers* **2022**, *14*, 223. [CrossRef]
26. Consortium, G.T. The Genotype-Tissue Expression (GTEx) project. *Nat. Genet.* **2013**, *45*, 580–585. [CrossRef]
27. Ward, L.D.; Kellis, M. HaploReg v4: Systematic mining of putative causal variants, cell types, regulators and target genes for human complex traits and disease. *Nucleic Acids Res.* **2016**, *44*, D877–D881. [CrossRef]
28. Eckel-Passow, J.E.; Serie, D.J.; Bot, B.M.; Joseph, R.W.; Cheville, J.C.; Parker, A.S. ANKS1B is a smoking-related molecular alteration in clear cell renal cell carcinoma. *BMC Urol.* **2014**, *14*, 14. [CrossRef]
29. Furge, K.A.; Chen, J.; Koeman, J.; Swiatek, P.; Dykema, K.; Lucin, K.; Kahnoski, R.; Yang, X.J.; Teh, B.T. Detection of DNA copy number changes and oncogenic signaling abnormalities from gene expression data reveals MYC activation in high-grade papillary renal cell carcinoma. *Cancer Res.* **2007**, *67*, 3171–3176. [CrossRef]
30. Gumz, M.L.; Zou, H.; Kreinest, P.A.; Childs, A.C.; Belmonte, L.S.; LeGrand, S.N.; Wu, K.J.; Luxon, B.A.; Sinha, M.; Parker, A.S.; et al. Secreted frizzled-related protein 1 loss contributes to tumor phenotype of clear cell renal cell carcinoma. *Clin. Cancer Res.* **2007**, *13*, 4740–4749. [CrossRef]
31. Jones, J.; Otu, H.; Spentzos, D.; Kolia, S.; Inan, M.; Beecken, W.D.; Fellbaum, C.; Gu, X.; Joseph, M.; Pantuck, A.J.; et al. Gene signatures of progression and metastasis in renal cell cancer. *Clin. Cancer Res.* **2005**, *11*, 5730–5739. [CrossRef]
32. Kort, E.J.; Farber, L.; Tretiakova, M.; Petillo, D.; Furge, K.A.; Yang, X.J.; Cornelius, A.; Teh, B.T. The E2F3-Oncomir-1 axis is activated in Wilms' tumor. *Cancer Res.* **2008**, *68*, 4034–4038. [CrossRef]
33. Lenburg, M.E.; Liou, L.S.; Gerry, N.P.; Frampton, G.M.; Cohen, H.T.; Christman, M.F. Previously unidentified changes in renal cell carcinoma gene expression identified by parametric analysis of microarray data. *BMC Cancer* **2003**, *3*, 31. [CrossRef]

34. Pena-Llopis, S.; Vega-Rubin-de-Celis, S.; Liao, A.; Leng, N.; Pavia-Jimenez, A.; Wang, S.; Yamasaki, T.; Zhrebker, L.; Sivanand, S.; Spence, P.; et al. BAP1 loss defines a new class of renal cell carcinoma. *Nat. Genet.* **2012**, *44*, 751–759. [CrossRef]
35. Stickel, J.S.; Weinzierl, A.O.; Hillen, N.; Drews, O.; Schuler, M.M.; Hennenlotter, J.; Wernet, D.; Muller, C.A.; Stenzl, A.; Rammensee, H.G.; et al. HLA ligand profiles of primary renal cell carcinoma maintained in metastases. *Cancer Immunol. Immunother.* **2009**, *58*, 1407–1417. [CrossRef]
36. von Roemeling, C.A.; Radisky, D.C.; Marlow, L.A.; Cooper, S.J.; Grebe, S.K.; Anastasiadis, P.Z.; Tun, H.W.; Copland, J.A. Neuronal pentraxin 2 supports clear cell renal cell carcinoma by activating the AMPA-selective glutamate receptor-4. *Cancer Res.* **2014**, *74*, 4796–4810. [CrossRef]
37. Wang, Y.; Roche, O.; Yan, M.S.; Finak, G.; Evans, A.J.; Metcalf, J.L.; Hast, B.E.; Hanna, S.C.; Wondergem, B.; Furge, K.A.; et al. Regulation of endocytosis via the oxygen-sensing pathway. *Nat. Med.* **2009**, *15*, 319–324. [CrossRef]
38. Wuttig, D.; Zastrow, S.; Fussel, S.; Toma, M.I.; Meinhardt, M.; Kalman, K.; Junker, K.; Sanjmyatav, J.; Boll, K.; Hackermuller, J.; et al. CD31, EDNRB and TSPAN7 are promising prognostic markers in clear-cell renal cell carcinoma revealed by genome-wide expression analyses of primary tumors and metastases. *Int. J. Cancer* **2012**, *131*, E693–E704. [CrossRef]
39. Yusenko, M.V.; Kuiper, R.P.; Boethe, T.; Ljungberg, B.; van Kessel, A.G.; Kovacs, G. High-resolution DNA copy number and gene expression analyses distinguish chromophobe renal cell carcinomas and renal oncocytomas. *BMC Cancer* **2009**, *9*, 152. [CrossRef] [PubMed]
40. Yusenko, M.V.; Zubakov, D.; Kovacs, G. Gene expression profiling of chromophobe renal cell carcinomas and renal oncocytomas by Affymetrix GeneChip using pooled and individual tumours. *Int. J. Biol. Sci.* **2009**, *5*, 517–527. [CrossRef] [PubMed]
41. Zhao, H.; Ljungberg, B.; Grankvist, K.; Rasmuson, T.; Tibshirani, R.; Brooks, J.D. Gene expression profiling predicts survival in conventional renal cell carcinoma. *PLoS Med.* **2006**, *3*, e13. [CrossRef]
42. Cifola, I.; Spinelli, R.; Beltrame, L.; Peano, C.; Fasoli, E.; Ferrero, S.; Bosari, S.; Signorini, S.; Rocco, F.; Perego, R.; et al. Genome-wide screening of copy number alterations and LOH events in renal cell carcinomas and integration with gene expression profile. *Mol. Cancer* **2008**, *7*, 6. [CrossRef]
43. Corbin, M.; de Reynies, A.; Rickman, D.S.; Berrebi, D.; Boccon-Gibod, L.; Cohen-Gogo, S.; Fabre, M.; Jaubert, F.; Faussillon, M.; Yilmaz, F.; et al. WNT/beta-catenin pathway activation in Wilms tumors: A unifying mechanism with multiple entries? *Genes Chromosomes Cancer* **2009**, *48*, 816–827. [CrossRef]
44. Cancer Genome Atlas Research, N. Comprehensive molecular characterization of clear cell renal cell carcinoma. *Nature* **2013**, *499*, 43–49. [CrossRef]
45. Vasaikar, S.V.; Straub, P.; Wang, J.; Zhang, B. LinkedOmics: Analyzing multi-omics data within and across 32 cancer types. *Nucleic Acids Res.* **2018**, *46*, D956–D963. [CrossRef]
46. Li, T.; Fan, J.; Wang, B.; Traugh, N.; Chen, Q.; Liu, J.S.; Li, B.; Liu, X.S. TIMER: A Web Server for Comprehensive Analysis of Tumor-Infiltrating Immune Cells. *Cancer Res.* **2017**, *77*, e108–e110. [CrossRef]
47. Storey, J.D.; Tibshirani, R. Statistical significance for genomewide studies. *Proc. Natl. Acad. Sci. USA* **2003**, *100*, 9440–9445. [CrossRef]
48. Tan, B.; Li, Y.; Zhao, Q.; Fan, L.; Wang, D.; Liu, Y. Inhibition of gastric cancer cell growth and invasion through siRNA-mediated knockdown of guanine nucleotide exchange factor Vav3. *Tumour Biol.* **2014**, *35*, 1481–1488. [CrossRef]
49. Jing, L.; Hua, X.; Yuanna, D.; Rukun, Z.; Junjun, M. Exosomal miR-499a-5p Inhibits Endometrial Cancer Growth and Metastasis via Targeting VAV3. *Cancer Manag. Res.* **2020**, *12*, 13541–13552. [CrossRef] [PubMed]
50. Xiao, Y.; Li, C.; Wang, H.; Liu, Y. LINC00265 targets miR-382-5p to regulate SAT1, VAV3 and angiogenesis in osteosarcoma. *Aging* **2020**, *12*, 20212–20225. [CrossRef] [PubMed]
51. Nayak, R.C.; Chang, K.H.; Singh, A.K.; Kotliar, M.; Desai, M.; Wellendorf, A.M.; Wunderlich, M.; Bartram, J.; Mizukawa, B.; Cuadrado, M.; et al. Nuclear Vav3 is required for polycomb repression complex-1 activity in B-cell lymphoblastic leukemogenesis. *Nat. Commun.* **2022**, *13*, 3056. [CrossRef]
52. Ojala, V.K.; Knittle, A.M.; Kirjalainen, P.; Merilahti, J.A.M.; Kortesoja, M.; Tvorogov, D.; Vaparanta, K.; Lin, S.; Kast, J.; Pulliainen, A.T.; et al. The guanine nucleotide exchange factor VAV3 participates in ERBB4-mediated cancer cell migration. *J. Biol. Chem.* **2020**, *295*, 11559–11571. [CrossRef]
53. Tsuboi, M.; Taniuchi, K.; Furihata, M.; Naganuma, S.; Kimura, M.; Watanabe, R.; Shimizu, T.; Saito, M.; Dabanaka, K.; Hanazaki, K.; et al. Vav3 is linked to poor prognosis of pancreatic cancers and promotes the motility and invasiveness of pancreatic cancer cells. *Pancreatology* **2016**, *16*, 905–916. [CrossRef]
54. Ruiz, S.; Santos, E.; Bustelo, X.R. The use of knockout mice reveals a synergistic role of the Vav1 and Rasgrf2 gene deficiencies in lymphomagenesis and metastasis. *PLoS ONE* **2009**, *4*, e8229. [CrossRef]
55. Cuadrado, M.; Robles-Valero, J. VAV Proteins as Double Agents in Cancer: Oncogenes with Tumor Suppressor Roles. *Biology* **2021**, *10*, 888. [CrossRef]

biomedicines

MDPI

Article

Generation of a Specific Fluorescence In Situ Hybridization Test for the Detection of Ovarian Carcinoma Cells

Amelie Limburg [1,†], Xueqian Qian [1,†], Bernice Brechtefeld [1], Nina Hedemann [1], Inken Flörkemeier [1], Christoph Rogmans [1], Leticia Oliveira-Ferrer [2], Nicolai Maass [1], Norbert Arnold [1], Dirk O. Bauerschlag [1] and Jörg Paul Weimer [1,*]

[1] Department of Gynaecology and Obstetrics, Christian-Albrechts-University and University Medical Center Schleswig-Holstein, 24105 Kiel, Germany; limburg.amelie@gmx.de (A.L.); nicolai.maass@uksh.de (N.M.); norbert.arnold@uksh.de (N.A.); dirk.bauerschlag@uksh.de (D.O.B.)
[2] Department of Gynaecology, University Hospital Hamburg-Eppendorf, 20246 Hamburg, Germany
* Correspondence: joerg-paul.weimer@uksh.de; Tel.: +49-431-500-21651
† These authors contributed equally to this work.

Abstract: Examinations of ovarian cancer cells require the ability to identify tumor cells. Array-based comparative genome hybridization (aCGH) on 30 ovarian carcinomas (OC) identified three genomic loci (8q24.23; 17p12; 18q22.3) over- or under-represented in OC. A fluorescence in situ hybridization (FISH) probe of these three loci is intended to identify tumor cells by their signal pattern deviating from a diploid pattern. Human DNA from these three loci is isolated from bacterial artificial chromosomes (BAC), amplified and labeled with fluorescent dyes. After a standard FISH procedure, 71 OC suspensions from primary tumors, three OC cell lines, three lymphocyte suspensions, and one mesenchymal cell line LP-3 are analyzed with a fluorescence microscope. On average, 15% of the lymphocytes deviate from the expected diploid signal pattern, giving a cut-off of 36%. If this value is exceeded, tumor cells are detected. The mesenchymal cell line LP-3 shows only 21% as a negative control. The OC cell lines as positive controls exceed this value at 38%, 67%, and 54%. Of the 71 OC primary cultures, four cases fell below this cut-off as false negatives. In the two-sample t-test, the percentages of conspicuous signal patterns differ significantly.

Keywords: ovarian cancer; FISH; aCGH; chromoanagenesis

1. Introduction

Ovarian cancer (OC) is one of the diagnoses with the worst prognosis in the range of gynecological–oncological diseases. The relative 5-year survival rate is about 40%. A key determining factor is the time of initial diagnosis; 76% of carcinomas are detected in late stage III/IV. The 5-year survival rate when detected in stage I is significantly higher at 88%, and in stage II, it is 79%. Hereditary mutations in the breast cancer genes *BRCA1* and *BRCA2* are the cause in one in ten cases, and if there is a known familial history, regular screening can facilitate earlier diagnosis [1,2]. There are three possible tissue origins of the OC: surface epithelium of the ovary, epithelium of the tube, and mesothelium covering the ovary and forming abdominal cavities [3]. Ninety percent arise from the surface epithelium of the ovary and represent epithelial ovarian carcinoma (EOC) [4]. The different types are divided into Type I and Type II [5]. Type I predominantly describes well-differentiated low-grade neoplasms, whereas Type II describes high-grade neoplasms that arise in the so-called de novo development without known precursor lesions. Type I includes low-grade serious, low-grade endometrioid, clear cell, mucinous, and transitional Brenner tumors. They do not show any *TP53* mutations and are characterized by their genetically relatively stable and indolent character [6]. Type II, on the other hand, mostly describes highly aggressive, poorly differentiated, and highly invasive carcinomas, which have mutations in the *TP53* gene in over 80% of cases. These are usually recognized at a late stage due to their increased formation of ascites, so understanding metastasis via this route is particularly important [5]. The colonization of OC cells in the abdominal cavity does not occur via an endothelial barrier, as is the case with most other solid tumors. In the case of OC, malignant ascites occur in more than a third of initial diagnoses and in every form of recurrent OC [7]. This malignant form plays an essential role in both metastasis and various forms of chemoresistance; the detailed and presumably interconnected processes are part of current research [8]. Primary and secondary tumor foci consist of complex cell types. In addition to tumor cells, there are also connective tissue cells, endothelial cells, and cells of the immune system in a tumor focus [9]. In order to increase an understanding of the complex processes of how these cells interact with each other, it is necessary to be able to differentiate the tumor cells from the other cell types. Because solid tumor cells, in contrast to non-tumor cells, accumulate genomic abnormalities, especially in the OC, genomic markers such as typical copy number variation (CNV) are ideal for distinguishing them from other cells [10,11]. As a result of this chromoanagenesis, typical CNVs can unmask tumor cells if it is known at which locations in the tumor genome chromoanagenesis particularly frequently produces changes. Such information can be explored using array-based comparative genome hybridization (aCGH). Particularly common CNVs can then be detected using a probe for fluorescence in situ hybridization (FISH) with corresponding DNA homology to the respective CNV. We deliberately do not detect tumor-relevant genes here, but rather want to make the genomic chaos in tumor cells visible by the simpler technique of FISH. Here, fluorescently labeled DNA, which corresponds to a specific locus in the genome, is melted into a single strand. Depending on the homology of their base pairing, these molecules hybridize to matching base sequences of the cell DNA, which is also denatured to form a single strand. FISH only indicates the presence of specific loci of the genome under study. Chromosomal changes in the genome of solid tumor cells lead to genomic imbalances. These are more likely to accumulate in some areas of the tumor genome than others. Loci in these more frequently altered areas can serve as markers for tumor cells and can be displayed using FISH. Such detection of tumor cells has already been shown on endometrial carcinoma cells [12]. The aim of this work is to find areas with the most common chromosomal changes in ovarian cancers and then generate a FISH probe homologous to these areas. This OC-FISH test is then intended to detect OC cells in that the hybridization pattern differs from the typical diploid pattern of non-neoplastic cells. In this study, 30 OCs were tested for genomic imbalances by aCGH. The three most common loci were used to generate homologous FISH probes. The validity of the OC-FISH test produced in this way was first checked on ovarian carcinoma cells, lymphocytes and the mesenchymal cell line LP-3. The strength of the OC-FISH test was then validated on 71 cell culture suspensions from primary ovarian carcinoma cell cultures.

2. Materials and Methods

Biomaterial: genomic imbalances in 30 ovarian cancers from patients treated at the Clinic for Gynecology and Obstetrics in Kiel between 1996 and 2013 were recorded using aCGH.

As a negative control for the OC-FISH test, we used normal male metaphases and interphases on CGH target slides (Abbot Molecular Inc., Des Plaines, IL, USA), a mesenchymal cell line LP-3, and specially isolated lymphocytes. As a positive control for OC-FISH test, we used three primary ovarian cancer cultures and ovarian cancer cell lines OVCAR 3, OVCAR 8, and SKOV 3. The authenticity of the cell lines was tested and confirmed using STR marker testing. The OC-FISH test was validated on 71 fixed primary cell cultures of ovarian cancer from 1999 to 2010 (Table 1). The use of these patient materials is based on their consent and a vote of the Ethics Committee of the Medical Faculty of the Christian-Albrechts University in Kiel (B327/10).

Table 1. All cells that were used as negative controls (green) and positive controls (red) and for validation (yellow) of the OC-FISH test are listed. The percentage of abnormal cells, the histological status, the FIGO value, the differentiation, and the score of the OC-FISH test are compared.

OC-FISH Test on:	Conspicuous Signal Pattern (%)	Histology	FIGO	Grading	Test Result
male lymphocytes	10				true negative
male lymphocytes	10				true negative
male lymphocytes	25				true negative
LP-3 mesenchyme	16				true negative
LP-3 mesenchyme	24				true negative
LP-3 mesenchyme	22				true negative
OvCa-cells	38	n.a.	n.a.	n.a.	true positive
OvCa-cells	67	n.a.	n.a.	n.a.	true positive
OvCa-cells	55	n.a.	n.a.	n.a.	true positive
OVCAR 3	100	serous	n.a.	3	true positive
OVCAR 8	100	serous	n.a.	3	true positive
SCOV 3	100	serous	n.a.	n.a.	true positive
RU-0001-OC	43	n.a.	n.a.	n.a.	true positive
SU-0002-OC	25	serous	IIIc	3	false negative
KA-0003-OC	65	serous	IIIb	borderline	true positive
WR-0004-OC	22	serous papillary	IIIc	3	false negative
BR-0005-OC	43	papillary	IIb	3	true positive
BI-0006-OC	39	serous	IIc	3	true positive
KS-0007-OC	32	serous	IIc	borderline	false negative
JH-0008-OC	50	serous papillary	IV	n.a.	true positive
BI-0009-OC	46	serous	IIc	3	true positive
HK-0011-OC	51	endometrioid	IIc	2	true positive
JE-0012-OC	49	endometrioid	IIIc	3	true positive
RH-0013-OC	58	papillary	IIIc	2	true positive
MH-0014-OC	43	serous papillary	n.a.	n.a.	true positive
SI-0015-OC	97	papillary clear cell	IIIc	3	true positive
DG-0016-OC	51	serous	IV	3	true positive
MA-0018-OC	37	serous papillary	n.a.	3	true positive
HJ-0019-OC	47	papillary	IIIc	3	true positive
KA-0020-OC	80	n.a.	IIIc	3	true positive
TW-0021-OC	53	serous papillary	IIIc	3	true positive
JD-0022-OC	85	serous papillary	IIIc	3	true positive
JS-0023-OC	38	serous papillary	IV	n.a.	true positive
KD-0024-OC	31	papillary	IIIc	2	false negative
SM-0028-OC	49	serous papillary	IIIc	3	true positive
JK-0030-OC	41	serous papillary	IIIc	2	true positive
ED-0031-OC	41	serous papillary	IIIb	3	true positive
SB-0032-OC	39	serous papillary	IIIb	3	true positive
TM-0033-OC	37	solid	IIIc	3	true positive

Table 1. *Cont.*

OC-FISH Test on:	Conspicuous Signal Pattern (%)	Histology	FIGO	Grading	Test Result
KA-0034-OC	53	serous papillary	IIIc	3	true positive
SD-0035-OC	75	mucinous	n.a.	2	true positive
KH-0036-OC	84	serous	n.a.	3	true positive
FF-0037-OC	67	papillary	IV	2	true positive
SD-0038-OC	55	mucinous	n.a.	2	true positive
PR-0039-OC	47	n.a.	Ic	2	true positive
RR-0040-OC	63	serous papillary	Iic	3	true positive
KR-0041-OC	61	papillary	IV	3	true positive
PK-0042-OC	47	serous	IV	3	true positive
DU-0043-OC	76	serous	n.a.	3	true positive
EA-0044-OC	96	serous papillary	IV	3	true positive
MI-0045-OC	99	n.a.	IV	n.a.	true positive
BE-0046-OC	52	n.a.	n.a.	n.a.	true positive
TB-0051-OC	70	serous papillary	IV	n.a.	true positive
SM-0053-OC	44	serous papillary	IV	n.a.	true positive
KK-0054-OC	99	endometrioid	Ia	1	true positive
BM-0055-OC	38	n.a.	n.a.	n.a.	true positive
AK-0056-OC	61	serous papillary	IV	1	true positive
MK-0057-OC	71	papillary	IIIc	3	true positive
TG-0058-OC	99	serous papillary	IIIc	3	true positive
JL-0059-OC	41	solid	IIIc	3	true positive
ZH-0061-OC	41	serous papillary	IV	n.a.	true positive
BF-0062-OC	48	papillary	IIIc	3	true positive
HH-0063-OC	51	serous papillary	IIc	3	true positive
SK-0064-OC	44	serous papillary	IIb	3	true positive
NG-0066-OC	43	serous papillary	n.a.	2	true positive
WP-0067-OC	62	serous	n.a.	borderline	true positive
PH-0068-OC	54	serous papillary	IV	3	true positive
BR-0069-OC	52	serous	IV	3	true positive
HM-0070-OC	95	endometrioid	Ic	2	true positive
SA-0071-OC	44	serous	IIIc	1	true positive
DR-0072-OC	45	mucinous	IV	1	true positive
KT-0073-OC	53	serous	IIc	borderline	true positive
AI-0075-OC	67	papillary	IV	1	true positive
KA-0076-OC	44	serous papillary	Ic	borderline	true positive
BKM-0077-OC	67	serous papillary	IV	3	true positive
WM-0078-OC	45	clear cell	n.a.	2	true positive
FG-0079-OC	71	serous papillary	IV	2	true positive
EL-0080-OC	99	n.a.	n.a.	n.a.	true positive
SB-0083-OiCa	72	serous papillary	IIIb	3	true positive

Table 1. *Cont.*

OC-FISH Test on:	Conspicuous Signal Pattern (%)	Histology	FIGO	Grading	Test Result
HK-0084-OC	67	serous endometrioid clear cell	IIIa	n.a.	true positive
BT-0085-OC	76	n.a.	n.a.	n.a.	true positive
HM-0086-OC	69	serous papillary	IIIc	2	true positive
ZI-0087-OC	99	serous papillary	IIIc	2	true positive

n.a. = not analyzed.

aCGH: following the Agilent protocol, 1 µg of isolated DNA from a tumor and an equivalent amount of reference Agilent female DNA (Agilent, Santa Clara, CA, USA) were used for aCGH. The DNA was digested with the restriction enzymes ALU I and RSA I. The tumor DNA was then labeled with Cy5-dUTP and the reference DNA with Cy3-dUTP (Agilent, Santa Clara, CA, USA). The labeled samples were purified according to the Agilent protocol and hybridized overnight. The hybridized and washed microarrays (Agilent 2x400k+SNP, design: 028081) were read out using a Dx Microarray Scanner G5761 from Agilent (Agilent, Santa Clara, CA, USA). The raw data were processed with the Agilent Feature Extraction software (Vers.: 3.0.5.1, Agilent Technologies Inc., Santa Clara, CA, USA) and then evaluated with the Agilent Cytogenomics (Vers.: 3.0.6.6) software (Agilent Technologies Inc., Santa Clara, CA, USA).

Preparation of the OC-FISH test: matching genomic sequences that most frequently exhibited CNV in OC were obtained from BACPAC Genomics, Inc. (BPG)—BACPAC Re-source Center; (BACPAC Genomics, Emeryville, CA, USA) bacterial artificial chromosomes (BAC) were used that had a homologous DNA sequence to the most common CNVs. These DH10B *Escherichia coli* clones were cultured overnight with 12.5 µg/mL chloramphenicol at 37 °C according to BACPAC instructions. The BAC DNA was isolated using a Qiagen® Plasmid Mini Kit (Qiagen, Hilden, Germany). As in Weimer et al. (1999), the BAC DNA is labeled with fluorescent dyes using a DOP-PCR [13]. The BAC clones RP11-17M8, RP11-347C14, RP11-449D3, RP11-911D14, and RP11-122H7 are homologous to 8q24.33 and are labeled with Green-dUTP (Enzo Life Science, NY, USA). The BAC clones RP11-455M13, RP11-1133K3, and RP11-504H5 are homologous to 18q22.3 and are labeled with aminoallyl-dUTP Cy3 (Jena Bioscience, Jena, Germany). The BAC clones RP11-837P21, RP11-746E8, and RP11-714I2 are homologous to 17p12 and are labeled with both fluorophores. The labeled DOP-PCR products are mixed with 40 µg Cot-1 DNA (GeneOn-BioScience, Ludwigshafen, Germany) and precipitated in 70% ethanol overnight. The precipitate is centrifuged at 4 °C, 13,000 RPM for 30 min. The dried pellet is dissolved in 50 µL hybridization mix (2×SSC, 50% formamide, 10% dextran sulphate, 1% Tween 20, and pH 7.0) [14,15].

OC-FISH test: the slides were defatted in ethanol (ETOH)/1% HCl for several days before hybridization. After the fixed cell suspensions were applied to the glass surface and buffered in Centipur phosphate buffer (Merck, Darmstadt, Germany) for 4 min, the cells were pretreated for hybridization by incubating the slides for 2 min at 37 °C in 2×SSC/0.5% Igepal, then incubated for 15 min in the 0.005% pepsin solution at 37 °C. The slides were then washed in DPBS for 3 min and fixed in 1% buffered formaldehyde solution for 10 min at room temperature. After a further 3 min in DPBS, the slide was dehydrated in an ascending alcohol series consisting of 70%, 90%, and 100% ETOH for 1 min each and then air-dried at room temperature. Both the target DNA in the prepared cells and the DNA of the OC-FISH test were co-denatured after covering with 11 µL OC-FISH test/slide half at 75 °C. Hybridization takes place overnight at 37 °C. After hybridization, coverslips were removed, and the slide was washed in 2×SSC, 0.1% Igepal for 2 min. This is followed by a stringent washing step in 0.4×SSC, 0.3% Igepal at 72 °C for 2 min. After another wash step in 2×SSC, 0.1% Igepal for 1 min, the slides are dehydrated in an ascending alcohol series (ethanol 70, 90, and 100%) and air-dried. Finally, the slides are capped with mounting medium containing DAPI. The observation was carried out on a Zeiss Axioplan 2 fluorescence microscope (Zeiss, Oberkochen, Germany), which is equipped with optical filter sets for FITC and Cy3. The documentation and evaluation are carried out using the ISIS software (Vers. 5.8, Metasystems, Altlusheim, Germany). One hundred and fifty interphases per case are counted in three series. Each recording to be evaluated is created as a seven-layer Z-stack so that no signals are lost in the three-dimensional core. Signal patterns that deviate from the typical diploid structure of two signals per loci are considered conspicuous. The signals to be considered for the evaluation must be within the core marked by DAPI. Signals are evaluated separately if they have a distance of at least one signal diameter between two signals.

Prospective primary cell culture: ovarian carcinoma material of four prospective patients (UF-478; UF-358; UF-384; UF-004) were cultured immediately after surgery as described by Kurbacher et al. (2011) [16]. Proliferation tests were carried out on the primary cultures, and 3D cell structures were cultured as described by Hedemann et al. (2021) [17].

3. Results

The evaluation of the aCGH data on 30 ovarian carcinomas revealed gains and losses that occur repeatedly in up to 60% of all cases at typical genomic loci (Figure 1).

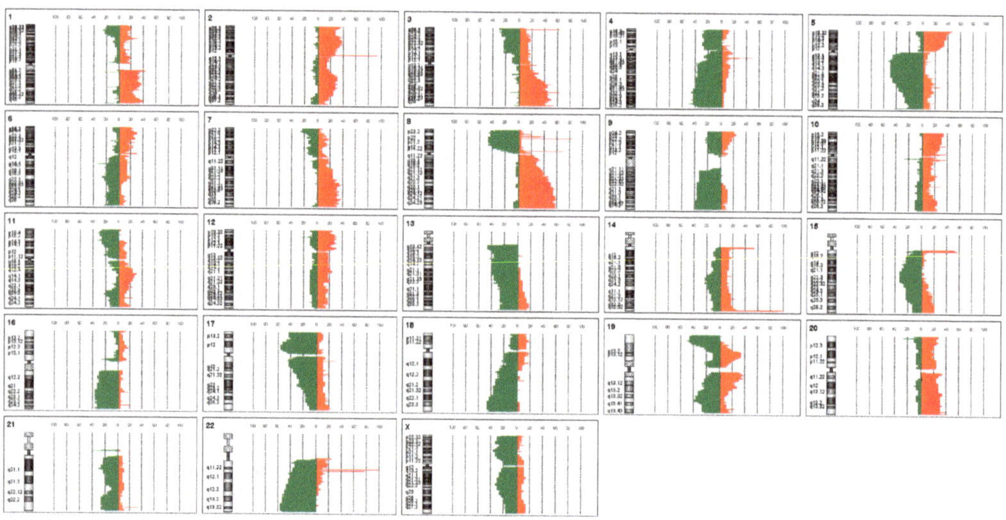

Figure 1. Shown is the relative proportion of copy number variations in 30 ovarian carcinomas for each human chromosome separately. Red bars represent gains, and green bars represent losses. The ideogram of the corresponding chromosome is shown on the left. The dashed lines show the percentage from 0 to 100% in increments of 10.

Particularly notable here are gains in chromosome 8q23 (60%), losses in 17p12 (57%), and losses in 18q22.3 in about half of all OCs examined with aCGH. These three genomic locations with the most common CNVs in ovarian cancer serve as a sequence template for a three-color OC-FISH test (Figure 2).

In order to determine a detection limit with which the proportion of deviations from the diploid state by the OC-FISH test can reliably detect ovarian cancer cells, a total of 91 lymphocyte nuclei were counted in three series. In 14 lymphocyte nuclei, the signal constellations deviated from the expected diploid pattern with two signals for each locus. In the three series, the non-diploid signal patterns had a mean of 15.38% and a standard deviation of 6.99%. Three times the standard deviation is added to the mean value found, resulting in the cut-off value of 36% for the OC-FISH test. If the count shows a proportion of non-diploid nuclei above the cut-off value, the existence of non-diploid cells is assumed to be given. This evaluation of the OC-FISH test was initially tested on the diploid mesenchymal cell line LP-3 as a negative control and on ovarian carcinoma cell lines as a positive control. The negative control showed an average proportion of non-diploid cells of 21% in three series, whereas the positive control had 53% nuclei with a deviation from the diploid signal pattern. To validate the OC-FISH test, it was carried out on fixed cells from 71 primary ovarian carcinoma cultures (see Table 1); 67 fixed primary cultures were above the cut-off and 4 below (Figure 3). The two-sample t-test shows a significant difference (t = 0.016) in the proportions of OC cells with an abnormal FISH pattern and cell suspensions that are not tumor cells.

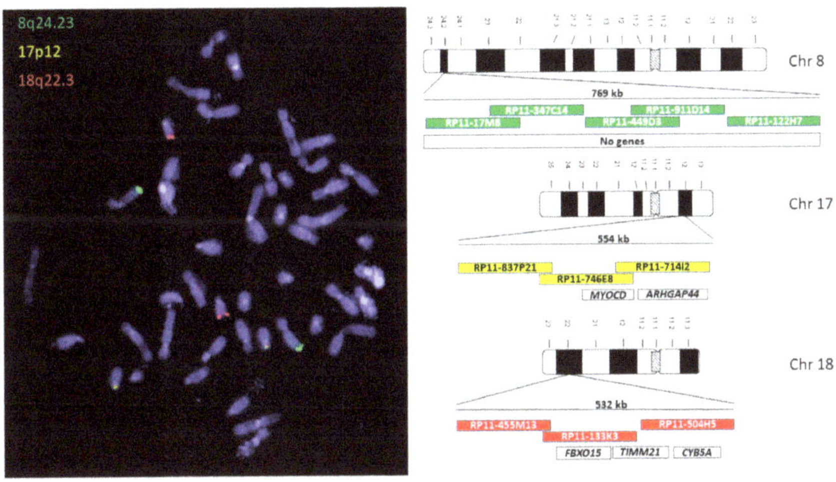

Figure 2. On the left is a lymphatic, diploid metaphase with the signals of the OC-FISH test. On the right are ideograms of the chromosomes of the OC-FISH test. The BACs that are involved in the respective loci are arranged in relation to each other in the colored boxes. In the uncolored boxes, genes are arranged in the respective OC-FISH test loci.

Considering the analysis of the lymphocytes, the negative control, the positive controls, and the validation, there are six true-negative findings, four false-negative findings, 73 true-positive findings, and no false-positive findings. Within this artificial case composition, which does not correspond to the natural population, we achieve a sensitivity of 0.94 and a specificity of 1 with the OC-FISH test. The average sensitivity value of the OC-FISH test for all possible specificity values is 0.84 (AUC), as Figure 4 shows.

In the OC-FISH test, all four prospective primary cultures produced proportional FISH signal patterns that deviated from the diploid pattern and were above the determined cut-off. The proportion of non-diploid signal patterns in UF-478 is 45.76%, in UF-358 is 68.42%, in UF-384 is 48.95%, and in UF-004 is 36.59%. We can therefore assume the existence of tumor cells in all primary cell cultures. Proliferation tests and 3D cell cultures confirm the existence of tumor cells in these prospective primary cultures.

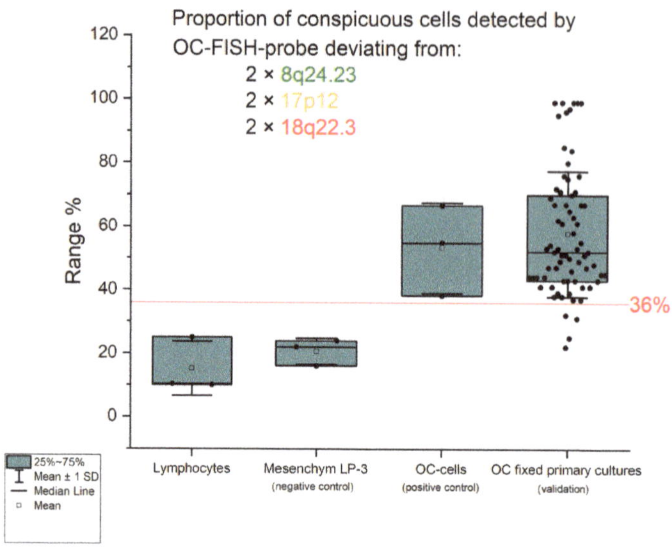

Figure 3. The graph shows the percentage of those interphases that deviate from the diploid pat-tern in the signal pattern. The green boxes correspond to the confidence interval (25%; 75%), the black solid line in the box corresponds to the median, and the transparent square in the box corresponds to the mean. The red solid line represents the cut-off of 36%. The standard deviation from the mean is shown by the antennas. The black dots are the percentages of interphases that are not diploid.

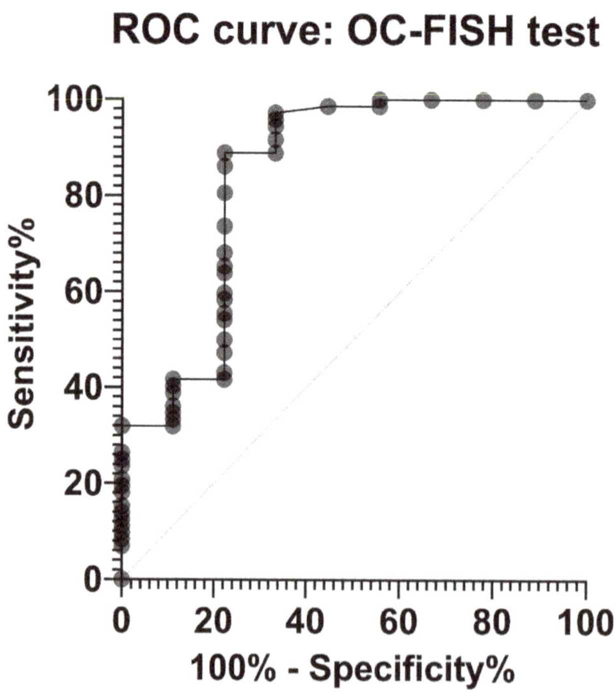

Figure 4. Receiver operating characteristic (ROC) curve of the OC-FISH test. The area under the curve is 0.8434 (95%CI: 0.672; $p = 0.0008$).

4. Discussion

Identifying tumor cells with individual genetic or specific surface markers is only possible to a limited extent [18,19]. The dynamic genetic changes in solid tumor cells also change these specific markers without the cell losing its tumor character. Román-Lladó et al. (2023) and Chrzanowska et al. (2020) have successfully shown that FISH is suitable for detecting tumor cells in different entities [20,21]. Unlike in this study, the authors used tumor-specific driver mutations as a target for the FISH probes. To use FISH as a far-reaching biomarker for tumor cells, the target of the FISH probe should concern tumor-specific DNA loci, which represent the diverse genomic changes in the form of genomic gains and losses. The loci that, on average, show the most deviations from a diploid state like CNVs in a tumor entity are suitable for this purpose.

The analysis of the most common CNVs in ovarian cancer partly corresponds to the data in the literature. Kim et al. (2007) have already shown genomic increases in 8q24 in serous OC, although these were located more distally in a gene-rich region in 8q24.3 [22]. Although our analysis also shows strong gains in this area, our peak of 60% is in 8q24.2 (Figure 1). In nearly 60% of the OCs we examined, we can also confirm losses in the chromosomal region 17p12, as also reported by Kim et al. (2007) and Lambros et al. (2005) [22,23]. The losses in 18q22 that we detected are also confirmed by Lambros et al. and Tan et al. [23,24]. Tan et al. (2011) confirm comparable gains and losses in clear cell ovarian carcinomas even in all three loci [24]. Despite different types of OC, the CGH results of these three authors largely correspond to our data, although we deliberately included all OC types in our study. The concordance of the CNVs suggests that the process of chromoanagenesis in OC results in comparable gains and losses [10,11]. Under this condition, a genomic marker that indicates the loci with the most frequent changes should be suitable for detecting OC cells. We were able to generate such a genomic marker calling OC-FISH test. To produce the OC-FISH test, we used the BACPAC genome bank, which offers *E-coli* clones with BACs. We ordered partially overlapping or at least adjacent clones and used their BACs to produce the OC-FISH test (Figure 2). During production, it turned out that two things are advantageous. On the one hand, staining three loci with only two colors (by staining two loci with only one color but staining the third loci evenly with both colors) has the advantage that the selection of colors with little background leads to clean and clear results. The more different colors are used, the higher the probability that one of the colors used will make the entire coloring unusable due to its own background. Furthermore, it is essential that the interphases to be analyzed are captured in their 3D structure by a focused Z-stack. This is the only way to ensure that all signals from the OC-FISH test are recorded. The signal length of the individual loci extends over a clearly visible 500 to 770 kb (Figure 2). Even if the genes *FBXO15*, *TIMM21*, and *CYB5A* are present in the loci 18q22 and the genes *MYOCD* and *ARHGAP44* in the loci 17p12, the selection of these loci for the OC-FISH test is not about these genes but primarily about the high probability that a CNV may be present in the three loci, which can be detected with the OC-FISH test. Other FISH tests in gynecology and senology are more about detecting the amplification of relevant genes, such as human epidermal growth factor receptor 2 (HER2/neu) [25]. This OC-FISH test is intended to detect typical genome changes, such as chromoanagenesis, as a biomarker proof. The basic functionality of this test is documented by hybridization on an inconspicuous metaphase shown in Figure 2. Here, it is also clear that the signals are detected at the intended location, and there are no cross-hybridizations. In principle, deviations from the diploid pattern are also possible in diploid, intact cells due to spatial overlays of signals. This level of misinterpretation must first be determined so that the existence of OC cells can actually be assumed in the quantity. The counting of signal constellations that deviated from the diploid pattern resulted in an average of 15.38%. The standard deviation was 6.99%. We added these three times to the average and thus arrived at a limit of 36%. The existence of true non-diploid cells can be assumed if a signal distribution that deviates from the diploid pattern occurs more frequently than in 36% of the interphases examined. We tested whether this regulation can also be used for cells other than lymphocytes using the mesothelial cell line LP-3 as a negative control and on a primary cell line of ovarian carcinoma as a positive control. Both LP3 and the primary OC cell line could be clearly differentiated using the OC-FISH test (Figure 3). The validation on 71 fixed primary cultures of ovarian cancer also showed very good differentiation by the OC-FISH test, with only four false-negative results, all of which were above the average for LP-3 and lymphocytes, compared to 67 true-positive results. At this point, it is important to realize that the retrospective compilation of the tested OC patients does not correspond to the natural prevalence but was artificially concentrated. An attempt to clarify the actual cell type of the four false-negative OC cell lines using immunohistochemical markers failed because the fixed cell suspensions were all over 10 years old, and the antibody epitopes were apparently too degenerated. The receiver operating characteristic curve (ROC) reflects an area under the ROC curve of 0.8434 and, thus, represents an acceptable quality of the OC-FISH test. The calculated sensitivity of the OC-FISH test is 0.94 (Figure 4).

For future studies of expression data and interactions in tumors, it will be important to determine the proportion of tumor cells and diploid cells in the microenvironment. This information will be particularly important when developing 3D cell culture models. The OC-FISH test can be helpful in an experimental approach for better and more targeted interpretation of the test results of further investigations. The OC-FISH test has the advantage over the FISH tests mentioned above in that it does not indicate specific gene mutations that are associated with tumor development. These can be very different and diverse. Rather, the OC-FISH test indicates very frequently occurring CNVs, which, unlike gene-specific mutations, can be detected relatively frequently.

5. Conclusions

With the OC-FISH test, we now have an instrument at our disposal that allows us to identify tumor cells, especially when it comes to questions involving cell networks involving different cell types. Clarifying the cell type is particularly interesting in research on 3D cell cultures of the OC when interactions between different cell types or drug effects in the microenvironment are to be researched [26]. Influencing immune cells or fibroblasts are likely to differ in their diploid character from the OC cells, whose chromoanagenesis can be detected by the OC-FISH test. In imaging, immunofluorescence detection of expressed proteins is possible in combination with FISH signals [27,28]. The differentiation of tumor cells with cells from the surrounding area can also be validated in formalin-fixed paraffin-embedded (FFPE) thin-layer preparations using the OC-FISH test, thus providing greater analytic certainty [29].

Author Contributions: Conceptualization, J.P.W.; methodology, A.L., X.Q., B.B. and J.P.W.; validation, J.P.W., L.O.-F. and A.L.; formal analysis, J.P.W., X.Q. and A.L.; investigation, J.P.W., A.L. and X.Q.; resources, N.M., D.O.B. and N.A.; writing—original draft preparation, J.P.W.; writing—review and editing, I.F., C.R. and N.H.; visualization, J.P.W.; supervision, J.P.W.; project administration, J.P.W. and N.A.; funding acquisition, N.M. All authors have read and agreed to the published version of the manuscript.

Funding: The biobank of the clinic of gynecology (BMB-Gyn) is a member of the PopGen 2.0 Biobank Network (P2N) Kiel and was funded by the German Federal Ministry of Education and Research (BMBF grand 01EY1103). Xueqian Qian's research stay was supported by the Medical Health Science and Technology Project of the Zhejiang Provincial Health Commission (2023KY89), China, and the National Key R&D Program of China (2022YFC2704200).

Institutional Review Board Statement: The study was conducted in accordance with the Declaration of Helsinki and approved by the ethics committee of the medical faculty of the Christian-Albrechts-University Kiel (B327/10; 11 January 2011).

Informed Consent Statement: Informed consent was obtained from all subjects involved in the study.

Data Availability Statement: The data presented in this study are available on request from the corresponding author.

Acknowledgments: We thank BMB-Gyn in Kiel for providing OC tissues for this study. We acknowledge financial support by DFG within the funding program "Open Access-Publikationskosten".

Conflicts of Interest: The authors declare no conflicts of interest. The funders had no role in the design of the study, in the collection, analyses, or interpretation of data, in the writing of the manuscript, or in the decision to publish the results.

References

1. Moschetta, M.; George, A.; Kaye, S.B.; Banerjee, S. BRCA somatic mutations and epigenetic BRCA modifications in serous ovarian cancer. *Ann. Oncol. Off. J. Eur. Soc. Med. Oncol.* **2016**, *27*, 1449–1455. [CrossRef] [PubMed]
2. Stewart, C.; Ralyea, C.; Lockwood, S. Ovarian Cancer: An Integrated Review. *Semin. Oncol. Nurs.* **2019**, *35*, 151–156. [CrossRef] [PubMed]
3. Lengyel, E. Ovarian cancer development and metastasis. *Am. J. Pathol.* **2010**, *177*, 1053–1064. [CrossRef] [PubMed]
4. Yousefi, M.; Dehghani, S.; Nosrati, R.; Ghanei, M.; Salmaninejad, A.; Rajaie, S.; Hasanzadeh, M.; Pasdar, A. Current insights into the metastasis of epithelial ovarian cancer—Hopes and hurdles. *Cell Oncol.* **2020**, *43*, 515–538. [CrossRef] [PubMed]
5. Shih Ie, M.; Kurman, R.J. Ovarian tumorigenesis: A proposed model based on morphological and molecular genetic analysis. *Am. J. Pathol.* **2004**, *164*, 1511–1518. [CrossRef] [PubMed]
6. Kurman, R.J.; Shih Ie, M. The origin and pathogenesis of epithelial ovarian cancer: A proposed unifying theory. *Am. J. Surg. Pathol.* **2010**, *34*, 433–443. [CrossRef] [PubMed]
7. Krugmann, J.; Schwarz, C.L.; Melcher, B.; Sterlacci, W.; Ozalinskaite, A.; Lermann, J.; Agaimy, A.; Vieth, M. Malignant ascites occurs most often in patients with high-grade serous papillary ovarian cancer at initial diagnosis: A retrospective analysis of 191 women treated at Bayreuth Hospital, 2006–2015. *Arch. Gynecol. Obstet.* **2019**, *299*, 515–523. [CrossRef] [PubMed]
8. Zhao, H.; Li, X.; Chen, D.; Cai, J.; Fu, Y.; Kang, H.; Gao, J.; Gao, K.; Du, N. Intraperitoneal administration of cisplatin plus bevacizumab for the management of malignant ascites in ovarian epithelial cancer: Results of a phase III clinical trial. *Med. Oncol.* **2015**, *32*, 292. [CrossRef] [PubMed]
9. Launonen, I.M.; Vähärautio, A.; Färkkilä, A. The Emerging Role of the Single-Cell and Spatial Tumor Microenvironment in High-Grade Serous Ovarian Cancer. *Cold Spring Harb. Perspect. Med.* **2023**, *13*, a041314. [CrossRef]
10. Cortes-Ciriano, I.; Lee, J.J.; Xi, R.; Jain, D.; Jung, Y.L.; Yang, L.; Gordenin, D.; Klimczak, L.J.; Zhang, C.Z.; Pellman, D.S.; et al. Comprehensive analysis of chromothripsis in 2,658 human cancers using whole-genome sequencing. *Nat. Genet.* **2020**, *52*, 331–341. [CrossRef]
11. Shorokhova, M.; Nikolsky, N.; Grinchuk, T. Chromothripsis-Explosion in Genetic Science. *Cells* **2021**, *10*, 1102. [CrossRef] [PubMed]
12. Weimer, J.; Huttmann, M.; Nusilati, A.; Andreas, S.; Roseler, J.; Tribian, N.; Rogmans, C.; Stope, M.B.; Dahl, E.; Mustea, A.; et al. Fluorescence in situ hybridization test for detection of endometrial carcinoma cells by non-invasive vaginal swab. *J. Cell. Mol. Med.* **2023**, *27*, 379–391. [CrossRef]
13. Weimer, J.; Kiechle, M.; Senger, G.; Wiedemann, U.; Ovens-Raeder, A.; Schuierer, S.; Kautza, M.; Siebert, R.; Arnold, N. An easy and reliable procedure of microdissection technique for the analysis of chromosomal breakpoints and marker chromosomes. *Chromosome Res. Int. J. Mol. Supramol. Evol. Asp. Chromosome Biol.* **1999**, *7*, 355–362. [CrossRef] [PubMed]
14. Acar-Perk, B.; Brautigam, K.; Grunewald, R.; Schmutzler, A.; Schem, C.; Arnold, N.K.; Jonat, W.; Weimer, J. The t(14,15) in mouse strain *CBA/CaH-T(14;15)6Ca/J* causes a break in the *ADAMTS12* gene. *Comp. Med.* **2010**, *60*, 118–122.
15. Weimer, J.; Kiechle, M.; Wiedemann, U.; Tonnies, H.; Neitzel, H.; Ruhenstroth, E.; Ovens-Raeder, A.; Arnold, N. Delineation of a complex karyotypic rearrangement by microdissection and CGH in a family affected with split foot. *J. Med. Genet.* **2000**, *37*, 442–445. [CrossRef]
16. Kurbacher, C.M.; Korn, C.; Dexel, S.; Schween, U.; Kurbacher, J.A.; Reichelt, R.; Arenz, P.N. Isolation and culture of ovarian cancer cells and cell lines. *Methods Mol. Biol.* **2011**, *731*, 161–180. [CrossRef] [PubMed]
17. Hedemann, N.; Herz, A.; Schiepanski, J.H.; Dittrich, J.; Sebens, S.; Dempfle, A.; Feuerborn, J.; Rogmans, C.; Tribian, N.; Flörkemeier, I.; et al. ADAM17 Inhibition Increases the Impact of Cisplatin Treatment in Ovarian Cancer Spheroids. *Cancers* **2021**, *13*, 2039. [CrossRef]
18. Hu, H.; Shikama, Y.; Shichishima, T.; Ikeda, K.; Akutsu, K.; Ono, T.; Kimura, H.; Ogawa, K.; Noji, H.; Takeishi, Y.; et al. A new method for maturity-dependent fractionation of neutrophil progenitors applicable for the study of myelodysplastic syndromes. *Biomark. Res.* **2014**, *2*, 2. [CrossRef] [PubMed]
19. Yamamoto, S.; Tsuda, H.; Honda, K.; Onozato, K.; Takano, M.; Tamai, S.; Imoto, I.; Inazawa, J.; Yamada, T.; Matsubara, O. Actinin-4 gene amplification in ovarian cancer: A candidate oncogene associated with poor patient prognosis and tumor chemoresistance. *Mod. Pathol. Off. J. United States Can. Acad. Pathol. Inc.* **2009**, *22*, 499–507. [CrossRef]
20. Román-Lladó, R.; Aguado, C.; Jordana-Ariza, N.; Roca-Arias, J.; Rodríguez, S.; Aldeguer, E.; Garzón-Ibañez, M.; García-Peláez, B.; Vives-Usano, M.; Giménez-Capitán, A.; et al. Fluorescence In Situ Hybridization (FISH) for the Characterization and Monitoring of Primary Cultures from Human Tumors. *J. Mol. Pathol.* **2023**, *4*, 57–68. [CrossRef]
21. Chrzanowska, N.M.; Kowalewski, J.; Lewandowska, M.A. Use of Fluorescence In Situ Hybridization (FISH) in Diagnosis and Tailored Therapies in Solid Tumors. *Molecules* **2020**, *25*, 1864. [CrossRef] [PubMed]

22. Kim, S.W.; Kim, J.W.; Kim, Y.T.; Kim, J.H.; Kim, S.; Yoon, B.S.; Nam, E.J.; Kim, H.Y. Analysis of chromosomal changes in serous ovarian carcinoma using high-resolution array comparative genomic hybridization: Potential predictive markers of chemoresistant disease. *Genes Chromosomes Cancer* **2007**, *46*, 1–9. [CrossRef] [PubMed]
23. Lambros, M.B.; Fiegler, H.; Jones, A.; Gorman, P.; Roylance, R.R.; Carter, N.P.; Tomlinson, I.P. Analysis of ovarian cancer cell lines using array-based comparative genomic hybridization. *J. Pathol.* **2005**, *205*, 29–40. [CrossRef] [PubMed]
24. Tan, D.S.; Iravani, M.; McCluggage, W.G.; Lambros, M.B.; Milanezi, F.; Mackay, A.; Gourley, C.; Geyer, F.C.; Vatcheva, R.; Millar, J.; et al. Genomic analysis reveals the molecular heterogeneity of ovarian clear cell carcinomas. *Clin. Cancer Res. Off. J. Am. Assoc. Cancer Res.* **2011**, *17*, 1521–1534. [CrossRef] [PubMed]
25. Patil Okaly, G.V.; Panwar, D.; Lingappa, K.B.; Kumari, P.; Anand, A.; Kumar, P.; Chikkalingaiah, M.H.; Kumar, R.V. FISH and HER2/neu equivocal immunohistochemistry in breast carcinoma. *Indian J. Cancer* **2019**, *56*, 119–123. [CrossRef] [PubMed]
26. Akerlund, E.; Gudoityte, G.; Moussaud-Lamodiere, E.; Lind, O.; Bwanika, H.C.; Lehti, K.; Salehi, S.; Carlson, J.; Wallin, E.; Fernebro, J.; et al. The drug efficacy testing in 3D cultures platform identifies effective drugs for ovarian cancer patients. *NPJ Precis. Oncol.* **2023**, *7*, 111. [CrossRef] [PubMed]
27. Weber-Matthiesen, K.; Deerberg, J.; Poetsch, M.; Grote, W.; Schlegelberger, B. Clarification of dubious karyotypes in Hodgkin's disease by simultaneous fluorescence immunophenotyping and interphase cytogenetics (FICTION). *Cytogenet. Cell Genet.* **1995**, *70*, 243–245. [CrossRef] [PubMed]
28. Martin-Subero, J.I.; Chudoba, I.; Harder, L.; Gesk, S.; Grote, W.; Novo, F.J.; Calasanz, M.J.; Siebert, R. Multicolor-FICTION: Expanding the possibilities of combined morphologic, immunophenotypic, and genetic single cell analyses. *Am. J. Pathol.* **2002**, *161*, 413–420. [CrossRef]
29. Summersgill, B.; Clark, J.; Shipley, J. Fluorescence and chromogenic in situ hybridization to detect genetic aberrations in formalin-fixed paraffin embedded material, including tissue microarrays. *Nat. Protoc.* **2008**, *3*, 220–234. [CrossRef]

biomedicines

MDPI

Review

Unlocking the Role of OCT4 in Cancer Lineage Plasticity: A Cross-Cancer Perspective with an Emphasis on Prostate Cancer

Mohammad Esfini Farahani [1], Yanquan Zhang [1,2], Amos Olalekan Akinyemi [1], Fatemeh Seilani [1], Md Rakibul Alam [1] and Xiaoqi Liu [1,2,*]

[1] Department of Toxicology and Cancer Biology, Collage of Medicine, University of Kentucky, Lexington, KY 40536, USA; mesfarahani@uky.edu (M.E.F.); yanquan.zhang@uky.edu (Y.Z.); amos.olalekan7@uky.edu (A.O.A.); fatemeh.seilani@uky.edu (F.S.); rakibul.alam@uky.edu (M.R.A.)

[2] Markey Cancer Center, University of Kentucky, Lexington, KY 40536, USA

* Correspondence: xiaoqi.liu@uky.edu

Abstract: Prostate cancer (PCa) is a highly heterogeneous disease, with castration-resistant prostate cancer (CRPC) and neuroendocrine prostate cancer (NEPC) representing its most aggressive and therapy-resistant forms. Emerging evidence indicates that lineage plasticity—driven by key transcription factors such as Octamer Binding Factor 4 (OCT4)—plays a crucial role in therapeutic resistance and disease progression. OCT4, in coordination with SOX2 and NANOG, acts as a master regulator of stemness and is frequently upregulated in prostate cancer stem cells (PCSCs). This upregulation contributes to tumor initiation, metastasis, and resistance to both androgen deprivation therapy (ADT) and chemotherapy. In this review, we explore the role of OCT4 in mediating lineage plasticity in prostate cancer, with particular emphasis on its involvement in treatment resistance and neuroendocrine differentiation. We also examine therapeutic strategies aimed at targeting OCT4 directly, such as microRNA-mediated suppression, small-molecule inhibitors, and suicide gene therapy, as well as indirect approaches that modulate OCT4 expression via FGFR and NF-κB signaling pathways. While these strategies offer promising avenues, challenges such as adaptive resistance and the intricate signaling networks within PCSCs remain significant hurdles. A deeper understanding of the molecular mechanisms underlying OCT4-driven plasticity may pave the way for novel therapeutic approaches and improved outcomes in advanced prostate cancer.

Keywords: octamer-binding transcription factor 4; prostate cancer stem cells; androgen deprivation therapy; castration-resistant prostate cancer; neuroendocrine prostate cancer

1. Introduction

PCa remains one of the most frequently diagnosed malignancies in men, ranking among the leading causes of cancer-related mortality worldwide [1]. The disease predominantly affects aging populations, with incidence rates rising significantly in men over 50 years old [2]. While early-stage PCa can often be effectively managed through localized interventions, such as surgery and radiation therapy, advanced cases present a major therapeutic challenge. Androgen deprivation therapy (ADT) has long been the cornerstone of treatment for metastatic prostate cancer [3,4]; however, most patients eventually develop castration-resistant prostate cancer (CRPC), an aggressive stage of the disease characterized by continued tumor growth despite androgen suppression [5,6]. A subset of CRPC cases undergoes further progression to neuroendocrine prostate cancer (NEPC), a highly aggressive and therapy-resistant variant with limited treatment options [7,8]. The molecular mechanisms driving this transition are complex and remain an area of intense research.

A key emerging concept in PCa progression is lineage plasticity, which refers to the ability of cancer cells to alter their differentiation state and adopt new cellular identities in response to therapeutic pressures [9]. This phenomenon has been recognized as a major driver of resistance to the androgen receptor (AR)-targeted therapies, such as enzalutamide and abiraterone, which are designed to block AR signaling and inhibit tumor growth [10,11]. However, some PCa cells evade these therapies by undergoing a lineage switch, losing their dependence on AR and transitioning into alternative states, including neuroendocrine-like or stem-like phenotypes. This process allows tumor cells to survive and proliferate even in the absence of androgen signaling, making them highly resistant to standard treatments [12,13].

Several molecular regulators contribute to lineage plasticity in PCa, including transcription factors, epigenetic modifiers, and oncogenic drivers. Pluripotency-associated factors such as OCT4 (POU5F1), SOX2, and NANOG are frequently implicated in dedifferentiation and cancer stem cell (CSC) maintenance, allowing tumor cells to regain developmental plasticity [14,15]. Concurrently, the emergence of neuroendocrine features is marked by the upregulation of synaptophysin (SYP), neuron-specific enolase (NSE/ENO2), and chromogranin A (CHGA), which are commonly used as biomarkers for NEPC. Additionally, epigenetic regulators such as enhancer of zeste homolog 2 (EZH2) and lysine-specific demethylase 1 (LSD1) have been shown to facilitate lineage reprogramming by altering chromatin states and repressing luminal differentiation programs. Oncogenic drivers, including Aurora kinase A (AURKA) and MYCN, further promote the transition from prostate adenocarcinoma to NEPC by stabilizing neuroendocrine transcriptional regulators and disrupting epithelial lineage commitment [16].

OCT4, a transcription factor best known for its essential role in maintaining pluripotency in embryonic stem cells, is among the key regulators of lineage plasticity. OCT4 functions as a master regulator of self-renewal and prevents differentiation, ensuring that stem cells retain their ability to give rise to multiple lineages [17,18]. While its developmental function is well established, accumulating evidence suggests that OCT4 is aberrantly re-expressed in various cancers, including PCa, where it contributes to tumor initiation, cancer stemness, therapy resistance, and disease progression. By sustaining CSC populations, OCT4 enables tumor cells to resist therapy, remain dormant, and later re-emerge as highly aggressive, treatment-resistant clones [19,20].

In prostate cancer, OCT4′s influence extends beyond cancer stem cell maintenance: its overexpression has been associated with increased tumor aggressiveness, enhanced metastatic potential, and resistance to both ADT and chemotherapy [21,22]. One mechanism by which OCT4 contributes to disease progression is through its regulation of epithelial–mesenchymal transition (EMT), a biological process that grants epithelial cells mesenchymal-like properties, including increased motility and invasiveness. EMT is a key driver of metastasis in several cancers, including PCa, and OCT4 has been shown to activate EMT-associated gene expression programs [23,24].

A particularly intriguing aspect of OCT4′s function in PCa is its interaction with the androgen receptor (AR)-signaling pathway, which is the primary driver of PCa growth. In early stages, tumors are highly dependent on AR signaling, rendering them sensitive to AR-targeted therapies. However, as the disease advances, cancer cells often develop mechanisms to bypass AR dependency. Emerging evidence shows that OCT4 plays a role in this transition by driving the loss of AR signaling and promoting androgen-independent growth, thereby contributing to therapy resistance [25]. More recently, studies have highlighted OCT4′s involvement in the development of treatment-induced NEPC, further underscoring its role in lineage plasticity and disease progression [15,26,27].

Given its multifaceted role in prostate cancer biology, OCT4 has emerged as both a potential biomarker and a therapeutic target [28,29]. Elevated OCT4 expression has been associated with poor clinical outcomes, including increased metastatic potential and reduced overall survival [30]. As such, OCT4 could serve as a valuable biomarker for identifying patients at a high risk of aggressive disease and therapy resistance [31,32]. Additionally, targeting OCT4 directly—or disrupting its associated pathways—represents a promising strategy to overcome therapy resistance [33]. Several experimental approaches, including small-molecule inhibitors, RNA-based therapies, and CRISPR-mediated gene editing, are currently under exploration [34–36].

This review aims to provide a comprehensive examination of OCT4′s role in PCa, with a particular focus on its contributions to lineage plasticity, disease progression, and therapy resistance. We will explore the molecular mechanisms by which OCT4 regulates cancer stemness, EMT, and AR independence, as well as its interactions with key oncogenic pathways. Additionally, we will discuss the potential of OCT4 as a biomarker for aggressive PCa and evaluate emerging therapeutic strategies aimed at targeting OCT4. By gaining a deeper understanding of OCT4′s role in PCa, we can uncover new opportunities for improving the diagnosis, prognosis, and treatment of this challenging disease.

2. OCT4 in Stemness and Plasticity

2.1. OCT4′s Function in Embryonic Stem Cells and Normal Tissue Development

OCT4, also known as POU5F1, is a pivotal transcription factor in embryonic stem cells (ESCs), essential for maintaining pluripotency and self-renewal [37,38]. It regulates genes critical for cell fate determination, such as NANOG and SOX2. In normal development, the OCT4 expression is tightly controlled and diminishes as cells differentiate [39]. However, aberrant reactivation of OCT4 in adult tissues has been linked to tumorigenesis and therapy resistance in various cancers, including PCa [15,20,24,31,40–44].

OCT4′s functional versatility is partly attributed to its interaction with multiple epigenetic regulators. A recent study by Ding et al. [45] identified several key binding partners of OCT4 involved in chromatin remodeling and gene regulation, including Supt16h, Zmym2, Ring1B/Rnf2, Msh2/6, Ash2l, Kif11, and Ppp1cc—all of which contribute to stem cell maintenance and somatic cell reprogramming. Additionally, OCT4 cooperates with other transcription factors, particularly SOX2, to recognize and bind to specific DNA elements, forming regulatory complexes that govern gene expression programs in both pluripotent and cancer cells [46].

Beyond transcriptional regulation, OCT4 is also subject to post-translational modifications (PTMs) that fine-tune its stability and activity. Notably, ubiquitination and phosphorylation have been shown to influence OCT4 protein turnover and function, providing another layer of control over its biological effects [47–49].

2.2. OCT4 in Cancer Stem-like Cells and Lineage Plasticity

Cancer stem-like cells (CSCs) represent a subpopulation of tumor cells with enhanced self-renewal capacity, plasticity, and resistance to therapy. These CSCs are believed to contribute to tumor initiation, progression, and metastasis. Therefore, they are considered cancer therapeutic targets [50,51]. OCT4 is a major regulator of CSC biology. It contributes to neovasculogenesis in vivo and sustains CSC populations by maintaining their undifferentiated state and promoting a stem-like transcriptional program [52].

In PCa, elevated OCT4 expression has been consistently linked with advanced and therapy-resistant disease states, including CRPC and NEPC [15], facilitating the transition from androgen-dependent adenocarcinoma to more aggressive, therapy-resistant forms. Consistently, a research group found that NEPC exhibits molecular features reminiscent of stem cells, further reinforcing the link between OCT4-driven stemness and lineage plasticity [53]. This plasticity enables cancer cells to evade androgen receptor (AR)-signaling dependence, contributing to the resistance against treatments like enzalutamide and abiraterone [10,54].

2.3. *OCT4-Associated Signaling Pathways in CSC and Plasticity*

2.3.1. Wnt/β-Catenin

The Wnt/β-catenin signaling pathway plays a critical role in regulating embryonic development, stem cell maintenance, and tissue homeostasis. However, dysregulation of this pathway is frequently implicated in tumorigenesis. In several cancers—including colorectal, breast, liver, and prostate cancer—mutations in key regulatory components, such as APC or β-catenin (CTNNB1), lead to aberrant pathway activation. Constitutive Wnt/β-catenin signaling results in uncontrolled cellular proliferation, enhanced tumor aggressiveness, and increased resistance to therapy. In the context of prostate cancer, aberrant activation of this pathway has been linked to disease progression, therapy resistance, and maintenance of cancer stem-like cells, potentially through interactions with pluripotency factors like OCT4 [55–57].

2.3.2. TGF-β

The TGF-β (transforming growth factor-beta) superfamily comprises a broad group of structurally related growth factors that regulate essential cellular processes, including development, proliferation, apoptosis, metabolism, and differentiation. In the context of cancer, TGF-β signaling exhibits a dual role, acting as a tumor suppressor in the early stages of the disease and as a tumor promoter in advanced cancers. During the initial stages of tumor development, TGF-β restricts the proliferation of epithelial and immune cells, preserves genomic stability, and suppresses mitogenic signaling, thereby functioning as a tumor suppressor. However, as cancer progresses, genetic and epigenetic alterations can subvert this pathway, shifting TGF-β's role from growth inhibition to tumor promotion. In later stages, TGF-β signaling facilitates tumor cell proliferation, invasion, epithelial–mesenchymal transition (EMT), and metastasis, contributing to disease progression and therapeutic resistance [58,59].

2.3.3. PI3K/AKT/mTOR

The PI3K/AKT/mTOR signaling pathway is a central regulator of cell survival, growth, metabolism, and proliferation, playing a crucial role in normal physiology and cancer progression. Under normal conditions, this pathway is activated by growth factors that bind to receptor tyrosine kinases (RTKs), leading to the phosphorylation of PI3K, which, in turn, activates AKT. Once activated, AKT promotes cell survival by inhibiting pro-apoptotic proteins and stimulating cell cycle progression. Further downstream, mTOR acts as a key effector, driving protein synthesis, metabolic reprogramming, and tumor growth. In cancer, aberrant activation of this pathway—often due to genetic mutations or loss of regulatory control—leads to uncontrolled proliferation, resistance to apoptosis, and enhanced metastatic potential. Moreover, PI3K/AKT/mTOR hyperactivation is associated with therapy resistance in various cancers, including parathyroid carcinoma, prostate, breast, colorectal, and lung cancer. Given its pivotal role in tumor progression, this pathway has emerged as a critical therapeutic target. Several inhibitors, such as PI3K inhibitors (Buparlisib, Alpelisib), AKT inhibitors (Capivasertib, Ipatasertib), and mTOR inhibitors (Everolimus, Temsirolimus), have been developed to block different components of the cascade. Additionally, combination therapies targeting PI3K/AKT/mTOR alongside conventional treatments, such as chemotherapy or immune checkpoint inhibitors, are being explored to improve patient outcomes [60–62].

2.3.4. Notch

The Notch signaling pathway is a highly conserved cell communication system that regulates critical cellular processes, including proliferation, differentiation, and apoptosis. Dysregulation of Notch signaling has been implicated in the progression of various cancers, largely due to its role in maintaining (CSCs) a subpopulation responsible for tumor initiation, metastasis, therapy resistance, and disease recurrence.

In prostate cancer and other solid tumors, aberrant Notch activity supports CSC survival and enhances tumor aggressiveness. Its interaction with key pluripotency regulators such as OCT4 may further reinforce stem-like properties and contribute to lineage plasticity, particularly under therapeutic pressure.

Given the central role of CSCs in treatment failure and tumor relapses, targeting Notch signaling has emerged as a promising strategy to eliminate these therapy-resistant populations. However, the context-dependent effects of Notch—acting as either an oncogene or tumor suppressor depending on the tissue type and disease stage—pose significant challenges for therapeutic targeting. Ongoing efforts aim to develop selective modulators of Notch activity that can effectively disrupt its oncogenic functions while minimizing unintended effects on normal tissues [63–65].

2.3.5. JAK1-STAT3

The JAK1-STAT3 signaling pathway is a key regulator of oncogenic processes, including cell proliferation, survival, and immune evasion. The aberrant and sustained activation of this pathway has been widely observed in multiple cancers and is particularly associated with the maintenance of cancer stem cells (CSCs), which drive tumor initiation, metastasis, and therapeutic resistance. STAT3 functions as a transcription factor that, when persistently activated, promotes an inflammatory tumor microenvironment, enhances stemness-related gene expression, and supports immune suppression. This immune evasion enables tumor cells to persist and expand despite host immune responses and therapeutic interventions.

In prostate cancer, chronic activation of the JAK1-STAT3 axis has been linked to lineage plasticity and disease progression. Its interaction with stemness regulators like OCT4 may further enhance the CSC properties, reinforcing therapy resistance and enabling phenotypic switching, such as neuroendocrine differentiation under androgen-deprived conditions [66–68].

2.3.6. ERK-MAPK

The ERK-MAPK signaling pathway is a critical regulator of cell proliferation, survival, differentiation, and apoptosis. Its dysregulation has been widely implicated in cancer progression, contributing to increased tumor aggressiveness, therapy resistance, and metastasis. This pathway is often hyperactivated in cancer due to mutations in upstream regulators such as receptor tyrosine kinases or RAS proteins. Notably, cancer stem cells (CSCs) exploit ERK-MAPK signaling to maintain their self-renewal capacity and resistance to conventional therapies. Given its central role in tumor biology, targeting ERKMAPK signaling has emerged as a promising therapeutic strategy to inhibit cancer progression and sensitize tumors to treatment [69–71].

Understanding the interplay between OCT4 and these signaling pathways provides insights into the mechanisms underlying cancer stemness and plasticity, offering potential therapeutic targets for combating aggressive and treatment-resistant cancers.

The following table (Table 1) and Figure 1 summarize the role of OCT4 in these signaling pathways:

Table 1. Key signaling pathways regulating OCT4 in CSCs.

Signaling Pathways	Key Role in Lineage Plasticity	Interaction with OCT4	Downstream Effector	Cancer Type	Therapeutic Implication	Clinical Evidence Level	References
Wnt/β-catenin	Elevation in CSC-like properties, promotes dedifferentiation, induces transcription, and enhances epithelial–mesenchymal transition, Angiogenesis, and Antiapoptotic effect, drug resistance	• Promote the promoter activity of OCT4 and upregulate its expression. • OCT4 overexpression increased the WNT signaling pathway. • OCT4 knockdown decreased Wnt/β-catenin pathway downstream genes. • OCT4 Activation • Expressed together • Forms complex with OCT4 and enhances its activity • Forms complex with OCT4 and modulates its activity • Activation of CSC marker, including OCT4 • OCT4 Activation • β-catenin stabilizes OCT4 expression in CSCs, and OCT4 is a critical mediator of CSC stemness in this pathway	• CagA (Cytotoxin-associated gene A). • LEF1 (lymphoid enhancer binding factor 1). • Wnt10b • Ang1, bFGF, HGF, VEGF, Bcl2 • Wnt1 • Nanog, Tbx3, Tcfcp2L1, and PDGFα • β-catenin, TAMs (Tumor-Associated Macrophages), IL6, OV6+ CSCs.	• Human Gastric Cancer • Hepatocellular Carcinoma • PBMSCs • ESCs • mESC • Human Ovarian Cancer • Breast Cancer • PCa	• Wnt/β-catenin inhibitor (xav939) • Curcumin, Wnt/β-catenin pathway inhibitor • GSK-3 inhibitor (CHIR99021) • CCL16 inhibition (GSK3β or STAT3-targeted inhibitor) • Targeting both CSCs and TAMs, using IL6R inhibitor (tocilizumab).	• Preclinical (XAV939, CHIR99021, CCL16 inhibition). • Clinical (Tocilizumab). • Preclinical/Clinical (Curcumin)	[72–80]

Table 1. *Cont.*

Signaling Pathways	Key Role in Lineage Plasticity	Interaction with OCT4	Downstream Effector	Cancer Type	Therapeutic Implication	Clinical Evidence Level	References
PI3K/AKT/mTOR	Enhance proliferation, EMT, and plasticity	• AKT phosphorylates OCT4. • Knockdown OCT4 downregulates the expression of p-PI3K, p-AKT, and p-mTOR. • AKT phosphorylates OCT4 and increases its stability and nuclear localization. • Reciprocal regulation with OCT4 (negative and positive feedback). • Induces OCT4 and SOX2 expression through WAVE3 signaling. • Promotes OCT4 and SOX2 expression.	• p-OCT4 • p-PI3K, p-AKT, and p-mTOR • p-OCT4, AKT1, SOX2, NANOG • mTOR CA125, WAVE3 • CD44, MMP-2, MMP-9	• Glioblastoma • Liver cancer • Ovarian Cancer • Embryonal Carcinoma • Ovarian Cancer • Nasopharyngeal Carcinoma (NPC)	• Inhibition of AKT (Akti-1/2) • Metformin (Inhibition of OCT4 Activity). • Inhibition of AKT (via LY294002). • mTOR signaling pathway inhibition (rapamycin)	• Preclinical (Akti-1/2, LY294002). • Clinical (Metformin, Rapamycin)	[23,81–85]
TGF-β	Induces EMT and plasticity	• OCT4 knockdown decreased TGF-β pathway downstream genes. • OCT4 could induce TGFBR2 transcription. • Expressed together	• ELF, Smad3, Smad4 • T-reg-like effector genes • Smad3 and Smad4	• Hepatocellular Carcinoma • GBM	• inhibition of TGFBR2	• Preclinical	[74,76, 86]

Table 1. *Cont.*

Signaling Pathways	Key Role in Lineage Plasticity	Interaction with OCT4	Downstream Effector	Cancer Type	Therapeutic Implication	Clinical Evidence Level	References
Notch1	Drives CSC maintenance, tumor aggressiveness promotes therapy resistance, and integrates EMT with CSC self-renewal	• Interacts with OCT4 and NANOG to expand CSC populations. • NOTCH1 is upregulated in EMT-like cells and contributes to stemness by increasing OCT4, NANOG, and SOX2. • NOTCH1 overexpression correlates with increased OCT4, NANOG, and SOX2, promoting cancer stem-like cell (CSC) features • Notch1 and OCT4 expression levels are positively associated. • miR-221/222 downregulates Reck and activates OCT4 expression through Notch1 signaling. • EGFR inhibition increases CSC-like properties via Notch1 activation, upregulating OCT4 and Bmi-1 • Notch1 activation correlates with increased expression of stemness markers like OCT4 • STC1 secreted by CAFs activates Notch1 signaling in HCC cells, promoting stemness • YAP1-Notch1 positive feedback loop enhances stem cell marker expression such as OCT4	• HES1, HEY1, NANOG. • Lin28B, miR-200, let-7, Polycomb Repressor Complex 2 (EZH2, SUZ12, EED), ZEB1, Vimentin • Snail, Slug, ZEB1/2, Vimentin (↑), E-cadherin (↓) • CD133 • NICD • HES1, Bmi-1 • Hes1, Hey1, Jagged1 • Hes1, Hey1, Cyclin D1, c-Myc • BMP4-SMAD1/5	• Prostate Cancer • Gastric Carcinoma • NSCLC • Salivary Adenoid Cystic Carcinoma • Hepatocellular Carcinoma • Breast Cancer	• MUC1-C or Notch1 inhibition. • Natural agents to downregulate miR-200. • GSI inhibitor (Notch inhibition) • Combined targeted therapy • Targeting miR-221/222 • γ-secretase inhibitor GSI to downregulate Notch1 Signaling • Notch1 inhibition using LY3039478 (a novel r-secretase inhibitor) • Suggesting inhibition of STC1 and/or Notch1 • Suggesting Targeting Notch1 signaling in combination with YAP1 and BMP4 pathways	• Preclinical (MUC1-C, miRNAs, STC1, YAP1/BMP4). • Clinical trials (GSI, LY3039478 in non-PCa tumors).	[87–95]

Table 1. *Cont.*

Signaling Pathways	Key Role in Lineage Plasticity	Interaction with OCT4	Downstream Effector	Cancer Type	Therapeutic Implication	Clinical Evidence Level	References
JAK1-STAT3	Promotes CSC plasticity and enhances tumor progression, viability, migration, and invasion. Contributes to chemoresistance and poor prognosis.	• OCT4 overexpression in HCC is correlated with increased survivin expression and STAT3 phosphorylation, indicating activation of the JAK/STAT pathway. • IL-6 activates JAK1/STAT3 signaling, leading to OCT4 upregulation and conversion of non-CSCs to CSCs. • Dox-induced Stat3 activation upregulates OCT4 and c-Myc, promoting CSC enrichment and drug resistance • LPS and TNF-α increase OCT4 expression, activating invasion pathways through Stat3 signaling. • MAPKi treatment activates STAT3, leading to the upregulation of OCT4 and SOX2, suppressing apoptosis and enhancing resistance to therapy. • STAT3 directly upregulates OCT4 expression, maintaining CSC properties	• Survivin • IL6, VEGF, MMP9 • c-Myc, CD44, and ABCG2 • JNK1, p65, and STAT3 • HIF-1α, Nanog, Sox2, CD44	• hHepatocellular Carcinoma • Breast Cancer • TNBC (Triple Negative Breast Cancer • OSCC (oral squamous cell carcinoma • Melanoma • Esophageal Adenocarcinoma Cells	• OCT4 Silencing • Stat3 inhibition via such as niclosamide and LLL12 or using anti-IL-6 antibody. • Stat3 inhibitor WP1066 • Alantolactone, a STAT3 inhibitor, combined with MAPKi.	• Preclinical (OCT4 silencing, LLL12, alantolactone). • Clinical trials (niclosamide, WP1066, anti-IL-6 antibody).	[96–101]

Table 1. *Cont.*

Signaling Pathways	Key Role in Lineage Plasticity	Interaction with OCT4	Downstream Effector	Cancer Type	Therapeutic Implication	Clinical Evidence Level	References
ERK/MAPK	Regulates tumor progression, differentiation, apoptosis, and EMT. Promotes CSC-like properties	• Co-activated with OCT4, SOX2, Myc, and Notch • Bach1 interacts with OCT4, Sox2, and Nanog to maintain CSC identity. • OCT4, NANOG, and SOX2 are upregulated in paclitaxel-resistant LUAD cells (A549/TAX) alongside MUC1, contributing to CSC maintenance and therapy resistance. • MK2 phosphorylates OCT4, enhancing its transcriptional activation of c-MYC and promoting tumor progression and therapy resistance. • FL3 activates p38 MAPK, leading to caspase-3-mediated apoptosis and suppression of OCT4 expression in cancer stem-like cells.	• E2F, Myc, SOX-2, TGF-β, OCT4 • CD44 • EGFR, IL-6, CD133 • c-MYC, MYCN, pMK2 • Caspase-3	• Gastric Cancer • Lung Cancer • LUAD (Lung Adenocarcinoma) • Neuroblastoma • Teratocarcinoma	• ERK/MAPK Kinase inhibitor PD98059 • MAPK inhibitor (LY2228820). • Suggest targeting MUC1 and MAPK pathways in combination with paclitaxel. • MK2 inhibition (PF3644022, MK2iIII). • MAPK inhibition by SB203580.	• Preclinical (PD98059, SB203580, MK2 inhibitors, MUC1 combo). • Clinical trials (LY2228820/ralimetinib)	[102–106]

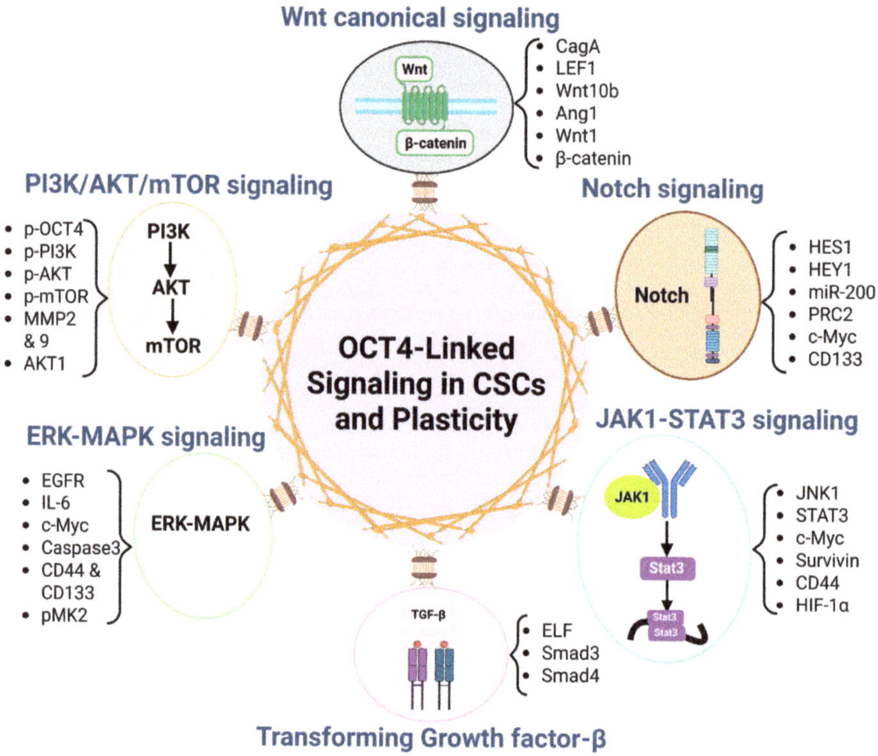

Figure 1. OCT4-associated signaling pathways driving cancer stemness and plasticity. This diagram illustrates the central role of OCT4 in regulating cancer stem cell (CSC) properties and phenotypic plasticity through its interaction with six key signaling pathways (Wnt/β-catenin, TGF-β, PI3K/AKT/mTOR, Notch, JAK1-STAT3, and ERK-MAPK) and their correlated down-stream effectors. These pathways contribute to the maintenance of stemness, promotion of epithelial–mesenchymal transition (EMT), therapy resistance, and tumor progression.

3. OCT4 in Prostate Cancer Progression and Lineage Plasticity

As discussed, OCT4 has been extensively studied for its role in maintaining pluripotency in embryonic stem cells. However, its aberrant expression in cancerous tissues—particularly in solid tumors—has been linked to tumorigenesis and aggressive disease progression, making it a potential target for eliminating cancer stem cells (CSCs) in various malignancies, including prostate cancer (PCa) [107]. In PCa, OCT4 is upregulated in tumor cells compared to normal prostate epithelium, suggesting its involvement in prostate cancer development.

3.1. OCT4 as a Driver of Prostate Cancer Initiation

The role of OCT4 in PCa initiation is closely tied to its ability to maintain cancer stem-like properties. As a key pluripotency factor, OCT4 works with SOX2 and NANOG to sustain an undifferentiated, stem-like state, preventing normal differentiation processes and driving tumor progression (Figure 2). The persistence of cancer stem-like cells (CSCs) in PCa is a significant contributor to tumor heterogeneity, therapeutic resistance, and disease recurrence.

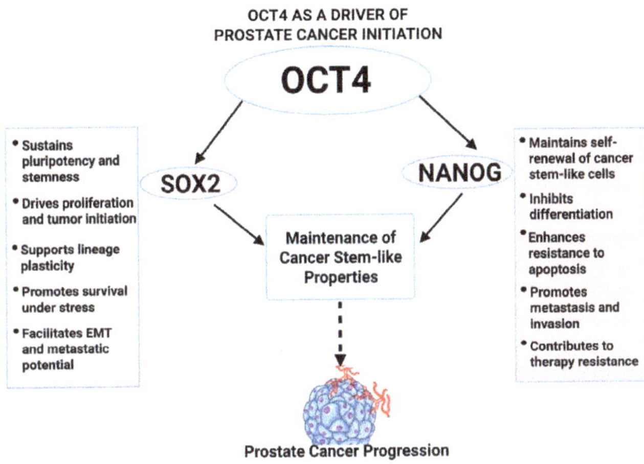

Figure 2. OCT4-mediated network in prostate cancer initiation. This diagram shows how OCT4 collaborates with SOX2 and NANOG to maintain cancer stem-like properties, block differentiation, and drives prostate cancer initiation and early progression.

Multiple studies, like the one by Roy et al. [108], have established a strong association between OCT4 expression and aggressive PCa phenotypes. Its presence has been detected in prostate hyperplasia and malignant tissues, indicating its potential role as a cancer stem cell marker in PCa [109]. High OCT4 expression has been linked to increased tumorigenicity in prostatic tissues, supporting its role in disease initiation and progression [41].

Moreover, OCT4 is upregulated via Nodal, a member of the TGF-β signaling family, further reinforcing its function in sustaining a stem-like state in PCa cells. Activating this pathway promotes a self-renewing and undifferentiated phenotype, contributing to the aggressiveness of the disease [110].

3.2. Association of OCT4 with Prostate Cancer Progression and Metastasis

The impact of OCT4 on the PCa progression extends beyond its role in tumor initiation. Elevated OCT4 expression is strongly associated with several clinical and pathological features that define aggressive PCa, including the following:

- Increased Tumor Grade and High Gleason Score

OCT4 isoforms demonstrate divergent associations with the prostate cancer prognosis. The OCT4A expression correlates with higher Gleason scores, increased proliferation, and reduced differentiation—features of a more aggressive tumor state. In contrast, OCT4B expression is linked to lower Gleason scores and improved biochemical recurrence-free survival, suggesting a potential role as a favorable prognostic biomarker [111].

- Enhanced Metastatic Potential

One of the most critical aspects of PCa progression is metastasis. OCT4 has been directly linked to increased motility, invasiveness, and metastatic spread. Studies have demonstrated the following:

OCT4+ CSCs are associated with visceral metastases, suggesting that cells expressing OCT4 have a greater ability to invade distant organs [22]. Nong et al. [112] reported that the OCT4 expression and OCT4-related polymorphisms were associated with a larger tumor size, lymph node involvement, and distant metastases, supporting a potential role for OCT4 in cancer dissemination and progression. OCT4 has been identified as a key driver of metastasis in a Galectin-dependent manner, indicating a novel regulatory mechanism through which it promotes PCa cell migration and invasion [113].

- Poor Patient Prognosis

Clinical studies have shown that patients with higher OCT4 expression levels tend to have poorer survival outcomes. Increased OCT4 expression correlates with the following:

- Higher recurrence rates following treatment and shortened overall survival in patients with advanced PCa [114].
- Resistance to conventional therapies, including androgen ADT, chemotherapy, and targeted therapies [115,116].

3.3. OCT4 and Therapy-Induced Lineage Plasticity in Prostate Cancer

A growing body of evidence suggests that androgen receptor (AR)-targeted therapies not only fail to fully eliminate prostate cancer (PCa) cells but may also promote lineage plasticity, contributing to the development of castration-resistant prostate cancer (CRPC)—a form of the disease that continues to progress despite androgen deprivation therapy [117]. This therapy-induced plasticity plays a pivotal role in treatment resistance and disease progression. Over time, some CRPC tumors may undergo further transdifferentiation, resulting in the emergence of neuroendocrine prostate cancer (NEPC), a highly aggressive and AR-independent subtype characterized by neuroendocrine features and poor prognosis [118–120].

OCT4, a key regulator of stemness and cellular plasticity, has been implicated in driving therapy-induced lineage transition in prostate cancer. Nuclear Oct4A expression has been observed in neuroendocrine prostate cancer cells [121], and pluripotency factors including OCT4 are upregulated during AR-negative/CRPC lineage reprogramming [15].

3.3.1. The Role of AR-Targeted Therapy in Driving Stemness and Plasticity

ADT- and AR-signaling inhibitors (ARSIs) like enzalutamide and abiraterone are standard treatments for advanced PCa [122,123]. While these therapies are initially effective in suppressing tumor growth, PCa cells often develop resistance by activating alternative survival pathways. One of the most well-documented responses to AR-targeted therapy is the upregulation of pluripotency-associated transcription factors, including OCT4, SOX2, and NANOG, which promote a stem-like transcriptional program [26,124,125].

PCSCs (Prostate Cancer Stem Cells) are largely AR-negative, allowing them to evade androgen deprivation therapy and sustain tumor growth through alternative survival pathways [126]. OCT4 enhances cellular plasticity by blocking differentiation pathways and maintaining a dedifferentiated, therapy-resistant state [127]. Also, AR-targeted therapies, particularly enzalutamide, have been shown to drive PCa stemness and lineage plasticity by enriching a therapy-resistant, stem-like-cell population [128,129]. Gene network and pathway analyses have identified OCT4, SOX2, and NANOG as key regulators of this process, promoting self-renewal and drug resistance through pluripotency-associated signaling pathways. Elevated OCT4 expression in enzalutamide-resistant cells reinforces its role in sustaining cancer stemness and driving therapy-induced lineage plasticity [130]. Additionally, CSC-enriched populations exhibit heightened resistance to therapy, further strengthening the role of OCT4 in sustaining cancer stemness [131]. The identification of OCT4-driven plasticity in enzalutamide-resistant cells highlights its role as a key mediator of therapy-induced lineage plasticity, making it a promising target for overcoming treatment resistance in PCa [36]. The interplay between cellular plasticity and stemness factors like OCT4, SOX2, and NANOG enables PCa cells to adapt under therapeutic pressure, contributing to tumor heterogeneity, EMT activation, and drug resistance [132]. In the context of NEPC, a research group suggests that OCT4A-expressing cells are increasingly detected in high-grade PCa and are associated with neuroendocrine differentiation, as they co-express chromogranin A and synaptophysin [121]. Formaggio N et al. [25] mentioned that OCT4 contributes to the dedifferentiation of PCa into an AR-negative state, promoting neuroendocrine differentiation and reducing sensitivity to AR-targeted therapies. Its expression is elevated in cells with RB1 and TP53 loss, though it alone may not be sufficient to drive enzalutamide resistance [133]. Recently, Kainulainen et al. [134] found that the inflammatory tumor microenvironment (TME), particularly tumor-associated macrophages (TAMs), significantly influences PCa plasticity. Pro-inflammatory M1 macrophages secrete factors that promote stemness by upregulating OCT4, SOX2, NANOG, KLF4, and CD44, while simultaneously suppressing AR signaling in PCa cells [134]. Additionally, OCT4 has been implicated in mediating resistance to chemotherapeutic agents like docetaxel and mitoxantrone, with drug-resistant PCa cells exhibiting increased OCT4 expression and tumor-initiating capacity. This resistance may arise through epigenetic reprogramming, including demethylation of the POU5F1/OCT4 locus, or the selection of pre-existing OCT4-positive subpopulations [135].

3.3.2. Chromatin Modifications in Driving Stemness and Plasticity in Prostate Cancer Contributing to Drug Resistance

PCa is highly sensitive to epigenetic regulation, which contributes significantly to tumor progression, therapy resistance, and lineage plasticity. A study by Chen et al. [136] revealed that oncogenes in PCa can acquire super-enhancers (SEs), leading to transcriptional addiction and enhanced tumorigenicity. These SEs regulate key pluripotency genes, such as OCT4, SOX2, and NANOG, thereby maintaining a stem-like cancer cell state.

OCT4, in particular, exerts epigenetic control through multiple mechanisms. AlAbdi et al. [137] demonstrated that OCT4 inhibits Lsd1 activity, preventing H3K4me1 demethylation and DNA methylation at developmental enhancers, creating a "primed" enhancer landscape. This state preserves chromatin accessibility for oncogenic transcription factors, thereby fueling tumorigenesis, metastasis, and resistance to therapy. Furthermore, OCT4 interacts with chromatin modifiers and transcriptional networks to block differentiation and sustain a dedifferentiated, stem-like phenotype, with its enhancer-promoter interactions and chromatin remodeling activities directly contributing to drug resistance [138]. Epigenetic modifications, particularly histone methylation and acetylation, also regulate the expression of pluripotency factors. For instance, active histone marks drive SOX2 and OCT4 transcription in PCa. Treatments with epigenetic drugs such as AZA, TSA, and DZNeP can reverse these chromatin changes, reduce OCT4 expression, and impair cancer cell viability [139].

In research published in Nature Cell Biology, the authors demonstrated that EZH2 plays a central role in driving lineage plasticity in prostate cancer, promoting neuroendocrine trans differentiation following androgen receptor (AR) inhibition. Within this framework, OCT4 was identified as a downstream effector contributing to cellular reprogramming. OCT4$^+$ cells, tracked using a dual-reporter system, acquired neuronal-like traits and co-expressed ASCL1. Transcriptomic analysis revealed that these cells were enriched for genes involved in plasticity and epigenetic regulation, with enhanced EZH2 activity observed in the OCT4$^+$ population [140]. Additionally, OCT4 plays a key role in transcription factor (TF) network formation in CRPC and NEPC by interacting with FOXA1/AR in AR-positive PCa and NRF1 in AR-negative cases. OCT4 occupies super-enhancer (SE) regions, where it helps organize transcription factor hubs and facilitates phase-separated transcriptional condensates—a process that amplifies oncogenic transcriptional output [15].

Beyond AR-targeted therapy resistance, chromatin remodeling plays a crucial role in PCa lineage plasticity, acting as an epigenetic "memory" that allows cells to transition between different states. A recent study by Logotheti et al. [141] identified distinct subtypes of CRPC with unique chromatin and transcriptional landscapes, including an OCT4-associated stem-like (CRPC-SCL) subtype defined by high CD44 expression. This suggests that OCT4-driven plasticity extends beyond AR-signaling suppression, contributing to broader dedifferentiation processes. In two studies by the same research group, MUC1-C was shown to promote lineage plasticity in NEPC by activating E2F1, which induces the PBAF chromatin remodeling complex, and by driving the MYC→BRN2→SOX2 pathway. These mechanisms collectively lead to the induction of pluripotency-associated transcription factors—including OCT4, SOX2, KLF4, and MYC—thereby reinforcing stemness and plasticity in prostate cancer [87,142]. Shokraii et al. [143] explained that in PCa stem-like cells (OCT4, SOX2, NANOG positive), epigenetic modifications, particularly histone alterations like increased H3K27me3 and decreased H3K4me3, drive CDH1 repression, enhancing metastasis. Saha et al. [144] claim that OCT4 plays a key role in PCa epigenetic regulation by influencing the stemness, lineage plasticity, and tumor progression. They mentioned that its variant, OCT4A, is crucial for self-renewal, while OCT4 pseudogenes (POU5F1P1, POU5F1P3, POU5F1P4) contribute to cancer development.

Epigenetic mechanisms, including histone modifications and DNA methylation, regulate OCT4 expression, affecting therapy resistance and clinical outcomes [137]. Moreover, epigenetic editing using dCas9 fusion proteins has demonstrated the ability to regulate gene expression in PCa. Notably, dCas9-CBP has been shown to upregulate OCT4 expression, highlighting its role in epigenetic reprogramming [145]. Transposable elements (TEs) also serve as epigenetically regulated hubs for transcription factors binding during fate transitions. In PCa, TEs are co-opted to support oncogenesis, shifting from pluripotency transcription factors like OCT4 to lineage-specific factors such as AR. Despite similarities with pluripotent stem cells, PCa cells hijack TE regulation to favor tumor progression. Epigenetic modifications at TEs, including chromatin state alterations, play a crucial role in this process [146].

3.4. *OCT4 as a Therapeutic Target in Prostate Cancer*

Androgen deprivation therapy promotes the expansion of cancer stem cells (CSCs) by altering the tumor microenvironment and upregulating key stem cell markers, including OCT4, SOX2, NANOG, CD133, and CD44, driving tumor initiation, progression, and recurrence in PCa [147,148]. While various therapeutic approaches targeting CSCs—such as small-molecule inhibitors, monoclonal antibodies, and combination therapies—have shown promise, long-term resistance remains a major challenge, emphasizing the need for improved treatment strategies. Inhibitors of signaling pathways such as Hedgehog, Wnt, Notch, and PI3K/AKT have shown potential, and targeting the CSC microenvironment—via VEGF or CXCR4 signaling—may further disrupt CSC maintenance [149]. Immunotherapy strategies, including CAR-T cells and dendritic cell vaccines targeting CSC markers like CD44, EpCAM, and CD133, represent emerging approaches to overcoming resistance and improving treatment outcomes [150]. However, no single approach has been fully effective, underscoring the importance of combination therapies that target both CSCs and bulk tumor cells to enhance therapeutic efficacy in PCa.

Given its critical role in tumor progression, therapy resistance, and metastatic potential, OCT4 has emerged as a compelling therapeutic target in PCa [15,151]. Strategies to inhibit

OCT4 expression or disrupt its downstream signaling pathways could provide novel treatment avenues, particularly in CRPC and NEPC, where current treatment options remain limited [119,152,153]. Recent studies have highlighted the role of the tumor microenvironment in regulating OCT4 expression. For instance, Kainulainen et al. [134] demonstrated that pro-inflammatory M1 macrophages enhance PCa cell plasticity by secreting factors that upregulate OCT4, NANOG, SOX2, KLF4, and CD44 via NFκB activation while suppressing AR signaling. Inhibition of NFκB signaling using the IKK16 inhibitor reversed this effect, reducing CSC marker expression and plasticity. MicroRNAs (miRNAs) have also been identified as key regulators of PCSCs. miR-100, miR-143, and miR-145 suppress PCa stemness by targeting essential transcription factors, including OCT4, KLF4, and c-Myc. Specifically, miR-100 downregulates AGO2, which influences stemness, while miR-143 and miR-145 directly inhibit OCT4 and other factors, thereby reducing tumorigenesis, migration, and invasion in PCa cells [154].

Natural compounds have shown promise in targeting PCSCs. Capsaicin treatment was found to reduce the expression of key PCSC markers, including CD44, CD133, ALDH1A1, SOX2, OCT4, and NANOG, in PC-3 and DU145 cells. This suppression of CSC traits was associated with the inhibition of the Wnt/β-catenin signaling pathway, ultimately leading to reduced cell growth [155]. Hormonal therapy has also been linked to CSC regulation. Guo et al. [29] found that enzalutamide modulates CSC marker expression by regulating SALL4, which influences OCT4 and SOX2 expression, thereby contributing to PCa progression. Targeting the AR/SALL4/OCT4-SOX2 pathway using sh-SALL4 may help mitigate enzalutamide-induced CSC expansion and invasion [29]. Similarly, TR4 has promoted chemoresistance to docetaxel in PCa by suppressing miR-145 expression, leading to increased OCT4 levels and enhanced resistance. Restoring miR-145 expression has been suggested as a potential strategy to counteract TR4-mediated chemoresistance [156,157]. Moreover, Fibroblast growth factor receptor 1 (FGFR1) has been identified as a crucial regulator of PCSCs. A study by Juyeon Ko et al. [28] demonstrated that OCT4-enriched 3D spheroids rely on FGFR signaling for survival. Inhibition of FGFR with BGJ398 or Dovitinib significantly reduced CSC proliferation, suggesting that targeting FGFR signaling could be a promising strategy for treating AR-independent CRPC.

Efforts to directly target OCT4-driven CSCs have led to innovative therapeutic strategies. Vaddi et al. [36] developed a SORE6-driven thymidine kinase (TK) suicide gene system designed to selectively eliminate SOX2/OCT4-overexpressing PCSCs. This system effectively blocked tumor progression and increased chemotherapy sensitivity, highlighting its potential as a therapeutic approach. Additionally, a study identified OCT4 as a key transcription factor in CRPC and NEPC, collaborating with FOXA1, AR, and NRF1 to drive the tumor progression. The antiviral agent Ribavirin was shown to disrupt these transcription factor interactions, sensitizing PCa cells to chemotherapy and slowing disease progression [15].

Together, these findings highlight the pivotal role of OCT4 in maintaining CSCs, promoting therapy resistance, and facilitating disease progression in PCa. Targeting OCT4 and its associated pathways, either directly or through combinatorial strategies, holds great potential for improving treatment outcomes in advanced PCa (Figure 3).

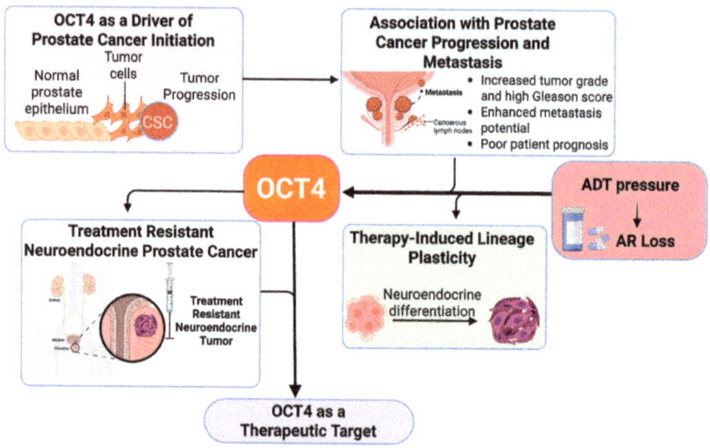

Figure 3. Role of OCT4 in prostate cancer progression and lineage plasticity. This figure shows how OCT4 helps prostate cancer cells change their identity, allowing the tumor to grow and become resistant to treatment. OCT4 promotes cell plasticity, which means cancer cells can switch to different types that survive even when hormone therapy is used.

4. Glimpse into the Future

Significant progress has been made in understanding OCT4's role in PCa, but many questions remain unanswered, presenting new avenues for future research. Given its critical involvement in lineage plasticity, therapy resistance, and the transition to NEPC, further investigation into OCT4's molecular regulation and therapeutic targeting is essential. Below, we outline several promising directions for future research on OCT4 in PCa (Figure 4).

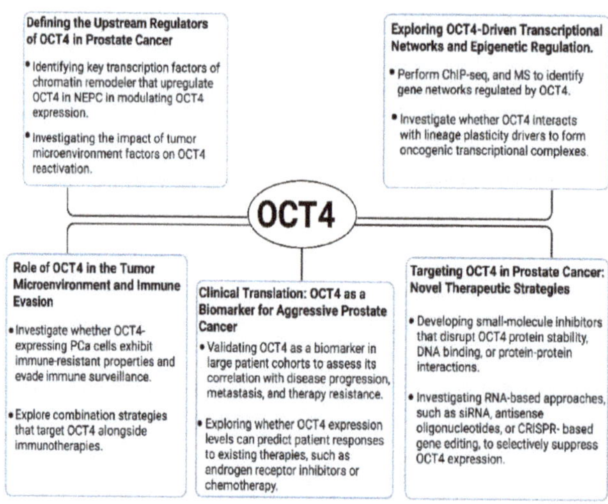

Figure 4. Future research directions for understanding and targeting OCT4 in prostate cancer. These schematics highlight five major areas of ongoing investigation: upstream regulators of OCT4 expression, its transcriptional and epigenetic networks, roles in immune evasion and the tumor microenvironment, potential as a clinical biomarker, and therapeutic strategies aimed at targeting OCT4 or its regulatory pathways.

1. *Defining the Upstream Regulators of OCT4 in Prostate Cancer*

Although OCT4 is well-established as a master regulator of pluripotency, its reactivation in PCa is still not fully understood. Investigating the signaling pathways and transcriptional regulators that drive OCT4 expression in PCa, particularly in response to ADT or other treatment pressures, could uncover novel mechanisms of therapy resistance. Potential areas of study include [158] the following:

- Identifying key transcription factors or chromatin remodelers that upregulate OCT4 in CRPC and NEPC.
- Investigating the role of long non-coding RNAs (lncRNAs) and microRNAs (miRNAs) in modulating the OCT4 expression.
- Investigating the impact of tumor microenvironment factors, including hypoxia, inflammatory cytokines, and stromal interactions, on the OCT4 reactivation.

2. *Exploring OCT4-Driven Transcriptional Networks and Epigenetic Regulation*

OCT4 functions as a transcription factor, orchestrating gene expression programs that maintain stemness and promote plasticity. However, its downstream targets and transcriptional co-factors in PCa remain largely unknown [159]. Future studies should

- Perform chromatin immunoprecipitation sequencing (ChIP-seq), RNA sequencing (RNA-seq), and mass spectrometry (MS) to identify the gene networks regulated by OCT4 in PCa.
- Investigate whether OCT4 interacts with other lineage plasticity drivers, such as SOX2, NANOG, EZH2, or AURKA, to form oncogenic transcriptional complexes.
- Examine the role of super-enhancers (SEs) in sustaining OCT4 expression and whether disrupting SEs could be a viable therapeutic approach.

3. *Role of OCT4 in the Tumor Microenvironment and Immune Evasion*

Emerging evidence suggests that cancer stem-like cells may contribute to immune evasion. These kinds of studies make the research field more clinically relevant because the tumor microenvironment and the immune system are included [160]. Future studies should

- Investigate whether OCT4-expressing PCa cells exhibit immune-resistant properties and evade immune surveillance.
- Determine whether OCT4 influences immune checkpoint expression (e.g., PD-L1) or modulates tumor-associated macrophages, myeloid-derived suppressor cells (MDSCs), or T cells in the tumor microenvironment.
- Explore combination strategies that target OCT4 and other key master regulators—such as SOX2, MYC, EZH2, and BRN2—alongside immunotherapies, to more effectively disrupt the stemness and immune-evasive phenotypes associated with lineage plasticity in prostate cancer.

4. *Clinical Translation: OCT4 as a Biomarker for Aggressive Prostate Cancer*

The clinical relevance of OCT4 in PCa, particularly in advanced subtypes such as CRPC and NEPC, is increasingly recognized but remains underexplored. Recent technological advances in liquid biopsy—including the analysis of circulating tumor cells (CTCs) and cell-free nucleic acids—offer promising non-invasive tools for tracking tumor evolution and treatment response [161]. Furthermore, elevated OCT4 expression has been linked to primary resistance to AR inhibitors, including enzalutamide and abiraterone. In patients with high pre-treatment OCT4 levels, poor response rates and early relapse have been reported. These findings support the potential of OCT4 as a predictive biomarker that could inform patient stratification and the selection of combination therapies aimed at delaying or circumventing resistance [10,147]. Future research should focus on the following:

- Validating OCT4 as a biomarker in large patient cohorts to assess its correlation with disease progression, metastasis, and therapy resistance.
- Developing non-invasive diagnostic tools (e.g., CTCs, exosomal OCT4 detection) to monitor disease progression in CRPC and NEPC patients.
- Exploring whether OCT4 expression levels can predict patient responses to existing therapies, such as androgen receptor inhibitors or chemotherapy.

5. *Targeting OCT4 in Prostate Cancer: Novel Therapeutic Strategies*

Given its role in therapy resistance, OCT4 represents an attractive target for drug development. However, direct inhibition of transcription factors remains challenging, and there is a lack in this area, especially in the clinic [162]. Future therapeutic strategies should explore the following:

- Developing small-molecule inhibitors that disrupt OCT4 protein stability, DNA binding, or protein–protein interactions.
- Investigating RNA-based approaches, such as siRNA, antisense oligonucleotides, or CRISPR-based gene editing, to selectively suppress OCT4 expression.
- Identifying upstream regulatory pathways (e.g., NFκB, FGFR, or Wnt/β-catenin) that indirectly modulate OCT4 and could be targeted with existing inhibitors.
- Exploring the potential of targeted protein degradation strategies, such as PROTACs (proteolysis-targeting chimeras), to selectively degrade OCT4 in PCa cells.

5. Conclusions

OCT4 plays a central role in the prostate cancer (PCa) progression by regulating stemness, plasticity, and resistance to therapy. Its activity is modulated by multiple oncogenic pathways, including Wnt/β-catenin, PI3K/AKT, STAT3, and NF-κB, as well as through chromatin remodeling and tumor microenvironmental cues [163–166].

In PCa, OCT4 emerges as a driver of lineage plasticity, therapy resistance, and the transition to aggressive subtypes such as CRPC and NEPC. By maintaining cancer stem cell populations and promoting epithelial–mesenchymal transition (EMT), OCT4 enables tumor cells to evade standard therapies and acquire more invasive and treatment-resistant characteristics. Its ability to suppress AR signaling and facilitate androgen-independent growth further underscores its significance in PCa pathophysiology. Given its broad impact on tumor evolution, OCT4 represents a compelling target for therapeutic intervention.

Given OCT4's intracellular localization and lack of enzymatic activity, directly targeting this transcription factor remains challenging. However, progress in developing RNA-based interventions (e.g., miRNAs, siRNA), CRISPR/dCas9 systems, and epigenetic therapies has opened new possibilities. These strategies either suppress the OCT4 expression or inhibit its downstream effects. Additionally, targeting regulators or microenvironmental factors that indirectly modulate OCT4—such as inflammatory macrophages or upstream oncogenic signals—offers another route to mitigate its pro-tumor functions. Combination therapies that integrate the targeting of OCT4 and other master regulators—such as SOX2, MYC, and EZH2—with standard treatments like ADT, chemotherapy, or immunotherapy may provide a more comprehensive strategy for overcoming resistance and improving patient outcomes.

Beyond its therapeutic potential, OCT4 also holds promise as a prognostic and predictive biomarker in PCa. Elevated OCT4 expression has been associated with poor clinical outcomes, including increased metastatic potential and reduced overall survival. Therefore, incorporating OCT4 assessment into clinical decision-making could help identify patients at a high risk of aggressive disease progression and therapy failure. Future studies should focus on validating OCT4 as a biomarker in large patient cohorts and exploring its utility in guiding treatment selection [22].

Ultimately, while targeting OCT4 and other stemness factors presents challenges, their central role in PCa lineage plasticity and therapy resistance makes it a key focus for future research. A deeper understanding of the molecular mechanisms governing stemness factor's function, as well as the development of more effective therapeutic strategies, could pave the way for novel treatment approaches aimed at overcoming resistance and improving survival outcomes for patients with advanced PCa.

Author Contributions: Conceptualization, M.E.F. and X.L.; software, M.E.F. and A.O.A.; writing—original draft preparation, M.E.F., Y.Z., A.O.A., F.S. and M.R.A.; writing—review and editing, M.E.F.; supervision, X.L. All authors have read and agreed to the published version of the manuscript.

Funding: This research received no external funding.

Conflicts of Interest: The authors declare no conflict of interest.

References

1. Siegel, R.L.; Kratzer, T.B.; Giaquinto, A.N.; Sung, H.; Jemal, A. Cancer statistics, 2025. *CA* **2025**, *75*, 10. [CrossRef]
2. Shih, H.J.; Fang, S.C.; An, L.; Shao, Y.H.J. Early-onset prostate cancer is associated with increased risks of disease progression and cancer-specific mortality. *Prostate* **2021**, *81*, 118–126. [CrossRef]
3. Teo, M.Y.; Rathkopf, D.E.; Kantoff, P. Treatment of advanced prostate cancer. *Annu. Rev. Med.* **2019**, *70*, 479–499. [CrossRef]
4. Swami, U.; McFarland, T.R.; Nussenzveig, R.; Agarwal, N. Advanced prostate cancer: Treatment advances and future directions. *Trends Cancer* **2020**, *6*, 702–715. [CrossRef]
5. Ma, Y.; Liu, Z.; Yu, W.; Huang, H.; Wang, Y.; Niu, Y. Investigating High-risk Factors, Precise Diagnosis, and Treatment of Castration-Resistant Prostate Cancer (CRPC). *Comb. Chem. High Throughput Screen.* **2024**, *27*, 2598–2608. [CrossRef]
6. Tashiro, K.; Kimura, S.; Tsuzuki, S.; Urabe, F.; Fukuokaya, W.; Mori, K.; Aikawa, K.; Murakami, M.; Sasaki, H.; Miki, K. Radiographic Progression at Castration-Resistant Prostate Cancer Diagnosis: A Prognostic Indicator of Metastatic Hormone-Sensitive Prostate Cancer. *Clin. Genitourin. Cancer* **2024**, *22*, 102075. [CrossRef]
7. Yamada, Y.; Beltran, H. Clinical and biological features of neuroendocrine prostate cancer. *Curr. Oncol. Rep.* **2021**, *23*, 15. [CrossRef]
8. Liu, S.; Alabi, B.R.; Yin, Q.; Stoyanova, T. Molecular mechanisms underlying the development of neuroendocrine prostate cancer. *Semin. Cancer Biol.* **2022**, *86*, 57–68. [CrossRef]
9. Storck, W.K.; May, A.M.; Westbrook, T.C.; Duan, Z.; Morrissey, C.; Yates, J.A.; Alumkal, J.J. The role of epigenetic change in therapy-induced neuroendocrine prostate cancer lineage plasticity. *Front. Endocrinol.* **2022**, *13*, 926585. [CrossRef]
10. Beltran, H.; Hruszkewycz, A.; Scher, H.I.; Hildesheim, J.; Isaacs, J.; Yu, E.Y.; Kelly, K.; Lin, D.; Dicker, A.; Arnold, J. The role of lineage plasticity in prostate cancer therapy resistance. *Clin. Cancer Res.* **2019**, *25*, 6916–6924. [CrossRef]
11. Ferguson, A.M.; Rubin, M.A. Lineage plasticity in prostate cancer: Looking beyond intrinsic alterations. *Cancer Lett.* **2022**, *548*, 215901. [CrossRef]
12. Zhu, J.; Liang, X.; Wu, D.; Chen, S.; Yang, B.; Mao, W.; Shen, D. Clinicopathological characteristics and survival outcomes in neuroendocrine prostate cancer: A population-based study. *Medicine* **2021**, *100*, e25237. [CrossRef]
13. Yao, J.; Liu, Y.; Liang, X.; Shao, J.; Zhang, Y.; Yang, J.; Zheng, M. Neuroendocrine carcinoma as an independent prognostic factor for patients with prostate cancer: A population-based study. *Front. Endocrinol.* **2021**, *12*, 778758. [CrossRef]
14. Rubin, M.A.; Bristow, R.G.; Thienger, P.D.; Dive, C.; Imielinski, M. Impact of lineage plasticity to and from a neuroendocrine phenotype on progression and response in prostate and lung cancers. *Mol. Cell* **2020**, *80*, 562–577. [CrossRef]
15. Takayama, K.-i.; Kosaka, T.; Suzuki, T.; Hongo, H.; Oya, M.; Fujimura, T.; Suzuki, Y.; Inoue, S. Subtype-specific collaborative transcription factor networks are promoted by OCT4 in the progression of prostate cancer. *Nat. Commun.* **2021**, *12*, 3766. [CrossRef]
16. Imamura, J.; Ganguly, S.; Muskara, A.; Liao, R.S.; Nguyen, J.K.; Weight, C.; Wee, C.E.; Gupta, S.; Mian, O.Y. Lineage plasticity and treatment resistance in prostate cancer: The intersection of genetics, epigenetics, and evolution. *Front. Endocrinol.* **2023**, *14*, 1191311. [CrossRef]

17. Swain, N.; Thakur, M.; Pathak, J.; Swain, B. SOX2, OCT4 and NANOG: The core embryonic stem cell pluripotency regulators in oral carcinogenesis. *J. Oral Maxillofac. Pathol.* **2020**, *24*, 368–373. [CrossRef]
18. Esch, D.; Vahokoski, J.; Groves, M.R.; Pogenberg, V.; Cojocaru, V.; Vom Bruch, H.; Han, D.; Drexler, H.C.; Arauzo-Bravo, M.J.; Ng, C.K. A unique Oct4 interface is crucial for reprogramming to pluripotency. *Nat. Cell Biol.* **2013**, *15*, 295–301. [CrossRef]
19. Robinson, M.; Gilbert, S.F.; Waters, J.A.; Lujano-Olazaba, O.; Lara, J.; Alexander, L.J.; Green, S.E.; Burkeen, G.A.; Patrus, O.; Sarwar, Z. Characterization of SOX2, OCT4 and NANOG in ovarian cancer tumor-initiating cells. *Cancers* **2021**, *13*, 262. [CrossRef]
20. Mohiuddin, I.S.; Wei, S.-J.; Kang, M.H. Role of OCT4 in cancer stem-like cells and chemotherapy resistance. *Biochim. Biophys. Acta (BBA)-Mol. Basis Dis.* **2020**, *1866*, 165432. [CrossRef]
21. Kosaka, T.; Nagamatsu, G.; Saito, S.; Oya, M.; Suda, T.; Horimoto, K. Identification of drug candidate against prostate cancer from the aspect of somatic cell reprogramming. *Cancer Sci.* **2013**, *104*, 1017–1026. [CrossRef]
22. Ma, Y. OCT4-positive circulating tumor cells may predict a poor prognosis in patients with metastatic castration-resistant prostate cancer treated with abiraterone plus prednisone therapy. *Oncol. Lett.* **2023**, *26*, 452. [CrossRef]
23. Xie, W.; Yu, J.; Yin, Y.; Zhang, X.; Zheng, X.; Wang, X. OCT4 induces EMT and promotes ovarian cancer progression by regulating the PI3K/AKT/mTOR pathway. *Front. Oncol.* **2022**, *12*, 876257. [CrossRef]
24. Bu, X.; Liu, Y.; Wang, L.; Yan, Z.; Xin, G.; Su, W. Oct4 promoted proliferation, migration, invasion, and epithelial-mesenchymal transition (EMT) in colon cancer cells by activating the SCF/c-Kit signaling pathway. *Cell Cycle* **2023**, *22*, 291–302. [CrossRef]
25. Formaggio, N.; Rubin, M.A.; Theurillat, J.-P. Loss and revival of androgen receptor signaling in advanced prostate cancer. *Oncogene* **2021**, *40*, 1205–1216. [CrossRef]
26. Nouruzi, S.; Ganguli, D.; Tabrizian, N.; Kobelev, M.; Sivak, O.; Namekawa, T.; Thaper, D.; Baca, S.C.; Freedman, M.L.; Aguda, A. ASCL1 activates neuronal stem cell-like lineage programming through remodeling of the chromatin landscape in prostate cancer. *Nat. Commun.* **2022**, *13*, 2282. [CrossRef]
27. Kaarijärvi, R.; Kaljunen, H.; Ketola, K. Molecular and functional links between neurodevelopmental processes and treatment-induced neuroendocrine plasticity in prostate cancer progression. *Cancers* **2021**, *13*, 692. [CrossRef]
28. Ko, J.; Meyer, A.N.; Haas, M.; Donoghue, D.J. Characterization of FGFR signaling in prostate cancer stem cells and inhibition via TKI treatment. *Oncotarget* **2021**, *12*, 22. [CrossRef]
29. Guo, C.; Kadier, A.; Zhang, Z.; Mao, S.; Yang, B.; Zheng, J.; Yao, X. ADT increases prostate cancer cell invasion via altering AR/SALL4/SOX2-OCT4 stem cell signaling. *Cell Biol. Toxicol.* **2025**, *41*, 107. [CrossRef]
30. Zhao, Y.; Li, C.; Huang, L.; Niu, S.; Lu, Q.; Gong, D.; Huang, S.; Yuan, Y.; Chen, H. Prognostic value of association of OCT4 with LEF1 expression in esophageal squamous cell carcinoma and their impact on epithelial-mesenchymal transition, invasion, and migration. *Cancer Med.* **2018**, *7*, 3977–3987. [CrossRef]
31. Li, H.; Wang, L.; Shi, S.; Xu, Y.; Dai, X.; Li, H.; Wang, J.; Zhang, Q.; Wang, Y.; Sun, S. The prognostic and clinicopathologic characteristics of OCT4 and lung cancer: A meta-analysis. *Curr. Mol. Med.* **2019**, *19*, 54–75. [CrossRef]
32. Kosaka, T.; Mikami, S.; Yoshimine, S.; Miyazaki, Y.; Daimon, T.; Kikuchi, E.; Miyajima, A.; Oya, M. The prognostic significance of OCT4 expression in patients with prostate cancer. *Hum. Pathol.* **2016**, *51*, 1–8. [CrossRef]
33. Zhang, Q.; Han, Z.; Zhu, Y.; Chen, J.; Li, W. The role and specific mechanism of OCT4 in cancer stem cells: A review. *Int. J. Stem Cells* **2020**, *13*, 312–325. [CrossRef]
34. Cui, Y.; Niu, Y.; Zhou, J.; Chen, Y.; Cheng, Y.; Li, S.; Ai, Z.; Chu, C.; Wang, H.; Zheng, B. Generation of a precise Oct4-hrGFP knockin cynomolgus monkey model via CRISPR/Cas9-assisted homologous recombination. *Cell Res.* **2018**, *28*, 383–386. [CrossRef]
35. Gao, L.; Yang, Y.; Xu, H.; Liu, R.; Li, D.; Hong, H.; Qin, M.; Wang, Y. MiR-335 functions as a tumor suppressor in pancreatic cancer by targeting OCT4. *Tumor Biol.* **2014**, *35*, 8309–8318. [CrossRef]
36. Vaddi, P.K.; Stamnes, M.A.; Cao, H.; Chen, S. Elimination of SOX2/OCT4-associated prostate cancer stem cells blocks tumor development and enhances therapeutic response. *Cancers* **2019**, *11*, 1331. [CrossRef]
37. Fogarty, N.M.; McCarthy, A.; Snijders, K.E.; Powell, B.E.; Kubikova, N.; Blakeley, P.; Lea, R.; Elder, K.; Wamaitha, S.E.; Kim, D. Genome editing reveals a role for OCT4 in human embryogenesis. *Nature* **2017**, *550*, 67–73. [CrossRef]
38. Hisey, E.; Ross, P.J.; Meyers, S.A. A review of OCT4 functions and applications to equine embryos. *J. Equine Vet. Sci.* **2021**, *98*, 103364. [CrossRef]
39. Niwa, H.; Miyazaki, J.-i.; Smith, A.G. Quantitative expression of Oct-3/4 defines differentiation, dedifferentiation or self-renewal of ES cells. *Nat. Genet.* **2000**, *24*, 372–376. [CrossRef]
40. Cai, W.; Wang, Z.; Wei, C.; Wu, M.; Zheng, W.; Zhang, H.; Liu, C.; Liu, L. Prognostic evaluation of NANOG and OCT4 expression for posttransplantation hepatocellular carcinoma recurrence. *J. Cell. Biochem.* **2019**, *120*, 8419–8429. [CrossRef]
41. Noel, K.; Ibraheem, M.M.; Ahmed, B.S.; Hameed, A.F.; Khamees, N.H.; Akkila, S.S. Expression of OCT4 stem cell marker in benign prostatic hyperplasia and normal tissue around the prostatic carcinoma in a sample of Iraqi patients. *Egypt. J. Histol.* **2020**, *43*, 245–254.

42. Su, B.-H.; Wang, C.-T.; Chang, J.-M.; Chen, H.-Y.; Huang, T.-H.; Yen, Y.-T.; Tseng, Y.-L.; Chang, M.-Y.; Lee, C.-H.; Cheng, L.-H. OCT4 promotes lung cancer progression through upregulation of VEGF-correlated chemokine-1. *Int. J. Med. Sci.* **2025**, *22*, 680. [CrossRef]
43. Lambis-Anaya, L.; Fernández-Ruiz, M.; Liscano, Y.; Suarez-Causado, A. High OCT4 expression might be associated with an aggressive phenotype in rectal cancer. *Cancers* **2023**, *15*, 3740. [CrossRef]
44. Pandian, J.; Panneerpandian, P.; Sekar, B.T.; Selvarasu, K.; Ganesan, K. OCT4-mediated transcription confers oncogenic advantage for a subset of gastric tumors with poor clinical outcome. *Funct. Integr. Genom.* **2022**, *22*, 1345–1360. [CrossRef]
45. Ding, J.; Xu, H.; Faiola, F.; Ma'ayan, A.; Wang, J. Oct4 links multiple epigenetic pathways to the pluripotency network. *Cell Res.* **2012**, *22*, 155–167. [CrossRef]
46. Ambrosetti, D.-C.; Basilico, C.; Dailey, L. Synergistic activation of the fibroblast growth factor 4 enhancer by Sox2 and Oct-3 depends on protein-protein interactions facilitated by a specific spatial arrangement of factor binding sites. *Mol. Cell. Biol.* **1997**, *17*, 6321–6329. [CrossRef]
47. Cho, Y.; Kang, H.G.; Kim, S.-J.; Lee, S.; Jee, S.; Ahn, S.G.; Kang, M.J.; Song, J.S.; Chung, J.-Y.; Yi, E.C. Post-translational modification of OCT4 in breast cancer tumorigenesis. *Cell Death Differ.* **2018**, *25*, 1781–1795. [CrossRef]
48. Sohn, E.J.; Moon, H.J.; Lim, J.K.; Kim, D.S.; Kim, J.H. Regulation of the protein stability and transcriptional activity of OCT4 in stem cells. *Adv. Biol. Regul.* **2021**, *79*, 100777. [CrossRef]
49. Dan, S.; Kang, B.; Duan, X.; Wang, Y.-J. A cell-free system toward deciphering the post-translational modification barcodes of Oct4 in different cellular contexts. *Biochem. Biophys. Res. Commun.* **2015**, *456*, 714–720. [CrossRef]
50. MacLean, M.R.; Walker, O.L.; Arun, R.P.; Fernando, W.; Marcato, P. Informed by cancer stem cells of solid tumors: Advances in treatments targeting tumor-promoting factors and pathways. *Int. J. Mol. Sci.* **2024**, *25*, 4102.
51. Weng, Z.; Lin, J.; He, J.; Gao, L.; Lin, S.; Tsang, L.L.; Zhang, H.; He, X.; Wang, G.; Yang, X. Human embryonic stem cell-derived neural crest model unveils CD55 as a cancer stem cell regulator for therapeutic targeting in MYCN-amplified neuroblastoma. *Neuro-Oncology* **2022**, *24*, 872–885. [CrossRef]
52. Liu, H.-L.; Tang, H.-t.; Yang, H.-l.; Deng, T.-T.; Xu, Y.-P.; Xu, S.-Q.; Peng, L.; Wang, Z.; Fang, Q.; Kuang, X.-Y. Oct4 regulates the transition of cancer stem-like cells to tumor endothelial-like cells in human liver cancer. *Front. Cell Dev. Biol.* **2020**, *8*, 563316. [CrossRef]
53. Smith, B.A.; Sokolov, A.; Uzunangelov, V.; Baertsch, R.; Newton, Y.; Graim, K.; Mathis, C.; Cheng, D.; Stuart, J.M.; Witte, O.N. A basal stem cell signature identifies aggressive prostate cancer phenotypes. *Proc. Natl. Acad. Sci. USA* **2015**, *112*, E6544–E6552. [CrossRef]
54. Beltran, H.; Prandi, D.; Mosquera, J.M.; Benelli, M.; Puca, L.; Cyrta, J.; Marotz, C.; Giannopoulou, E.; Chakravarthi, B.V.; Varambally, S. Divergent clonal evolution of castration-resistant neuroendocrine prostate cancer. *Nat. Med.* **2016**, *22*, 298–305. [CrossRef]
55. Song, P.; Gao, Z.; Bao, Y.; Chen, L.; Huang, Y.; Liu, Y.; Dong, Q.; Wei, X. Wnt/β-catenin signaling pathway in carcinogenesis and cancer therapy. *J. Hematol. Oncol.* **2024**, *17*, 46. [CrossRef]
56. Liu, J.; Xiao, Q.; Xiao, J.; Niu, C.; Li, Y.; Zhang, X.; Zhou, Z.; Shu, G.; Yin, G. Wnt/β-catenin signalling: Function, biological mechanisms, and therapeutic opportunities. *Signal Transduct. Target. Ther.* **2022**, *7*, 3. [CrossRef]
57. Pandey, P.; Khan, F.; Seifeldin, S.A.; Alshaghdali, K.; Siddiqui, S.; Abdelwadoud, M.E.; Vyas, M.; Saeed, M.; Mazumder, A.; Saeed, A. Targeting Wnt/β-catenin pathway by flavonoids: Implication for cancer therapeutics. *Nutrients* **2023**, *15*, 2088. [CrossRef]
58. Leonardo-Sousa, C.; Barriga, R.; Florindo, H.F.; Acúrcio, R.C.; Guedes, R.C. Structural Insights and Development of Small Molecule Inhibitors Targeting TGF-β Receptor I: A Comprehensive Review of Clinical Advances. *Mol. Ther. Oncol.* **2025**, *33*, 200945. [CrossRef]
59. Du, L.; Zhu, W. Research Progress on TGF-B Gene Family. *Octa J. Environ. Res.* **2024**, *12*, 1–10.
60. Ebrahimi, M.; Nourbakhsh, E.; Hazara, A.Z.; Mirzaei, A.; Shafieyari, S.; Salehi, A.; Hoseinzadeh, M.; Payandeh, Z.; Barati, G. PI3K/Akt/mTOR signaling pathway in cancer stem cells. *Pathol.-Res. Pract.* **2022**, *237*, 154010.
61. Song, J.-x.; Dong, Y.-q.; Han, R.-l.; Xie, J.; Zhu, A.-y.; Chen, X.; Yang, Y.-y.; Sheng, C.-x.; Jiang, T.; Zhao, H.-y. PI3K/AKT/mTOR Activation is Associated with Malignant Severity and Poorer Prognosis in Parathyroid Carcinomas. *J. Clin. Endocrinol. Metab.* **2025**, dgaf042. [CrossRef]
62. Versari, I.; Salucci, S.; Bavelloni, A.; Battistelli, M.; Traversari, M.; Wang, A.; Sampaolesi, M.; Faenza, I. The Emerging Role and Clinical Significance of PI3K-Akt-mTOR in Rhabdomyosarcoma. *Biomolecules* **2025**, *15*, 334. [CrossRef]
63. Iluta, S.; Nistor, M.; Buruiana, S.; Dima, D. Notch and Hedgehog Signaling Unveiled: Crosstalk, Roles, and Breakthroughs in Cancer Stem Cell Research. *Life* **2025**, *15*, 228. [CrossRef]

64. Lou, L.; Peng, K.; Ouyang, S.; Ding, W.; Mo, J.; Yan, J.; Gong, X.; Liu, G.; Lu, J.; Yue, P. Periostin-mediated NOTCH1 activation between tumor cells and HSCs crosstalk promotes liver metastasis of small cell lung cancer. *J. Exp. Clin. Cancer Res.* **2025**, *44*, 6. [CrossRef]
65. Chen, C.; Du, Y.; Nie, R.; Wang, S.; Wang, H.; Li, P. Notch signaling in cancers: Mechanism and potential therapy. *Front. Cell Dev. Biol.* **2025**, *13*, 1542967. [CrossRef]
66. Huang, Y.; Wang, Y.; Wu, H.; Wang, Y.; Deng, Y.; Chang, Y.; Su, K.; Yang, L.; Tao, W.; Liu, W. Exploring the mechanism of Jianpi Lishi Jiedu Granules against postoperative recurrence of colorectal adenoma based on IL-6/JAK/STAT3 signaling pathway. *Cell. Signal.* **2025**, *127*, 111535. [CrossRef]
67. Ma, L.; Liu, X.; Roopashree, R.; Kazmi, S.W.; Jasim, S.A.; Phaninder Vinay, K.; Fateh, A.; Yang, F.; Rajabivahid, M.; Dehghani-Ghorbi, M. Long non-coding RNAs (lncRNAs) in cancer development: New insight from STAT3 signaling pathway to immune evasion. *Clin. Exp. Med.* **2025**, *25*, 53. [CrossRef]
68. Gao, Y.; Lan, L.; Wang, C.; Wang, Y.; Shi, L.; Sun, L. Selective JAK1 inhibitors and the therapeutic applications thereof: A patent review (2016–2023). *Expert Opin. Ther. Pat.* **2025**, *35*, 181–195. [CrossRef]
69. Duan, J.; Wang, Y.; Chen, Y.; Wang, Y.; Li, Q.; Liu, J.; Fu, C.; Cao, C.; Cong, Z.; Su, M. Silencing LY6D expression inhibits colon cancer in xenograft mice and regulates colon cancer stem cells' proliferation, stemness, invasion, and apoptosis via the MAPK pathway. *Molecules* **2023**, *28*, 7776. [CrossRef]
70. Emelyanova, A.; Zolotovskaia, M.; Poddubskaya, E.; Modestov, A.; Buzdin, A.; Kuzmin, D. Activation of P38 MAPK Signaling Cascade is Linked with Clinical Outcomes and Therapeutic Responses in Human Cancers. *Biochemistry* **2024**, *89*, 2155–2173. [CrossRef]
71. Liu, Y.-C.; Lin, T.-J.; Chong, K.-Y.; Chen, G.-Y.; Kuo, C.-Y.; Lin, Y.-Y.; Chang, C.-W.; Hsiao, T.-F.; Wang, C.-L.; Shih, Y.-C. Targeting the ERK1/2 and p38 MAPK pathways attenuates Golgi tethering factor golgin-97 depletion-induced cancer progression in breast cancer. *Cell Commun. Signal.* **2025**, *23*, 22. [CrossRef]
72. Yong, X.; Tang, B.; Xiao, Y.-F.; Xie, R.; Qin, Y.; Luo, G.; Hu, C.-J.; Dong, H.; Yang, S.-M. Helicobacter pylori upregulates Nanog and Oct4 via Wnt/β-catenin signaling pathway to promote cancer stem cell-like properties in human gastric cancer. *Cancer Lett.* **2016**, *374*, 292–303. [CrossRef]
73. Sun, L.; Liu, T.; Zhang, S.; Guo, K.; Liu, Y. Oct4 induces EMT through LEF1/β-catenin dependent WNT signaling pathway in hepatocellular carcinoma. *Oncol. Lett.* **2017**, *13*, 2599–2606. [CrossRef]
74. Yuan, F.; Zhou, W.; Zou, C.; Zhang, Z.; Hu, H.; Dai, Z.; Zhang, Y. Expression of Oct4 in HCC and modulation to wnt/β-catenin and TGF-β signal pathways. *Mol. Cell. Biochem.* **2010**, *343*, 155–162. [CrossRef]
75. Wang, P.; Deng, Z.; Li, A.; Li, R.; Huang, W.; Cui, J.; Chen, S.; Li, B.; Zhang, S. β-Catenin promotes long-term survival and angiogenesis of peripheral blood mesenchymal stem cells via the Oct4 signaling pathway. *Exp. Mol. Med.* **2022**, *54*, 1434–1449. [CrossRef]
76. Bassiouny, A. Regulation of Oct4 signaling on tumorigenesis and modulation of wnt/β-catenin and TGF-β signal pathways in hepatocellular carcinoma cells. *J. Clin. Oncol.* **2011**, *29* (Suppl. 15), e13551.
77. Kelly, K.F.; Ng, D.Y.; Jayakumaran, G.; Wood, G.A.; Koide, H.; Doble, B.W. β-catenin enhances Oct-4 activity and reinforces pluripotency through a TCF-independent mechanism. *Cell Stem Cell* **2011**, *8*, 214–227.
78. Guo, Y.; Li, B.; Yan, X.; Shen, X.; Ma, J.; Liu, S.; Zhang, D. Bisphenol A and polychlorinated biphenyls enhance the cancer stem cell properties of human ovarian cancer cells by activating the WNT signaling pathway. *Chemosphere* **2020**, *246*, 125775.
79. Shen, W.; Zhang, X.; Tang, J.; Zhang, Z.; Du, R.; Luo, D.; Liu, X.; Xia, Y.; Li, Y.; Wang, S. CCL16 maintains stem cell-like properties in breast cancer by activating CCR2/GSK3β/β-catenin/OCT4 axis. *Theranostics* **2021**, *11*, 2297.
80. Huang, H.; Wang, C.; Liu, F.; Li, H.-Z.; Peng, G.; Gao, X.; Dong, K.-Q.; Wang, H.-R.; Kong, D.-P.; Qu, M. Reciprocal network between cancer stem-like cells and macrophages facilitates the progression and androgen deprivation therapy resistance of prostate cancer. *Clin. Cancer Res.* **2018**, *24*, 4612–4626.
81. Zhao, Q.W.; Zhou, Y.W.; Li, W.X.; Kang, B.; Zhang, X.Q.; Yang, Y.; ChENG, J.; Yin, S.Y.; Tong, Y.; He, J.Q. Akt-mediated phosphorylation of Oct4 is associated with the proliferation of stem-like cancer cells. *Oncol. Rep.* **2015**, *33*, 1621–1629. [CrossRef]
82. Lin, Y.; Yang, Y.; Li, W.; Chen, Q.; Li, J.; Pan, X.; Zhou, L.; Liu, C.; Chen, C.; He, J. Reciprocal regulation of Akt and Oct4 promotes the self-renewal and survival of embryonal carcinoma cells. *Mol. Cell* **2012**, *48*, 627–640. [CrossRef]
83. Li, W.; Zhou, Y.; Zhang, X.; Yang, Y.; Dan, S.; Su, T.; She, S.; Dong, W.; Zhao, Q.; Jia, J. Dual inhibiting OCT4 and AKT potently suppresses the propagation of human cancer cells. *Sci. Rep.* **2017**, *7*, 46246. [CrossRef]
84. Park, G.B.; Kim, D. TLR5/7-mediated PI3K activation triggers epithelial-mesenchymal transition of ovarian cancer cells through WAVE3-dependent mesothelin or OCT4/SOX2 expression. *Oncol. Rep.* **2017**, *38*, 3167–3176. [CrossRef]

85. Yang, C.; Zhang, Y.; Zhang, Y.; Zhang, Z.; Peng, J.; Li, Z.; Han, L.; You, Q.; Chen, X.; Rao, X. Downregulation of cancer stem cell properties via mTOR signaling pathway inhibition by rapamycin in nasopharyngeal carcinoma. *Int. J. Oncol.* **2015**, *47*, 909–917. [CrossRef]
86. Johnson, A.; Korleski, J.; Laterra, J.; Lopez-Bertoni, H. Abstract PR013: Oct4 and Sox2 induce cellular transition of glioma stem cells to an immune suppressive, regulatory T cell-like state. *Cancer Res.* **2022**, *82* (Suppl. 10), PR013. [CrossRef]
87. Hagiwara, M.; Yasumizu, Y.; Yamashita, N.; Rajabi, H.; Fushimi, A.; Long, M.D.; Li, W.; Bhattacharya, A.; Ahmad, R.; Oya, M. MUC1-C activates the BAF (mSWI/SNF) complex in prostate cancer stem cells. *Cancer Res.* **2021**, *81*, 1111–1122. [CrossRef]
88. Kong, D.; Banerjee, S.; Ahmad, A.; Li, Y.; Wang, Z.; Sethi, S.; Sarkar, F.H. Epithelial to mesenchymal transition is mechanistically linked with stem cell signatures in prostate cancer cells. *PLoS ONE* **2010**, *5*, e12445. [CrossRef]
89. Zhang, L.; Sha, J.; Yang, G.; Huang, X.; Bo, J.; Huang, Y. Activation of Notch pathway is linked with epithelial-mesenchymal transition in prostate cancer cells. *Cell Cycle* **2017**, *16*, 999–1007. [CrossRef]
90. Ibrahim, D.A.; Elsebai, E.A.; Fayed, A.; Abdelrahman, A.E. Prognostic value of NOTCH1 and OCT4 in gastric carcinoma. *Indian J. Pathol. Microbiol.* **2022**, *65*, 328–335. [CrossRef]
91. Guo, Y.; Wang, G.; Wang, Z.; Ding, X.; Qian, L.; Li, Y. Reck-notch1 signaling mediates miR-221/222 regulation of lung cancer stem cells in NSCLC. *Front. Cell Dev. Biol.* **2021**, *9*, 663279. [CrossRef]
92. Wang, Y.; Han, Y.; Xu, S.; Zhang, L.; Zhang, X.; Deng, J.; Ye, W.; Liu, S. Targeting EGFR enriches stem cell-like properties in salivary adenoid cystic carcinoma by activating the Notch1 pathway. *Cancer Manag. Res.* **2020**, *12*, 6655–6663. [CrossRef]
93. Cheng, J.-w.; Duan, L.-x.; Yu, Y.; Wang, P.; Feng, J.-l.; Feng, G.-z.; Liu, Y. Bone marrow mesenchymal stem cells promote prostate cancer cell stemness via cell–cell contact to activate the Jagged1/Notch1 pathway. *Cell Biosci.* **2021**, *11*, 87. [CrossRef]
94. Bai, S.; Zhao, Y.; Chen, W.; Peng, W.; Wang, Y.; Xiong, S.; Aruna; Li, Y.; Yang, Y.; Chen, S. The stromal-tumor amplifying STC1-Notch1 feedforward signal promotes the stemness of hepatocellular carcinoma. *J. Transl. Med.* **2023**, *21*, 236. [CrossRef]
95. Zhao, L.; Lei, J.; Gu, S.; Zhang, Y.; Jing, X.; Wang, L.; Zhang, L.; Ning, Q.; Luo, M.; Qi, Y. A yes-associated protein 1-Notch1 receptor positive feedback loop promotes breast cancer lung metastasis by attenuating the bone morphogenetic protein 4-SMAD family member 1/5 signaling. *Carcinogenesis* **2022**, *43*, 1162–1175. [CrossRef]
96. Wang, G.; Zhou, H.; Gu, Z.; Gao, Q.; Shen, G. Oct4 promotes cancer cell proliferation and migration and leads to poor prognosis associated with the survivin/STAT3 pathway in hepatocellular carcinoma. *Oncol. Rep.* **2018**, *40*, 979–987. [CrossRef]
97. Kim, S.-Y.; Kang, J.W.; Song, X.; Kim, B.K.; Yoo, Y.D.; Kwon, Y.T.; Lee, Y.J. Role of the IL-6-JAK1-STAT3-Oct-4 pathway in the conversion of non-stem cancer cells into cancer stem-like cells. *Cell. Signal.* **2013**, *25*, 961–969. [CrossRef]
98. Cheng, C.-C.; Shi, L.-H.; Wang, X.-J.; Wang, S.-X.; Wan, X.-Q.; Liu, S.-R.; Wang, Y.-F.; Lu, Z.; Wang, L.-H.; Ding, Y. Stat3/Oct-4/c-Myc signal circuit for regulating stemness-mediated doxorubicin resistance of triple-negative breast cancer cells and inhibitory effects of WP1066. *Int. J. Oncol.* **2018**, *53*, 339–348. [CrossRef]
99. Sun, S.; Yang, H.; Wang, F.; Zhao, S. Oct4 downregulation-induced inflammation increases the migration and invasion rate of oral squamous cell carcinoma. *Acta Biochim. Biophys. Sin.* **2021**, *53*, 1440–1449. [CrossRef]
100. Zhao, K.; Zhao, Q.; Dai, X.; Wen, X.; Luo, X.; Duan, Y.; Yang, Z.; Dai, Q. Alantolactone enhances the sensitivity of melanoma to MAPK pathway inhibitors by targeting inhibition of STAT3 activation and down-regulating stem cell markers. *Cancer Cell Int.* **2024**, *24*, 191. [CrossRef]
101. Chen, M.; Ye, A.; Wei, J.; Wang, R.; Poon, K. Deoxycholic acid upregulates the reprogramming factors KFL4 and OCT4 through the IL-6/STAT3 pathway in esophageal adenocarcinoma cells. *Technol. Cancer Res. Treat.* **2020**, *19*, 1533033820945302. [CrossRef]
102. Pandian, J.; Ganesan, K. Delineation of gastric tumors with activated ERK/MAPK signaling cascades for the development of targeted therapeutics. *Exp. Cell Res.* **2022**, *410*, 112956. [CrossRef]
103. Jiang, P.; Li, F.; Liu, Z.; Hao, S.; Gao, J.; Li, S. BTB and CNC homology 1 (Bach1) induces lung cancer stem cell phenotypes by stimulating CD44 expression. *Respir. Res.* **2021**, *22*, 320. [CrossRef]
104. Xu, H.; Du, Z.; Li, Z.; Liu, X.; Li, X.; Zhang, X.; Ma, J. MUC1-EGFR crosstalk with IL-6 by activating NF-κB and MAPK pathways to regulate the stemness and paclitaxel-resistance of lung adenocarcinoma. *Ann. Med.* **2024**, *56*, 2313671. [CrossRef]
105. Wei, S.-J.; Nguyen, T.H.; Yang, I.-H.; Mook, D.G.; Makena, M.R.; Verlekar, D.; Hindle, A.; Martinez, G.M.; Yang, S.; Shimada, H. MYC transcription activation mediated by OCT4 as a mechanism of resistance to 13-cis RA-mediated differentiation in neuroblastoma. *Cell Death Dis.* **2020**, *11*, 368. [CrossRef]
106. Emhemmed, F.; Azouaou, S.A.; Thuaud, F.; Schini-Kerth, V.; Désaubry, L.; Muller, C.D.; Fuhrmann, G. Selective anticancer effects of a synthetic flavagline on human Oct4-expressing cancer stem-like cells via a p38 MAPK-dependent caspase-3-dependent pathway. *Biochem. Pharmacol.* **2014**, *89*, 185–196. [CrossRef]
107. Yang, L.; Shi, P.; Zhao, G.; Xu, J.; Peng, W.; Zhang, J.; Zhang, G.; Wang, X.; Dong, Z.; Chen, F. Targeting cancer stem cell pathways for cancer therapy. *Signal Transduct. Target. Ther.* **2020**, *5*, 8.

108. Roy, A.; Mishra, J.; Chakraborty, S.; Singh, S.P.; Patra, S.K. Epigenetic regulation of pluripotency inducer genes NANOG and SOX2 in human prostate cancer. *Prog. Mol. Biol. Transl. Sci.* **2023**, *197*, 241–260.
109. Costa, C.D.; Justo, A.A.; Kobayashi, P.E.; Story, M.M.; Palmieri, C.; Amorim, R.L.; Fonseca-Alves, C.E. Characterization of OCT3/4, Nestin, NANOG, CD44 and CD24 as stem cell markers in canine prostate cancer. *Int. J. Biochem. Cell Biol.* **2019**, *108*, 21–28. [CrossRef]
110. Qi, Y.-F.; Wu, L.; Li, Z.-Q.; Wu, M.-L.; Wang, H.-F.; Chan, K.-Y.; Lu, L.-L.; Cai, S.-H.; Wang, H.-S.; Du, J. Nodal signaling modulates the expression of Oct-4 via nuclear translocation of β-catenin in lung and prostate cancer cells. *Arch. Biochem. Biophys.* **2016**, *608*, 34–41. [CrossRef]
111. De Resende, M.F.; Chinen, L.T.D.; Vieira, S.; Jampietro, J.; Da Fonseca, F.P.; Vassallo, J.; Campos, L.C.; Guimarães, G.C.; Soares, F.A.; Rocha, R.M. Prognostication of OCT4 isoform expression in prostate cancer. *Tumor Biol.* **2013**, *34*, 2665–2673. [CrossRef]
112. Nong, S.; Guan, Y.; Wang, Z.; Wei, Z.; Zhang, Y.; Ni, J.; He, C.; Ma, L.; Zhou, S.; Li, W. Significant association between IL-18 and OCT4 gene polymorphisms in susceptibility and clinical characteristics of prostate cancer. *Oncol. Transl. Med.* **2019**, *5*, 123–130. [CrossRef]
113. Caputo, S.; Grioni, M.; Brambillasca, C.S.; Monno, A.; Brevi, A.; Freschi, M.; Piras, I.S.; Elia, A.R.; Pieri, V.; Baccega, T. Galectin-3 in prostate cancer stem-like cells is immunosuppressive and drives early metastasis. *Front. Immunol.* **2020**, *11*, 540641. [CrossRef]
114. Wang, Q.; Zhang, J.; Wang, W. Expression and significance of S100P, CD147, and OCT4 in different prostate cancer tissue TNM stages. *Genet. Mol. Res.* **2015**, *14*, 6844–6851. [CrossRef]
115. Hepburn, A.; Steele, R.; Veeratterapillay, R.; Wilson, L.; Kounatidou, E.; Barnard, A.; Berry, P.; Cassidy, J.; Moad, M.; El-Sherif, A. The induction of core pluripotency master regulators in cancers defines poor clinical outcomes and treatment resistance. *Oncogene* **2019**, *38*, 4412–4424. [CrossRef]
116. Miyashita, M.; Tomogane, M.; Nakamura, Y.; Shimizu, T.; Fujihara, A.; Ukimura, O.; Ashihara, E. Sphere-derived prostate cancer stem cells are resistant to γδ T cell cytotoxicity. *Anticancer Res.* **2020**, *40*, 5481–5487. [CrossRef]
117. Federer-Gsponer, J.R.; Müller, D.C.; Zellweger, T.; Eggimann, M.; Marston, K.; Ruiz, C.; Seifert, H.H.; Rentsch, C.A.; Bubendorf, L.; Le Magnen, C. Patterns of stemness-associated markers in the development of castration-resistant prostate cancer. *Prostate* **2020**, *80*, 1108–1117. [CrossRef]
118. Liu, B.; Jiang, H.-Y.; Yuan, T.; Luo, J.; Zhou, W.-D.; Jiang, Q.-Q.; Wu, D. Enzalutamide-induced upregulation of PCAT6 promotes prostate cancer neuroendocrine differentiation by regulating miR-326/HNRNPA2B1 axis. *Front. Oncol.* **2021**, *11*, 650054. [CrossRef]
119. Fujimoto, N.; Tsubonuma, Y.; Nagata, Y.; Minato, A.; Tomisaki, I.; Harada, K.; Miyamoto, H. Second-line systemic therapy for highly aggressive neuroendocrine prostate cancer. *Anticancer Res.* **2023**, *43*, 3841–3847. [CrossRef]
120. Bishop, J.L.; Thaper, D.; Vahid, S.; Davies, A.; Ketola, K.; Kuruma, H.; Jama, R.; Nip, K.M.; Angeles, A.; Johnson, F. The master neural transcription factor BRN2 is an androgen receptor–suppressed driver of neuroendocrine differentiation in prostate cancer. *Cancer Discov.* **2017**, *7*, 54–71. [CrossRef]
121. Sotomayor, P.; Godoy, A.; Smith, G.J.; Huss, W.J. Oct4A is expressed by a subpopulation of prostate neuroendocrine cells. *Prostate* **2009**, *69*, 401–410. [CrossRef]
122. Gillessen, S.; Turco, F.; Davis, I.D.; Efstathiou, J.A.; Fizazi, K.; James, N.D.; Shore, N.; Small, E.; Smith, M.; Sweeney, C.J. Management of patients with advanced prostate cancer. Report from the 2024 Advanced Prostate Cancer Consensus Conference (APCCC). *Eur. Urol.* **2025**, *87*, 157–216.
123. Thomson, A.; Al Saffar, H.; Tempo, J.; Lawrentschuk, N.; Murphy, D.G.; Perera, M. Time to castrate the cost? the rising expense of chemical castration for the management of prostate cancer. *Prostate Int.* **2025**. [CrossRef]
124. Liu, X.; Li, W.; Puzanov, I.; Goodrich, D.W.; Chatta, G.; Tang, D.G. Prostate cancer as a dedifferentiated organ: Androgen receptor, cancer stem cells, and cancer stemness. *Essays Biochem.* **2022**, *66*, 291–303.
125. Sanchez, B.G.; Bort, A.; Vara-Ciruelos, D.; Diaz-Laviada, I. Androgen deprivation induces reprogramming of prostate cancer cells to stem-like cells. *Cells* **2020**, *9*, 1441. [CrossRef]
126. Quintero, J.C.; Díaz, N.F.; Rodríguez-Dorantes, M.; Camacho-Arroyo, I. Cancer stem cells and androgen receptor signaling: Partners in disease progression. *Int. J. Mol. Sci.* **2023**, *24*, 15085. [CrossRef]
127. Tiwari, R.; Manzar, N.; Ateeq, B. Dynamics of cellular plasticity in prostate cancer progression. *Front. Mol. Biosci.* **2020**, *7*, 130. [CrossRef]
128. Ge, R.; Wang, Z.; Montironi, R.; Jiang, Z.; Cheng, M.; Santoni, M.; Huang, K.; Massari, F.; Lu, X.; Cimadamore, A. Epigenetic modulations and lineage plasticity in advanced prostate cancer. *Ann. Oncol.* **2020**, *31*, 470–479. [CrossRef]
129. Al Salhi, Y.; Sequi, M.B.; Valenzi, F.M.; Fuschi, A.; Martoccia, A.; Suraci, P.P.; Carbone, A.; Tema, G.; Lombardo, R.; Cicione, A. Cancer stem cells and prostate cancer: A narrative review. *Int. J. Mol. Sci.* **2023**, *24*, 7746. [CrossRef]

130. Verma, S.; Shankar, E.; Kalayci, F.N.C.; Mukunda, A.; Alassfar, M.; Singh, V.; Chan, E.R.; MacLennan, G.T.; Gupta, S. Androgen deprivation induces transcriptional reprogramming in prostate cancer cells to develop stem cell-like characteristics. *Int. J. Mol. Sci.* **2020**, *21*, 9568. [CrossRef]
131. Banerjee, P.; Kapse, P.; Siddique, S.; Kundu, M.; Choudhari, J.; Mohanty, V.; Malhotra, D.; Gosavi, S.W.; Gacche, R.N.; Kundu, G.C. Therapeutic implications of cancer stem cells in prostate cancer. *Cancer Biol. Med.* **2023**, *20*, 401–420. [CrossRef]
132. Fatma, H.; Siddique, H.R. Cancer cell plasticity, stem cell factors, and therapy resistance: How are they linked? *Cancer Metastasis Rev.* **2024**, *43*, 423–440. [CrossRef]
133. Mu, P.; Zhang, Z.; Benelli, M.; Karthaus, W.R.; Hoover, E.; Chen, C.-C.; Wongvipat, J.; Ku, S.-Y.; Gao, D.; Cao, Z. SOX2 promotes lineage plasticity and antiandrogen resistance in TP53-and RB1-deficient prostate cancer. *Science* **2017**, *355*, 84–88. [CrossRef]
134. Kainulainen, K.; Niskanen, E.A.; Kinnunen, J.; Mäki-Mantila, K.; Hartikainen, K.; Paakinaho, V.; Malinen, M.; Ketola, K.; Pasonen-Seppänen, S. Secreted factors from M1 macrophages drive prostate cancer stem cell plasticity by upregulating NANOG, SOX2, and CD44 through NFκB-signaling. *Oncoimmunology* **2024**, *13*, 2393442. [CrossRef]
135. Linn, D.E.; Yang, X.; Sun, F.; Xie, Y.; Chen, H.; Jiang, R.; Chen, H.; Chumsri, S.; Burger, A.M.; Qiu, Y. A role for OCT4 in tumor initiation of drug-resistant prostate cancer cells. *Genes Cancer* **2010**, *1*, 908–916. [CrossRef]
136. Chen, X. Super-enhancer in prostate cancer: Transcriptional disorders and therapeutic targets. *npj Precis. Oncol.* **2020**, *4*, 31. [CrossRef]
137. AlAbdi, L.; Saha, D.; He, M.; Dar, M.S.; Utturkar, S.M.; Sudyanti, P.A.; McCune, S.; Spears, B.H.; Breedlove, J.A.; Lanman, N.A. Oct4-mediated inhibition of Lsd1 activity promotes the active and primed state of pluripotency enhancers. *Cell Rep.* **2020**, *30*, 1478–1490.e6. [CrossRef]
138. Feng, Y.; Liu, X.; Pauklin, S. 3D chromatin architecture and epigenetic regulation in cancer stem cells. *Protein Cell* **2021**, *12*, 440–454. [CrossRef]
139. Kar, S.; Niharika, N.; Roy, A.; Patra, S.K. Overexpression of SOX2 gene by histone modifications: SOX2 enhances human prostate and breast cancer progression by prevention of apoptosis and enhancing cell proliferation. *Oncology* **2023**, *101*, 591–608. [CrossRef]
140. Davies, A.; Nouruzi, S.; Ganguli, D.; Namekawa, T.; Thaper, D.; Linder, S.; Karaoğlanoğlu, F.; Omur, M.E.; Kim, S.; Kobelev, M. An androgen receptor switch underlies lineage infidelity in treatment-resistant prostate cancer. *Nat. Cell Biol.* **2021**, *23*, 1023–1034. [CrossRef]
141. Logotheti, S.; Papadaki, E.; Zolota, V.; Logothetis, C.; Vrahatis, A.G.; Soundararajan, R.; Tzelepi, V. Lineage Plasticity and Stemness Phenotypes in Prostate Cancer: Harnessing the Power of Integrated "Omics" Approaches to Explore Measurable Metrics. *Cancers* **2023**, *15*, 4357. [CrossRef]
142. Yasumizu, Y.; Rajabi, H.; Jin, C.; Hata, T.; Pitroda, S.; Long, M.D.; Hagiwara, M.; Li, W.; Hu, Q.; Liu, S. MUC1-C regulates lineage plasticity driving progression to neuroendocrine prostate cancer. *Nat. Commun.* **2020**, *11*, 338. [CrossRef]
143. Shokraii, F.; Moharrami, M.; Motamed, N.; Shahhoseini, M.; Totonchi, M.; Ezzatizadeh, V.; Firouzi, J.; Khosravani, P.; Ebrahimi, M. Histone modification marks strongly regulate Cdh1 promoter in prostospheres as a model of prostate cancer stem like cells. *Cell J.* **2019**, *21*, 124.
144. Saha, S.K.; Jeong, Y.; Cho, S.; Cho, S.-G. Systematic expression alteration analysis of master reprogramming factor OCT4 and its three pseudogenes in human cancer and their prognostic outcomes. *Sci. Rep.* **2018**, *8*, 14806. [CrossRef]
145. Pacheco, M.B.; Camilo, V.; Henrique, R.; Jerónimo, C. Epigenetic editing in prostate cancer: Challenges and opportunities. *Epigenetics* **2022**, *17*, 564–588. [CrossRef]
146. Grillo, G.; Keshavarzian, T.; Linder, S.; Arlidge, C.; Mout, L.; Nand, A.; Teng, M.; Qamra, A.; Zhou, S.; Kron, K.J. Transposable elements are co-opted as oncogenic regulatory elements by lineage-specific transcription factors in prostate cancer. *Cancer Discov.* **2023**, *13*, 2470–2487. [CrossRef]
147. Kushwaha, P.P.; Verma, S.; Kumar, S.; Gupta, S. Role of prostate cancer stem-like cells in the development of antiandrogen resistance. *Cancer Drug Resist.* **2022**, *5*, 459. [CrossRef]
148. Escudero-Lourdes, C.; Alvarado-Morales, I.; Tokar, E.J. Stem cells as target for prostate cancer therapy: Opportunities and challenges. *Stem Cell Rev. Rep.* **2022**, *18*, 2833–2851. [CrossRef]
149. Verma, P.; Shukla, N.; Kumari, S.; Ansari, M.; Gautam, N.K.; Patel, G.K. Cancer stem cell in prostate cancer progression, metastasis and therapy resistance. *Biochim. Biophys. Acta (BBA)-Rev. Cancer* **2023**, *1878*, 188887.
150. Wolf, I.; Gratzke, C.; Wolf, P. Prostate cancer stem cells: Clinical aspects and targeted therapies. *Front. Oncol.* **2022**, *12*, 935715. [CrossRef]
151. Murakami, S.; Ninomiya, W.; Sakamoto, E.; Shibata, T.; Akiyama, H.; Tashiro, F. SRY and OCT4 are required for the acquisition of cancer stem cell-like properties and are potential differentiation therapy targets. *Stem Cells* **2015**, *33*, 2652–2663. [CrossRef]
152. Zhu, X.; Ding, C.-K.C.; Aggarwal, R.R. Emerging Therapeutic Targets of Neuroendocrine Prostate Cancer. *Curr. Oncol. Rep.* **2025**, *27*, 362–374. [CrossRef]

153. Agarwal, N.; Azad, A.; Carles, J.; Fay, A.P.; Matsubara, N.; Szczylik, C.; De Giorgi, U.; Joung, J.Y.; Fong, P.C.; Voog, E. Final overall survival (OS) with talazoparib (TALA)+ enzalutamide (ENZA) as first-line treatment in unselected patients with metastatic castration-resistant prostate cancer (mCRPC) in the phase 3 TALAPRO-2 trial. *Am. Soc. Clin. Oncol.* **2025**, *43*, 5. [CrossRef]
154. Ramesh, S.; Selvakumar, P.; Ameer, M.Y.; Lian, S.; Abdullah Alzarooni, A.I.M.; Ojha, S.; Mishra, A.; Tiwari, A.; Kaushik, A.; Jung, Y.D. State-of-the-art therapeutic strategies for targeting cancer stem cells in prostate cancer. *Front. Oncol.* **2023**, *13*, 1059441. [CrossRef]
155. Zhu, M.; Yu, X.; Zheng, Z.; Huang, J.; Yang, X.; Shi, H. Capsaicin suppressed activity of prostate cancer stem cells by inhibition of Wnt/β-catenin pathway. *Phytother. Res.* **2020**, *34*, 817–824. [CrossRef]
156. Zhu, J.; Qin, P.; Cao, C.; Dai, G.; Xu, L.; Yang, D. Use of miR-145 and testicular nuclear receptor 4 inhibition to reduce chemoresistance to docetaxel in prostate cancer. *Oncol. Rep.* **2021**, *45*, 963–974. [CrossRef]
157. Zhang, S. The mechanism of TR4 participate in prostate cancer metastasis and therapy. *Theor. Nat. Sci.* **2024**, *61*, 21–26.
158. Mehravar, M.; Ghaemimanesh, F.; Poursani, E.M. An overview on the complexity of OCT4: At the level of DNA, RNA and protein. *Stem Cell Rev. Rep.* **2021**, *17*, 1121–1136. [CrossRef]
159. Panayiotou, T.; Eftychiou, M.; Patera, E.; Promponas, V.J.; Strati, K. A paradigm for post-embryonic Oct4 re-expression: E7-induced hydroxymethylation regulates Oct4 expression in cervical cancer. *J. Med. Virol.* **2023**, *95*, e29264. [CrossRef]
160. Lei, M.M.L.; Lee, T.K.W. Cancer stem cells: Emerging key players in immune evasion of cancers. *Front. Cell Dev. Biol.* **2021**, *9*, 692940. [CrossRef]
161. Skvortsov, S.; Skvortsova, I.-I.; Tang, D.G.; Dubrovska, A. Concise review: Prostate cancer stem cells: Current understanding. *Stem Cells* **2018**, *36*, 1457–1474. [CrossRef]
162. Su, H.; Huang, L.; Zhou, J.; Yang, G. Prostate cancer stem cells and their targeted therapies. *Front. Cell Dev. Biol.* **2024**, *12*, 1410102. [CrossRef]
163. Deng, X.; Jiao, Y.; Hao, H.; Guo, Z.; An, G.; Zhang, W.; Xue, D.; Han, S. Dandelion extract suppresses the stem-like properties of triple-negative breast cancer cells by regulating CUEDC2/β-catenin/OCT4 signaling axis. *J. Ethnopharmacol.* **2025**, *342*, 119408. [CrossRef]
164. Lin, T.-C.; Wang, K.-H.; Chuang, K.-H.; Kao, A.-P.; Kuo, T.-C. Oct-4 induces cisplatin resistance and tumor stem cell-like properties in endometrial carcinoma cells. *Taiwan. J. Obstet. Gynecol.* **2023**, *62*, 16–21. [CrossRef]
165. Kasaju, M.; Mihailescu, M.-R. BPS2025-Investigation of miR-145-5p and FMRP binding to the 3′-UTR Oct4 mRNA G-quadruplex forming sequence. *Biophys. J.* **2025**, *124*, 87a. [CrossRef]
166. Zou, J.; Chen, J.; Deng, L.; Xu, B.; Yu, T.; Wang, J.; He, C. Mechanistic Insights into SENP1 and OCT4 Interaction in Promoting Drug Resistance and Stem Cell Features in Colon Cancer. *Am. J. Physiol.-Cell Physiol.* **2025**, *328*, C1260–C1278. [CrossRef]

biomedicines

MDPI

Review

Molecular Biomarkers of Glioma

Punsasi Rajakaruna [1,†], Stella Rios [1,†], Hana Elnahas [1,†], Ashley Villanueva [1], David Uribe [1], Sophia Leslie [1], Walaa A. Abbas [1], Larissa Barroso [1], Stephanie Oyervides [1], Michael Persans [1], Wendy Innis-Whitehouse [2] and Megan Keniry [1,*]

1 School of Integrative Biological and Chemical Sciences, The University of Texas Rio Grande Valley, 1201 W. University Dr., Edinburg, TX 78539, USA; punsasi.rajakaruna@utrgv.edu (P.R.); stella.rios01@utrgv.edu (S.R.); hana.elnahas01@utrgv.edu (H.E.); ashley.villanueva03@utrgv.edu (A.V.); david.uribe01@utrgv.edu (D.U.); sophia.leslie01@utrgv.edu (S.L.); walaa.abbas01@utrgv.edu (W.A.A.); larissa.barroso01@utrgv.edu (L.B.); stephanie.oyervides01@utrgv.edu (S.O.); michael.persans@utrgv.edu (M.P.)

2 Burrell College of Osteopathic Medicine, 3501 Arrowhead Dr, Las Cruces, NM 88001, USA; winnis@burrell.edu

* Correspondence: megan.keniry@utrgv.edu; Tel.: +956-665-7463

† These authors contributed equally to this work.

Abstract: In this review, we discuss how mutations in glioma are associated with prognosis and treatment efficacy. A fascinating characteristic of glioma and all cancers is that while common growth and developmental pathways are altered, the characteristic mutations are distinct depending on the specific type of tumor with concomitant prognoses. Next-generation sequencing, precision medicine, and artificial intelligence are boosting the employment of molecular biomarkers in cancer diagnosis and treatment. Understanding the biological underpinnings of distinct mutations on critical signaling pathways is crucial for developing novel therapies for glioma.

Keywords: glioma; glioblastoma; IDH; oligodendroglioma; astrocytoma

1. Introduction

Glioma encompasses many types of brain tumors originating from glial cells, such as astrocytes, oligodendrocytes, and ependymomas [1–3]. Glioblastoma accounts for 50% of primary, malignant brain tumors and has a median survival of 12–14 months [1]. Glioblastoma is highly infiltrative, invading neighboring structures, and vascularized [1]. Histologically related malignant brain tumors that harbor mutations in *IDH1*/*IDH2* were formerly described as glioblastoma, but since the 2021 World Health Organization classification of central nervous system tumors, they are now denoted as *IDH*-mutant astrocytoma (even if high-grade) or oligodendroglioma (*IDH*-mutant with 1p/19q co-deletion) [1–3]. This review discusses progress in developing glioma molecular biomarkers that inform prognosis and treatment strategies.

2. *IDH1* and *IDH2* Mutations Are Crucial Biomarkers for Glioma

A seismic shift in glioblastoma classification occurred based on the molecular biomarkers *IDH1* (*isocitrate dehydrogenase 1*) and *IDH2* (*isocitrate dehydrogenase 2*). Mutations in *IDH1*/*IDH2* (abbreviated *IDH*) were found in 10–12% of brain tumors that were histologically classified as glioblastoma [4,5]. The *IDH* mutations were associated with a much better prognosis than non-mutant *IDH* glioblastoma [4]. Mutations associated with *IDH1* and *IDH2* ultimately led to the reclassification of gliomas, changing them from being glioblastomas to astrocytomas (even if high grade) and oligodendrogliomas by the World Health Organization (WHO) in 2021 [1,3]. In the presence of *IDH* mutations, a hypermethylation phenotype is observed [6]. IDH1 normally catalyzes the conversion of isocitrate to alpha-ketoglutarate. The IDH1-R132H mutant protein catalyzes alpha-ketoglutarate conversion to D-2-hydroxyglutarate (D-2-HG) in an NADPH-dependent manner [7]. The accumulation of D-2-HG alters metabolism (such as the Krebs cycle and glycolysis) and blocks the demethylation of histones and nucleotides, resulting in the silencing of tumor suppressor genes and halting cellular differentiation [6,7]. Similar impacts on the Krebs cycle and gliomagenesis were found with *FH* and *SDH* mutations, as shown in Figure 1 [8,9].

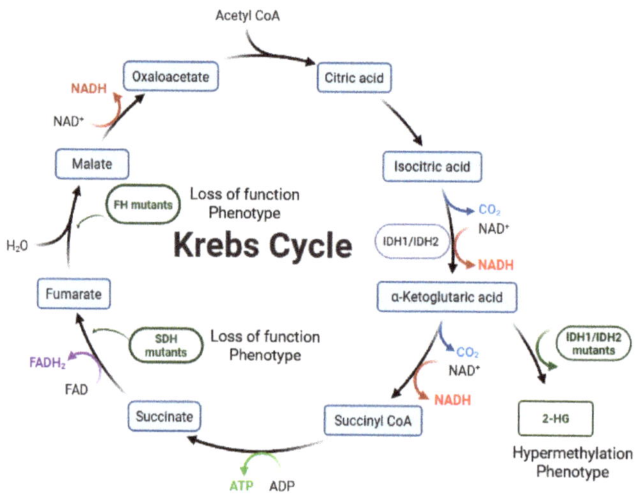

Figure 1. Krebs cycle mutations in glioma. *IDH1/IDH2* mutants convert α-Ketoglutarate to 2-Hydroxyglutarate (2-HG). Loss-of-function mutations in *Succinate Dehydrogenase* (*SDH*) and *Fumarate Hydratase* (*FH*) lead to the accumulation of succinate and fumarate, which inhibit JMJD demethylases to contribute to glioma oncogenesis [8,9].

2.1. The Frequency of IDH Mutations in Glioma

Mutations in the *IDH1* and *IDH2* genes are present in glioma at varying rates. In the cases analyzed, *IDH1* mutations were detected in 10–15%, and *IDH2* mutations were 1–5% [4,5,10]. Lower-grade gliomas, such as grades II and III, had a higher *IDH1/2* mutation frequency of 70–80% [4,5,10]. Alternatively, wildtype *IDH* (primary glioblastomas) showed a low occurrence of these mutations [11,12]. This significant difference highlights the important role that *IDH* mutations play in identifying distinct types of gliomas.

2.2. IDH Mutations Associated with Immature Glial Differentiation Programs

IDH mutations are found in younger patients and are associated with tumors with a specific genetic profile [13]. *IDH* mutations are typically of the proneural glioma subtype, associated with the glioma-CpG island methylator phenotype (G-CIMP) [6,14]. At a gene expression level, *IDH*-mutant gliomas harbor programs that resemble the recycling of early glial developmental programs, favoring either the early stages of astrocytic or oligodendrocyte cell fate specification [15,16]. Interestingly, single-cell sequencing revealed that very similar populations of cells were found in *IDH*-mutant astrocytoma (*IDH*-A) and oligodendroglioma (*IDH*-O). Both have a population of undifferentiated, proliferative stem-like cells, as well as non-proliferative populations resembling astrocyte and the oligodendrocyte lineages [15,16].

2.3. *IDH Mutation and Prognosis in Glioma*

Observations indicate that patients with *IDH* mutations have more extended survival periods than glioma patients with the wildtype *IDH* gene [4,14]. Yamauchi et al. (2018) describe the median progression-free survival (PFS) for *IDH* mutants as 4.7 years, with a 5-year life expectancy rate of 42%. In glioblastoma (without these mutations), patients had a PFS of 1.4 years and a 5-year life expectancy rate of 14% [17]. Metellus et al. (2010) indicated that *IDH* mutations were associated with prolonged patient survival and therapeutic response [18]. This finding shows that *IDH* mutation status is an essential predictor of glioma prognosis. Circulating cell-free DNA (cfDNA) can be used in liquid biopsies to detect *IDH1* mutations in glioma patients (especially *IDH1*-R132H) [19–22]. This mutational information has a significant impact on the tumor classification of oligodendroglioma, and of *IDH* mutant astrocytoma or glioblastoma with associated prognoses. The National Comprehensive Cancer Network (NCCN) considers *IDH* mutations important in assessing risks and treating gliomas. The NCCN recommends testing for these mutations as a standard diagnostic procedure [22]. Further studies on prognostic indicators in *IDH*-mutant glioma are underway. Recently, it was found that copy number variations and methylation changes were associated with deregulated miRNA expression in *IDH*-mutant glioma [23]. The knockdown of *miR-155-5p*, *miR-196a-5p*, *miR196b-5p*, *miR-200a-3p*, *miR-503-5p*, and *miR-15b-5p* significantly reduced the expression of immune evasion proteins PD-L1, CTLA4, and FOXP3 [23].

2.4. *Association Between Drug Efficacy and IDH Mutation*

There are multiple research avenues exploiting *IDH* mutations and drug efficacy. *IDH* mutants influence how tumors react to specific treatments [24–26]. Patients' responses to treatments with temozolomide (TMZ) change with the presence or absence of *IDH* mutations [24–26]. Although TMZ is an effective treatment for gliomas with *IDH* mutations, determining the best dosage to use and understanding the tumor response to TMZ is complex. New strategies that use TMZ in combination with other drugs may be needed for more effective outcomes [25]. This emphasizes that *IDH* mutation is a potential factor in tailoring patient treatment plans. *IDH* mutations are initial factors in glioma development, leading to the buildup of D-2-hydroxyglutarate (D-2-HG), which alters the energy usage of cells and affects DNA within cells. These are crucial factors in understanding how tumors behave and react to therapy [26].

The NOA16 clinical trial examined the *IDH1* peptide vaccine in patients with *IDH1*-R132H mutation; see Table 1. A 64% three-year progression-free survival (PFS) rate and an overall survival rate (OS) of 84% were reported, indicating the success of immunotherapy methods [27]. The *IDH* inhibitors, ivosidenib, which targets *IDH1*, and vorasidenib, which targets *IDH1* and *IDH2*, showed a favorable response in individuals with *IDH1*-mutant Grade IV astrocytoma; see Table 1 [27]. This suggests that targeted *IDH* inhibitors are valuable in treating specific tumors [24]. Research is ongoing about how *IDH* mutations affect survival. Further information is needed from ongoing clinical studies to draw more conclusions. As we gain knowledge about the molecular mechanisms behind these mutations, personalized treatment strategies and effective care for patients become more feasible.

Table 1. Biomarkers with associated drug treatments.

Biomarker	Drug Treatment
IDH	• IDH1 peptide vaccine [27]
	• IDH1 inhibitor ivosidenib [24]
	• IDH1/IDH2 inhibitor vorasidenib [24]
PTEN	• TMZ and poly (ADP-ribose) polymerase (PARP) inhibitors [28]
	• IFN-β/TMZ combination treatment [29]
	• Bcl-2 inhibitors (e.g., venetoclax, navitoclax, and sabutoclax) [30]
	• TNF-α treatment [31]
	• p110α inhibitors (e.g., Alpelisib; BYL719) [32]
PIK3CA	• EGFR inhibitor (AZD-9291), dual PI3K/mTOR inhibitor (GDC-0084) [33]
	• Pan-PI3K inhibitor (e.g., Buparlisib; BKM120 and Pilaralisib; XL147), p110α inhibitor (Alpelisib; BYL719), and dual PI3K/mTOR inhibitors (e.g., Dactolisib; NVP-BEZ235 and GDC-0084) [34]
	• PI3K inhibitor (GDC-0941) and MEK inhibitor (GDC-0973) [35]
	• Dual PI3K/mTOR inhibitors (BEZ235 and BKM120), MEK inhibitors (GSK1120212 and PD0325901) [36]
	• mTOR inhibitor (Everolimus), pan-PI3K inhibitor (e.g., BKM120, XL147, PX866, and GDC-0941), p110α inhibitor (such as BYL719), dual PI3K/mTOR inhibitor (such as BEZ235, XL765) [37]
PIK3R1	• AKT inhibitor (MK2206) [37,38]
	• PI3K inhibitors and a combination of PI3K and MAPK signaling inhibition [38]
	• [39] MEK inhibitors (PD0325901, AZD6244, GSK1120212B) and JNK inhibitors (SP600125 and BI78D3) [40]
EGFR	• Small molecule EGFR inhibitors: Afatinib, Dacomitinib, Osimertinib, Rociletinib, Gefitinib, Erlotinib, Lapatinib [41–43]
	• Monoclonal antibody to EGFR: Cetuximab [41–43]
NOTCH1	• Gamma secretase inhibitors: DAPT and MRK003 [44,45]

3. Molecular Markers on the PI3K Pathway in Glioma

The PI3K/AKT pathway is crucial in cell growth, survival, and metabolism. When bound by a ligand, receptor tyrosine kinases (RTKs) become activated, leading to a cascade of signaling events. Phosphatidylinositol 3-kinase (PI3K) becomes activated by RTKs, which then phosphorylates phosphatidylinositol (4,5)-bisphosphate (PIP2) to become the second messenger, phosphatidylinositol (3, 4, 5)-trisphosphate (PIP3) [4,5,46]. Afterward, PIP3 recruits AKT (protein kinase B) to the cellular membrane, which becomes phosphorylated and activated by phosphoinositide-dependent kinase, PDK1 [46,47].

The PI3K/AKT pathway promotes cellular growth and proliferation in part via the downstream mTOR complexes, mTORC1, and mTORC2. The activation of mTOR begins by the phosphorylation of tuberous sclerosis complex 2 (TSC2) by AKT, leading to cytosol sequestration [46,47]. This sequestration hinders the ability of TSC2 to interact with Rheb. Next, Rheb accumulates at the lysosome, which then activates mTORC1, allowing for the regulation of anabolic processes such as the synthesis of proteins, lipids, and nucleotides [46,47].

3.1. PTEN (Phosphatase and TENsin) Loss of Function Mutations in Glioblastoma

PTEN, or Phosphatase and TENsin homolog, is a tumor suppressor gene located on chromosome 10q23, encoding a dual specificity phosphatase (403 amino acids) that down-regulates the PI3K pathway by diminishing PIP3 [48]. PTEN induces apoptosis, hinders cancer proliferation, and promotes genomic stability [28]. In glioblastoma, *PTEN* mutations are frequently found in primary tumors, at approximately 32%, compared to secondary tumors (4%) [49,50]. Wang et al. analyzed 34 primary glioblastoma cases, observing *PTEN* mutations in 44% (15 out of 34) and 74% (25 out of 34), exhibiting LOH at the *PTEN* locus [25]. Additionally, 60% of primary glioblastomas that exhibited LOH carried a somatic *PTEN* mutation [51].

PTEN mutation is associated with the mesenchymal subtype of glioblastoma and a poor prognosis due to an increase in tumor aggressiveness, proliferation, and treatment resistance [52,53]. There is a significantly lower survival rate in patients who present with *PTEN* mutations (62.5% 36-week survival rate) compared to those who do not present (92.9% 36-week survival rate) [54]. The *PTEN* mutation incidence significantly differs between WHO Grade III and Grade IV glioma classifications ($p = 0.024$) [46]. *PTEN* null mutations induce the PI3K/AKT pathway, which can drastically reduce the efficacy of targeted treatments and chemotherapy [29]. Tumors with *PTEN* mutations respond less favorably to standard therapies such as TMZ [29].

Deficiency in *PTEN* disrupts cell cycle checkpoints, allowing damaged cells to mutate further and avoid apoptosis [29]. This disruption of cell cycle mechanisms contributes to treatment resistance [30]. The *BCL2* family regulates intrinsic apoptotic pathways and includes anti-apoptotic members, *BCL2*, *BCL-xL*, *MCL1*, and pro-apoptotic members, *BAX* and *BAK* [30]. *PTEN*-deficient cells with elevated levels of anti-apoptotic proteins, such as *BCL2*, resist TMZ-induced apoptosis [30,31].

Currently, *PTEN* mutations can be identified preoperatively via MRI. Through gene ontology analysis, researchers have discovered that radiomic signatures were significantly associated with processes commonly seen in *PTEN* mutations [51]. The transcriptome data of 64 patients obtained from the Cancer Genome Atlas were analyzed in a Pearson correlation test to select genes that were significantly related to radiomic signature—of which 200 genes were found to be significantly positively correlated [55]. The gene ontology analysis revealed that the radiomic signature was significantly associated with *PTEN*-related biological processes such as cell migration, cell motion, and anti-apoptotic [39]. These results imply that radiomic signatures can predict *PTEN* mutation status non-invasively, as the underlying genetic characteristics of the tumor can be reflected [56].

In another study, data from 244 glioma patients were collected from a local database (n = 77) and the Cancer Imaging Archive (n = 167), and they were randomly divided into a training set (n = 170) and a validation set (n = 74) [57]. Three models were developed to determine the prediction of *PTEN* mutations in patients: a convolutional neural network (CNN) model, a radiomics model, and an integrated model (radiomics and CNN) [57]. Of the three models, the integrated model showed the highest accuracy (86.5%) compared to the CNN (81.1%) and radiomics (66.2%) model [57].

PTEN mutations were detected via liquid biopsy through circulating cell-free DNA (cfDNA) and tumor DNA (tDNA) in GBM patients [58]. A total of 75 samples (25 GBM blood samples, 25 GBM tumor samples, and 25 healthy control blood samples) were studied; the cfDNA characteristics were compared between GBM patients and the control group [58]. *PTEN* mutations were found in 33% of tumor samples and 30% of cfDNA samples, suggesting that liquid biopsy could serve as a non-invasive diagnostic tool for GBM [58].

3.2. *PIK3CA-Activating Mutations in Glioma*

Phosphatidylinositol 3 Kinase (PI3K) is a heterodimer composed of a catalytic subunit, such as the *p110a* isoform, encoded by *PIK3CA*, which converts phosphatidylinositol 4,5 bisphosphate (PIP2) into phosphatidylinositol 3,4,5 trisphosphate (PIP3), and a regulatory subunit, p85, encoded by the *PIK3R1* (*phosphatidylinositol-4,5-bisphosphate 3-kinase regulatory subunit alpha*) gene. The regulatory subunit stabilizes the catalytic subunit and is critical for maintaining various cellular processes, including cell growth, survival, and proliferation. *PIK3CA* mutations have been reported in between 5 and 30%; this variation in the range can be attributed to different methodologies for analyzing mutation frequency in glioblastoma [32]. *PIK3CA* is mutated in hotspots on exons 10 and 21, encoding the constitutively active mutants H1047R, E542K, and E545K [32]. These activating mutations trigger an aberrant downstream signaling cascade of the AKT/mTOR pathway, which increases cell proliferation, survival, and contributes to oncogenesis.

Studies have shown that *PIK3CA* mutations are observed in tumors with concurrent mutations in the isocitrate dehydrogenase (*IDH1* and *IDH2*) genes [32]. *IDH*-mutant glioma had a mutation rate of 9% compared to *IDH* wildtype glioblastoma, which had a mutation rate of 3% [32]. *IDH1*-mutant glioma is associated with the proneural subtype and a better prognosis. *PIK3CA* mutations expressed in *IDH* wildtype tumors had shorter overall survival [32].

Mutations in *PIK3CA* contribute to resistance mechanisms via the β-catenin and Hedgehog signaling pathways [32]. The selective PI3K inhibitor Alpelisib is being investigated to deter constitutive *PIK3CA* mutations in cancer [33]. Additionally, combination therapies that target the PI3K/AKT pathway in conjunction with MEK or EGFR inhibitors can provide synergistic effects compared to monotherapies [33,34]. Preclinical studies combining PI3K and MEK inhibitors showed effectiveness in cancer models with *RAS* mutations in basal-like breast cancer. One study found synergistic effects in *K-RAS*-mutant cancer models with the PI3K inhibitor, GDC-0941, and the MEK inhibitor, GDC-0973. This synergistic effect is also reflected in glioblastoma models, where an orthotopic mouse model treated with both GDC-0941 and GDC-0973 displayed substantial tumor reduction [35,36]. Additionally, the combination of these inhibitors effectively targets critical components in the PI3K/AKT and EGFR/MEK/ERK pathways, resulting in enhanced apoptosis, reduced tumor growth, and bypassing compensatory activation. *PIK3CA*-mutant tumors treated with PI3K/AKT and EGFR/MEK/ERK dual inhibition displayed significant regression in experimental mouse models; see Table 1 [35,37].

Recently, researchers suggested that *PIK3CA* mutations can be detected preoperatively via dual-time-point [18F]FET PET/CT imaging [59]. Patients aged 18 and older suspected to have a primary brain tumor were recruited between June 2021 and January 2024 (n = 76) [59]. Of these patients, 51 had *IDH* wildtype glioblastoma, 13 had *IDH*-mutant astrocytoma, and 12 had *IDH*-mutant oligodendroglioma [59]. Of the 13 astrocytoma patients, 2 were classified as Grade II, 6 were classified as Grade III, and 5 were classified as Grade IV. In contrast, the oligodendroglioma patients were evenly distributed between Grades II and III [59]. Two PET/CT scans were performed after [18F]FET injection, the first 20 min post-injection and the second 80 min post-injection [59]. The maximum standardized uptake value (SUV) was measured for each scan, with results showing that patients with *PIK3CA* mutations had a significantly higher max SUV compared to patients with no mutations; the difference remained significant even after an adjustment for MRI enhancement, tumor grade, pathology type, and age [59].

Additionally, *PIK3CA* mutations can be detected through liquid biopsy [58]. Palande et al. found that *PIK3CA* mutations were detected in 9% of tumor samples and 7.8% of cfDNA samples [58]. These results offer a promising non-invasive method for preoperatively detecting *PIK3CA* mutation status in glioma patients.

3.3. *PIK3R1 Mutations in Glioblastoma*

PIK3R1 encodes alternatively spliced isoforms of the regulatory subunit involved in the Class IA PI3K lipid kinase heterodimer; p85a is the most commonly expressed regulatory subunit variant from the *PIK3R1* gene [60]. The p85a regulatory subunit associates with the catalytic subunit p110, encoded by *PIK3CA*, to stabilize and, to some degree, inhibit kinase activity, leading to a low level of PI3K pathway activity. In cancer, the p85a subunit is frequently reduced in expression or mutated, leading the catalytic subunit p110 to associate with another regulatory subunit p85b, encoded by the gene *PIK3R2*, leading to high levels of PI3K lipid kinase activity [60–63].

PIK3R1 mutation rates vary within the context of glioblastoma, but according to the Cancer Genome Atlas, the mutation frequency of *PIK3R1* in glioma is 9.9% [62]. Mutations in *PIK3R1* alter the regulatory subunit's ability to interact with p110α, resulting in aberrant hyperactivation of the AKT/mTOR signaling pathway, leading to uncontrolled cell growth and survival [60–62]. Within the iSH2 domain, mutations such as DKRMNS560del, R574fs, and T576del have been discovered to have a gain-of-function mutation, showing increased kinase activity of the PI3K complex, which results in increased independent phosphorylation of PIP2 to PIP3, activating AKT signaling [61]. Furthermore, truncating mutations, such as R348* and L370fs, can localize into the nucleus, activating other pathways, such as JNK, thus promoting tumor progression and bypassing apoptosis [38]. Additionally, loss-of-function mutations within *PIK3R1* have been shown to impair the inhibitory regulation of the catalytic subunit p110α and even disrupt the ability to stabilize *PTEN* [40,61]. Mutations such as E160* impair *PTEN* stability, resulting in hyperactivation of the AKT signaling pathway [40]. Research has found a connection between specific glioblastoma subtypes and *PIK3R1* mutations, with most observed in the mesenchymal subtype [64]. *IDH* wildtype gliomas have also shown a high frequency of *PIK3R1* mutations [65]. Mutations in *PIK3R1* are almost mutually exclusive with *PIK3CA* mutations and often coexist with other mutations, such as *TERT* promotor mutations and/or *PTEN* mutations [65].

PIK3R1 mutations are associated with poor prognosis due to their disruption of crucial signaling pathways, such as the PI3K/AKT pathway and Wnt/β-catenin [64]. These signaling pathways become hyperactivated, thus increasing tumor invasiveness and aggressiveness. Patients presenting with *PIK3R1* mutations often have poor progression-free survival (PFS) and OS [60]. One study that identified potential markers correlated to poor prognosis in diffuse glioma patients validated that patients presenting with a *PIK3R1* mutation had an overall poorer prognosis than individuals with *PIK3R1* wildtype tumors, with a median survival of 2.4 years and 5.4 years, respectively [60,66]. Another study found that *PIK3R1* mutation was associated with poor prognosis in the mesenchymal subtype of glioblastoma. These characteristics result from the *PIK3R1* mutation, leading to constitutive activation of PI3K signaling [64].

Studies have shown that tumors harboring *PIK3R1* mutations have an increased sensitivity to PI3K pathway inhibitors, such as the AKT inhibitor MK2206, as shown in Table 1 [61,62]. This increased sensitivity poses the potential to build on and create targeted therapeutic approaches. Furthermore, therapeutic combinations using PI3K inhibitors in conjunction with EGFR inhibitors have shown synergistic efficacy [61]. Overall, *PIK3R1* mutations trigger a hyperactive PI3K/AKT pathway, leading to increased cellular proliferation, resistance to apoptosis, and enhanced migration and invasion, allowing metastasis and tumor cells to invade surrounding tissues [67].

PIK3R1 mutations can be detected via liquid biopsy, as 7.8% of mutations were found in tumor samples and 7.0% were found in cfDNA samples [58]. Although these mutations were detected less frequently in comparison to *PTEN* and *PIK3CA* mutations, the detection rate of *PIK3R1* mutations was similar in both tumor and cfDNA samples (only a 0.8% difference), which implies that these mutations can be reliably detected when present in GBM patients [58].

4. Biomarkers on the RAS Pathway in Glioma

The RAS pathway is aberrantly activated by mutations in cancers, including glioblastoma [68]. The molecular circuitry of the RAS pathway includes the binding of ligands to receptor tyrosine kinases such as Epidermal Growth Factor Receptor (EGFR) or Platelet-Derived Growth Factor Receptor (PDGFR), which leads to GTP binding/activation of the G-protein RAS. RAS-GTP activates serine/threonine kinase BRAF, which phosphorylates MEK. Then, MEK phosphorylates MAPK kinases to promote growth, survival, and loss of contact inhibition to promote tumorigenesis [69]. RAS signaling also impacts the cytoskeleton and other targets, such as the PI3K pathway [70].

The mutation rates of RAS pathway components vary, depending on the gene. The three RAS encoding genes *N-RAS, H-RAS,* and *K-RAS* are mutated at a low frequency in glioblastoma (approximately 2% of cases) [71]. The occurrence of *BRAF* mutations is about 3% in adult glioblastoma [72,73]. *EGFR, NF1,* and *PDGFRA* mutations are more frequent in glioblastoma [74]. *EGFR* mutations are over-expressed in glioblastoma tumors (50–60% of the time) [74,75]. *PDGFRA* mutations are common in glioblastoma; one study found that 40% of glioblastomas had *PDGFRA* mutations [76]. *NF1* is mutated in approximately 13% of glioblastoma [55]. Interestingly, *ATRX* mutations are associated with Ras pathway mutations in glioblastoma; *ATRX* mutation is associated with a better prognosis [77].

RAS pathway mutants are differentially associated with glioblastoma subtypes. *EGFR* amplification/mutation is strongly associated with the classical subtype of glioma [14,41]. *NF1* mutations are primarily associated with the mesenchymal glioblastoma subtype [55,78], and *PDGFRA* is correlated with the proneural glioma subtype [14,79]. Additionally, *BRAF* mutations are common in epithelioid glioma [80–82].

There is evidence that *EGFR* amplification or mutation is associated with poor prognosis. *EFGR* amplification was detected by fluorescent in situ hybridization (FISH) [68]. To analyze the *EFGR* copy number status, SNP Array analysis was used by extracting high-molecular-weight genomic DNA from glioblastoma patients [68]. Patients with *EGFR* alteration had the shortest survival rate, supporting a contribution to poor prognosis [83]. *PDGFRA* was detected using next-generation sequencing (NGS) by extracting DNA from formalin-fixed paraffin-embedded (FFPE) tumor samples [69]. However, these results were obtained after they performed gross or subtotal tumor removal on 56 patients and partial tumor removal (PTR) or biopsy on 51 patients, including treating them with temozolomide during radiotherapy [69]. Their defined levels of biomarker gain were 3–5 copies, and amplification was greater than five copies [69]. The median overall survival of patients with and without *PDGFRA* gain-of-function mutations/amplification was 15.2 and 29.5 months, which showed a significantly improved prognosis for patients without the *PDGFR* gain-of-function mutations/amplification [84].

EGFR mutation and expression are crucial in drug efficacy for treating glioblastoma [42,85–87]. Studies have examined several small molecular kinase inhibitors and antibodies to target EGFR, including Afatinib, Dacomitinib, Osimertinib, Rociletinib, Gefitinib, Erlotinib, and Lapatinib, as well as the monoclonal antibody Cetuximab [42,86,87]. However, the main drawbacks of these drugs are that they cannot outcompete ATP, and the heterogeneity in *EGFR* mutations successfully affects their efficacy, feedback mechanisms, low specificity, and increases side effects (diarrhea) [78,86,87]. Researchers demonstrated that the expression of *PDGFRA* is associated with drug efficacy in treating glioblastoma [88]. The experiment was performed on *Nod.Scid.Il2rg*^{0} (NSG) mice using HIF1α inhibitor delivered by intracranial implantation [88].

BRAF and *NF1* mutations correlate with poor prognosis [89,90]. DCC 0.1.0 Software was used to detect circRNAs (cirBRAFs) obtained from the Illumina HiSeq Sequencer [87]. A protocol called Volcano Plot filtering was used to identify differentially expressed circRNAs [76]. *NF1* mutations were significantly associated with poor prognosis in glioblastoma [55,72]. In this investigation, researchers assembled a retrospective cohort of 542 *IDH*-wildtype GBM to study detected *NF1* mutations [37]. *NF1* immunohistochemistry was used to identify *NF1* alterations [37]. Two NF1 antibodies were used for this technique, which were NFC, Sigma-Aldrich, St. Louis, MO, USA (recognizes the last 281 amino acids of human neurofibromin), and iNF-07E, iNFixion (recognizes amino acids 863–867 of *NF1*) [37]. Bioscience combination therapies that target multiple steps of the RAS signaling pathway are under study to develop new interventions [91].

The Capicua Transcriptional Repressor as a Glioma Biomarker on the Ras Pathway

The Capicua transcriptional repressor (*CIC*) gene encodes for a large protein [92] that represses downstream RTK/RAS/ERK signaling [93]. The *CIC* gene is located at the cytoband 19q13.2 and encodes a high-mobility group-box transcriptional repressor. Under normal circumstances, the CIC protein represses proliferation genes [92,94]. *CIC* mutations lead to protein inactivation, which results in upregulation of the CIC target genes, activation of proliferative pathways, inhibition of differentiation, and a statistically significant poorer outcome in patients with co-deletion 1p/19q [92]. Chromosome 19q13.2 has somatic mutations, comprising insertions/deletions encompassing the *CIC* gene, which has been validated by deep sequencing in recurrent oligodendrogliomas [56].

A study researching *CIC* inactivating mutations sequenced DNA from 127 oligodendroglial tumors and found *CIC* mutations in 47% of the patients, with 59 out of 60 also having *IDH* mutations. It was also noted during this sequencing that chromosomes 4, 9p, and 10q were often lost [92]. Another study characterizing *CIC* mutations hypothesized that because *CIC* mutations were highly associated with *IDH* mutation, the hemizygous presentation of mutant *CIC* may be correlated with oligodendroglioma pathogenesis in *IDH* mutants [56]. NGS, IHC, and WTS studies performed on *CIC*-mutated formalin-fixed paraffin-embedded (FFPE) tissue samples showed that mutations in *CIC* resulted in an increased rate of 1p/19q co-deletion, *TERT* promoter mutations, *MGMT* promoter methylation, and deficient mismatch repair resulting in microsatellite instability [94]. The Catalogue of Somatic Mutations in Cancer (COSMIC) showed a total mutation rate of 7.69% of the *CIC* gene in all central nervous system cancers [95]. Most *CIC* mutations occur in the 1p/19q co-deletion, associated with a worse prognosis, but when disregarding the co-deletion cases, *CIC* mutations in astrocytoma and oligodendroglioma were 2% [56,92]. A study that classified glioma samples according to the 2021 WHO CNS5 criteria showed that *CIC* had a mutation rate of 52.1% in oligodendroglioma, 1.7% in astrocytoma, and 0.6% in glioblastoma [94].

A common form of mutation to the *CIC* gene is an unbalanced translocation resulting in the loss of one copy of chromosome 1p and 19q. This occurs in up to 80% of oligodendrogliomas and 15% of oligoastrocytomas. Most co-deleted gliomas are also mutated on *IDH1/IDH2*, which is associated with a better prognosis than *IDH* wildtype [92].

Work on Hs683 cells found that a *CIC* mutation resulted in a defect in the nuclear targeting of this protein [92]. These mutations occur homogeneously in the coding sequence and have been seen upstream and in the protein/protein interaction domain [92]. Most truncation mutations resulted in the loss of the nuclear localization sequence (NLS) and the C1 domain, with the rest only involving the loss or partial loss of the C1 domain.

Despite many advances in cancer treatment, glioma remains challenging to treat, partly due to its inherent characteristics, such as location and aggressiveness, but also because of the natural defense of the blood–brain barrier. Many researchers have begun to dissect molecular mechanisms and gene therapies that may bring a better prognosis. Some of these new research areas are non-invasive, such as radiomic techniques that blend magnetic resonance images with a program scanning 11 features that can predict *CIC* mutation in glioma with an accuracy of 94.2% at a 95% confidence interval [96]. Circulating tumor DNA (ctDNA) from patients' blood can also be evaluated for the *CIC* co-deletion biomarker with 55% sensitivity and 100% specificity via microsatellite analysis [97]. The standard of care for glioblastoma usually includes resection and treatment with TMZ, an alkylating agent [94]. Treatment with TMZ in patients with *CIC* mutation showed an increased median overall survival rate of 1874 days versus 602 days [94]. Besides the current treatment protocols, studies have shown that MEK/MAPK inhibitors are viable treatment options for malignancies with MAPK dysfunctions, such as gliomas with *CIC* mutations [94]. Trametinib, binimetinib, selumetinib, and cobimetinib are four inhibitors already approved for use in adult and pediatric solid tumors [94]. The observed degradation of CIC in RAS/ERK-driven tumors may increase ERK inhibitors' efficacy for treating glioma [93]. Another method of gene therapy targeting the deletion of the ERK binding interface for CIC stability in vivo may be a subject of further investigation for the extended survival of patients [93].

5. *TP53* as a Glioma Biomarker

The *Tumor Suppressor 53* (*TP53*) gene on chromosome 17 encodes the p53 protein. This gene is critical in controlling cell division, DNA repair, apoptosis (programmed cell death), and cell cycle arrest [98,99]. It is an important part of the regulatory network involved in tumorigenesis. It can be functionally categorized into several areas: stemness, cell metabolism, inflammatory responses, the tumor microenvironment, and the immune response [100].

Mutations in the *TP53* gene have been strongly linked to cancer cell proliferation and metastasis, with over 50% of human tumors expressing mutant *TP53* [98]. *TP53* mutations occur in approximately 30% of primary glioblastoma cases, 65–90% of secondary glioblastoma cases, and 46.7% of pediatric glioma cases [95,101]. Many of the mutations mentioned above occur in the DNA-binding domain, a prominent hotspot for *TP53* mutations [102].

TP53 mutation causes altered sensitivity to 27 known drugs, including MIRA-1, a drug that targets TP53 through the p53 pathway; Dabrafenib, which targets the protein kinase BRAF through the ERK MAPK signaling pathway [103], and Selumetinib, which targets MEK1 and MEK2 mitogen-activated protein kinases through the ERK MAPK signaling pathway [103].

The knockdown of mutated *TP53* in glioblastoma cells leads to a five-fold increase in chemosensitivity to the drug TMZ due to O^6-methyltransferase (MGMT) expression. Reduced expression of mutant *TP53* leads to decreased MGMT expression [104]. The IC_{50} of temozolomide in T98G cells was 575.32 μg/mL before mutant *TP53* silencing and 112.15 μg/mL after. In U138 cells, the IC_{50} was 510.79 μg/mL before knockdown and 127.79 μg/mL after [104]. Since MGMT counteracts the effects of TMZ by repairing TMZ-induced DNA damage, it can be concluded that the chemosensitivity of glioblastoma to TMZ decreases with mutant *TP53* and increases with the knockdown of mutant *TP53* [104]. In another study, Kaplan–Meier survival analysis of 512 glioma patients (248 with TP53 alterations, 264 without) showed that the *TP53* altered group had a shorter median survival of 79.99 months as compared to the *TP53* unaltered group with a median survival of 95.57 months, indicating that *TP53* alterations are associated with poorer overall survival [100]. *TP53* status is significantly associated with disease progression and patient survival in glioblastoma during radio- and chemotherapy [105,106].

TP53 mutation status is currently evaluated through blood tests, bone marrow tests, or tumor tissue biopsies and it can be incorporated into diagnostic panels for glioma classification. Although not yet widely implemented in liquid biopsy for glioma, *TP53* mutations are detectable in circulating tumor DNA in other cancers, suggesting future potential [107]. The WHO CNS5 recognizes *TP53* alterations as common in both primary and secondary glioblastoma, and *TP53* mutation status may impact therapeutic decision making, for example, regarding temozolomide sensitivity and clinical trial eligibility [3].

6. *LRP1B* Is a Key Tumor Suppressor in Glioma

The *LDL receptor-related protein 1B* (*LRP1B*) gene encodes a member of the low-density lipoprotein (LDL) receptor family [108]. LRP1B has a wide range of biological functions, from cargo transport to cell signaling. It is among the top 10 altered genes in human cancer, suggesting it plays a vital role as a tumor suppressor gene [108].

Inactivation of LRP1B promotes cell migration and invasion, primarily through the activation of the RhoA/Cdc42 signaling pathway or the upregulation of urokinase plasminogen activator receptor (uPAR), a receptor involved in extracellular matrix degradation [109]. This activation leads to the reorganization of the actin cytoskeleton, which is essential for cell movement. In glioblastoma, approximately 4% of cases harbor mutations in *LRP1B*.

Research indicates a strong link between *LRP1B* deletion and the development of glioma, particularly in patients with wildtype *IDH1/2* [110]. Studies reveal that 10% of *IDH1/2* wildtype glioblastoma tissues contain *LRP1B* deletions, significantly reducing expression in tumor samples compared to healthy tissue. *LRP1B* deletion has been strongly associated with poor prognosis in glioblastoma patients [109].

Furthermore, mutations in *LRP1B* are linked to altered sensitivity to specific chemotherapeutic drugs, including AZD4877, which targets EG5, and MK-1775, which inhibits WEE1 and PLK1 [102].

Although *LRP1B* mutations are not yet routinely evaluated in standard clinical practice, they can be identified through next-generation sequencing (NGS) panels performed on biopsy specimens. LRP1B's association with poor prognosis in *IDH*-wildtype glioblastoma shows its emerging potential as a prognostic biomarker and a possible therapeutic target for drugs.

7. The *SMARCB1* Gene as a Glioma Biomarker

The *SMARCB1* gene, also known as SWI/SNF (*SWItch/Sucrose Non-Fermentable-related Matrix-associated Actin-dependent Regulator of Chromatin subfamily B member 1*), encodes a protein subunit of the SWI/SNF protein complexes. These complexes regulate gene expression through chromatin remodeling [111]. This process alters nucleosome positioning on the DNA, affecting gene activity during expression.

SWI/SNF complexes participate in various cellular processes, including DNA repair, replication, and cell growth regulation. As a part of these complexes, the SMARCB1 protein is believed to function as a tumor suppressor, helping to prevent uncontrolled cell growth. Research indicates that SMARCB1 suppresses *CCND1* transcription and inhibits CDK 4/6 activity by binding to and recruiting HDAC in the G1 phase of the cell cycle, ultimately affecting cell cycle progression [112,113].

Although mutations in the *SMARCB1* gene are found in only 2–3% of glioblastoma cases, studies suggest these mutations are linked to an earlier disease onset [102,113]. This indicates that SMARCB1 may play a critical role in glioma's early development and presentation. Additionally, *SMARCB1* mutations are associated with altered sensitivity to one known drug, Axitinib, which targets receptors PDGFR, KIT, and VEGFR [95].

While the relationship between *SMARCB1* mutations and glioblastoma prognosis is not well researched, *SMARCB1* loss has been identified in several rare pediatric and adult cancers, termed *SMARCB1*-deficient cancers, most of which have a poor prognosis [114].

SMARCB1 mutations can also be detected using NGS assays on tumor tissue [115]. While SMARCB1 is not yet a formal requirement for glioma classification in WHO CNS5, a loss of SMARCB1 function is increasingly recognized in pediatric and early-onset gliomas [113]. It is being investigated as a marker for prognosis and therapeutic vulnerabilities, particularly for resistance mechanisms related to cell cycle regulation [116].

8. *TERT* Mutations Drive Telomerase in Glioma

Telomerase reverse transcriptase (*TERT*) is one of the top genes mutated in glioblastoma. Mutations in the promoter region of the *TERT* gene occur in 70–80% of all glioblastomas [117–119]. Higher-grade glioma tissues were seen to have more *TERT* mutations than low-grade glioma [117]. *TERT* promoter mutations result in a gain of function of TERT protein production, increasing telomere length and resulting in immortality due to the cell dividing but not undergoing senescence [120]. One study found that in 35 of the 37 glioblastoma cell lines studied, there was either a C228T or C250T promoter mutation [119]. These *TERT*-mutated cell lines had elevated levels of telomerase expression, but the amount of telomerase produced varied between cell lines [119]. Furthermore, in another study, in 55% of the 358 glioblastomas analyzed, *TERT* promoter mutations (C228T, C250T) were detected; of the 55%, 73% had a C228T mutation, and 27% had a C250T mutation; only one glioblastoma had both mutations [2]. Within that study, it was found that mutations in the *TERT* promoter occurred significantly more often in *IDH1* wildtype glioblastomas (187 out of 322; 58%) compared to *IDH1*-mutated gliomas (10 out of 36; 28%; $p = 0.0056$) [39,118].

Glioblastoma patients with *TERT* mutations had a shorter survival period and an overall poorer prognosis than those without the mutations. A study concluded that the *TERT* mut is an independent factor for poor prognosis [121]. In a study, 359 plasma samples were taken from 110 glioma patients, and by using droplet digital polymerase chain reaction (ddPCR), the DNA was isolated and analyzed for three key gene mutations, including *TERTp*. It was found that the *TERTp* C228T mutation was detected in 88% of the plasma ctDNA. Therefore, detecting *TERTp* by ddPCR demonstrates the potential use of the technique for glioma liquid biopsy, indicating a method of preoperational detection [122].

TERT may be a chemotherapeutic target for glioblastoma. Specifically, mycophenolic acid (MPA) is a known inhibitor of IMP dehydrogenase (IMPDH). The inhibition of IMPDH is a new target therapy for glioblastoma. MPA was found to lower TERT levels in both

U87MG and U251MG cell lines while also reducing O6-methylguanine-DNA methyltransferase (MGMT) expression in U251 cells [123]. Furthermore, MPA treatment resulted in a decline in telomere repeat numbers in both cell lines. Additionally, MPA induced a dose-dependent increase in p53 and CCCTC-binding factor (CTCF), both known to repress *TERT*, in U87MG and U251 cell lines [123].

9. *KMT2C* Gene Mutation and Glioma

The *Lysine Methyltransferase 2* (*KMT2C*) gene, which is known for mixed-lineage leukemia protein 3 (MLL3), mediates the histone methyltransferase activity of Histone H3 on lysine 4 (H3K4) [124]. It controls the regulation of gene expression and DNA accessibility with a strong association with epigenetic modifications [125]. Zhang et al. explored the role of *KMT2C* gene mutations at both the protein level and genetic alterations. They examined 171 genes encoding epigenetic modifier proteins from 283 lower-grade gliomas (LGG). Their findings showed that the *KMT2C* gene was one of the epigenetic modifier genes with mutations and frequent copy number alterations (11%) in lower-grade gliomas and a rare mutation frequency in primary glioblastoma (5%) [126]. Notably, *KMT2C* mutations have been identified in several aggressive cancer types with mutation frequencies, including prostate (6–9%), breast (12%), melanoma (45%), and colon cancer (14%) [124,127,128]. According to the Catalogue Of Somatic Mutations In Cancer (COSMIC), the *KMT2C* gene is mutated in 4% of glioblastomas [95]. In a recent study, the *KMT2C* gene was identified as mutated and was associated with cancer stem cells in four glioblastoma patients using comparative analysis and the exome sequencing [129]. The study was based on the genetic variants of the tumor core and peritumor tissue, and it indicates that the heterozygous indel was recognized at the chr7:151945071 position and was associated with p.Tyr816Ter [129].

Sarker et al. found that glioblastoma-mutated oncodriver receptor genes (derived from astrocyte-like neural stem cells) could be promising drug target candidates [130]. They examined several receptor genes across NCBI whole-exome sequencing (WES) profiles and CGGA databases. They found that the *KMT2C* gene was among the top 20 glioblastoma-mutated genes among other missense-mutated genes. Accordingly, it was defined as one of the 16 glioblastoma top-ranked oncodriver genes derived from the somatically mutated gene set [130]. The *KMT2C* mutations in glioblastoma disrupt DNA damage repair mechanisms, dysregulating genomic stability [131]. Wang et al. demonstrated that the knockout of the *KMT2* gene in urothelial carcinoma resulted in disrupted differentiation and genetic instability, which led to increased inflammatory signals and heightened oncogenic transformation [132].

10. *H3F3A* Is a Biomarker for Pediatric Glioma

The *H3F3A* is commonly mutated at two positions (K27M, G34R/G34V) in 31% of pediatric glioblastoma [133]. The H3F3A K27M-mutant pediatric glioblastoma is a distinct entity that transcends the established proneural/mesenchymal/classical adult glioma class. While adult gliomas are subtyped on these lines, with the proneural type having better prognosis and the mesenchymal type being therapy-resistant, pediatric H3K27M-mutant tumors are developing an emerging 'diffuse midline glioma' profile with admixed features from these classes [133].

H3K27M-mutant tumors have significantly poorer outcomes (12–15-month survival) compared to wildtype pediatric gliomas due to their unfavorable biology and drug resistance [134]. *H3K27M*-mutants are associated with altered H3K27me3 marks and PRC2 complex dysregulation [135]. *H3K27M*-mutant tumors are also resistant to conventional therapies due to their destabilized chromatin structure and stem-cell-like phenotype. Surprisingly, this subtype is differentially sensitive to targeted agents relative to adult gliomas or pediatric H3 wildtype tumors, and thus subtype-specific treatment is needed [136]. Due to the mechanistic complexity of H3F3A, a single treatment option is not recommended; instead, a combination of HDAC inhibitors and radiotherapy has shown promising results in clinical trials. Other clinical trials focus on other pathways like the dopamine receptor DRD2, which promotes tumor growth and stem cell phenotypes in *H3K27M* tumors.

H3F3A-mutated pediatric glioblastoma is mechanistically distinct from adult glioblastoma [137]. While adult glioblastoma resistance typically develops from *EGFR* amplification or *MGMT* promoter methylation, pediatric *H3K27M*-mutant tumors evade treatment by employing chromatin remodeling and disrupted developmental processes (e.g., PRC2 dysfunction) [138]. Individually, the *H3F3A* K27M mutation is a vital molecular biomarker of triple clinical significance: (1) it is a diagnostic subtype (diffuse midline glioma), (2) it predicts aggressive clinical behavior and dismal prognosis independent of histologic grade, and (3) it labels tumors with distinct therapeutic vulnerabilities through its epigenetic reprogramming effects [133,134,139,140].

11. Wnt Pathway as Glioma Biomarkers

11.1. The Wnt Pathway in Glioblastoma

The Wnt/β-catenin signaling pathway is integral to embryogenesis and tissue homeostasis [141]. Signaling permits the regulation of cell proliferation, migration, fate determination, and differentiation [142,143]. Evidence suggests that aberrant activation of this pathway encourages tumorigenesis [143,144].

β-catenin, encoded by *CTNNB1,* plays a dual role in cell maintenance by behaving as a key mediator in intracellular adhesion and an integral downstream regulator of the Wnt/β-catenin pathway [145]. In the presence of Wnt signaling, a Wnt ligand binds to a complex consisting of Frizzled and LRP5/6. Phosphorylation of LRP6 then leads to Disheveled protein recruitment [145]. This protein prevents the destruction complex, consisting of APC, AXIN, CKIa, and GSK-3β, from phosphorylating and ubiquitinating β-catenin. β-catenin can then propagate the cytoplasmic signal into the nucleus [145]. Within the nucleus, β-catenin works directly with transcription factors, such as TCF and LEF [145]. Without the Wnt ligand, the destruction complex phosphorylates β-catenin, which becomes ubiquitinated by SCF, leads to proteasomal degradation [145].

11.2. CTNNB1 Mutations Are Rare in Glioblastoma

CTNNB1 mutations are rare in glioblastoma, unlike other cancers [146]. Mutations in the *CTNNB1* oncogene are present in medulloblastoma, hepatocellular carcinoma, colon and ovarian cancers [147]. In previous studies, fifteen percent of cases analyzed underwent Wnt activation among medulloblastomas, and seventy-three percent of those cases had *CTNNB1* mutations [148]. According to the COSMIC catalog, all medulloblastoma patients displaying a *CTNNB1* mutation within their catalog underwent a missense substitution mutation at the gene [95]. Within the same catalog, out of 5793 hepatocellular carcinoma samples, 20% displayed *CTNNB1* mutations, out of which 83.78% experienced missense substitution mutations, as seen in medulloblastoma patients [95]. The prevalence of *CTNNB1* mutations and their manifestation as missense substitutions is a crucial to factor in when considering how this type of mutation leads to increased proliferation, immunosuppression, and metabolic regulation disruptions, indicating that *CTNNB1* has a role in tumorigenesis [147]. The upregulation of canonical Wnt pathway signaling is associated with mesenchymal glioblastoma, leading to a more motile and invasive behavior compared to proneural or classical subtypes [149,150].

11.3. Prognosis

β-catenin mutations promote poor prognosis in neural progenitor cells, based on previous studies on mice conducted by Chenn et al. in 2002 and Zechnar et al. in 2003 [151,152]. Within these studies, a constitutively activated β-catenin causes an increase in proliferative ability in mouse progenitor cells; meanwhile, deletion leads to a decrease in the same cells [153]. Additionally, in biopsies collected from 96 patients, immunohistochemical staining showed several Wnt pathway factors, such as β-catenin, to have protein levels with a positive correlation between the World Health Organization (WHO) glioma grading system and Karnofsky performance scale [154]. Therefore, β-catenin has been considered a potential biomarker in glioblastoma [155,156].

A study conducted by Nager et al. in 2017 found that inhibiting *CTNNB1* in human glioblastoma cell lines, U251MG and U87MG (through shRNA/siRNA), induced autophagy followed by apoptosis [146]. Through this study, it is evident that targeting the CTNNB1/TCF and autophagy pathways behaves as a potential therapeutic option, indicating the importance of β-catenin and, ultimately, *CTNNB1* in glioblastoma cell viability [146].

11.4. The Impact of the Wnt Pathway on Drug Efficacy in Glioblastoma

The blockade of the Wnt/β-catenin signal is an active area of research, as it was observed that inhibiting β-catenin in the glioblastoma cell lines, A172, U373, LN18, and LN229 leads to a decrease in the expression of genes associated with proliferation and differentiation. When glioblastoma cell lines were exposed to TMZ and the Wnt/β-catenin inhibitor LGK974, an increase in drug treatment efficacy was observed when compared to TMZ alone [157].

12. The NOTCH Pathway Is Commonly Activated in Glioma

The NOTCH signaling pathway is essential for cell differentiation, developing embryos, and tissue homeostasis [158]. The NOTCH pathway uses ligand receptors such as Delta-like-1 and subsequent NOTCH receptor cleavage to send the intracellular domain directly to the nucleus, influencing gene expression [158]. Mechanisms like negative feedback and ubiquitination tightly regulate the NOTCH pathway in a healthy context [158]. This cell-to-cell circuitry allows NOTCH signaling to control key developmental and homeostatic processes like cell maintenance and fate [159]. Notably, NOTCH dysregulation is seen across aggressive cancers such as breast, prostate, and pancreatic cancer, and melanoma [160]. In glioblastoma, NOTCH1 participates in mechanisms such as cell proliferation and increased vascularization [159]. Furthermore, *NOTCH1* mutations are found in approximately 8.5% of gliomas, with higher mutation frequencies in lower-grade gliomas [161,162]. NOTCH1 activation contributes to therapeutic resistance, at least in part, by activating the NFκβ pathway [163]. Moreover, upregulation of the NOTCH1 protein is seen in the clonal cells of glioblastoma, accentuating aggressive local tumor progression and distant relapse [146]. Mutation of *NOTCH1* was found to be associated with a shorter progression-free survival and local relapse in glioblastoma [164]. Current clinical trials include inhibitors of γ-secretase blocking NOTCH signaling [44,45]. Yet, mechanistic value is essential as signal blocking can lead to chemoresistance in some instances.

13. Future Directions

At the leading edge of glioma molecular subtyping are evolving omics approaches such as single-cell and spatial transcriptomics, moving quickly into spatial proteomics [15,164–167]. Transcriptional profiling of single cells and small groups of cells (approximately 50 μm in diameter) has allowed for the sophisticated visualization of glioblastoma tumor heterogeneity. Single-cell sequencing revealed four basic cell states in glioblastoma—neural progenitor-like (NPC), oligodendrocyte progenitor-like (OPC), astrocyte-like (AC), and mesenchymal-like (MES)—and three basic cell states for *IDH*-mutant gliomas: including astrocytic-like, oligodendrocyte-like and undifferentiated, stem cell-like [15,166]. The resolution of spatial transcriptomics is not yet at the single-cell stage but at the level of a small cluster of cells [165,167]. This allows for the investigation of cell–cell contacts within the tumor and with the tumor microenvironment. Proteomics are now also employed in concert with spatial transcriptomics to develop integrative, comprehensive models for how glioma tumors are organized (or not organized in some instances) and interact with the tumor microenvironment [165,167]. Hypoxia drove the organization of cellular states within a tumor in a gradient-like manner in glioblastoma tumors [165]. Hypoxia in glioblastoma is associated with therapeutic resistance and poor immune cell infiltration [168]. Understanding tumor organization, cellular plasticity, and heterogeneity will direct future therapeutic interventions.

14. Conclusions

Glioma accounts for 80% of malignant brain tumors and includes glioblastoma, *IDH*-mutant astrocytoma, oligodendroglioma, and ependymoma [1–3]. *IDH*-wildtype glioblastoma is associated with poor prognosis (median survival of 14 months) and *PTEN*, *TP53*, *TERT*, *EGFR*, and *PIK3R1* mutations, as shown in Figure 2 [11,31,39,49,50,60,61,75,83,85,99,100,104,117–119,121]. Glioblastoma commonly harbors activated PI3K, RAS, Wnt, and NOTCH pathways that drive the highly aggressive phenotype [37,71,147,150,153,163,169,170]. *IDH*-mutant astrocytoma and oligodendroglioma are associated with a better prognosis than glioblastoma, with a median survival of 5–10 years [5,14,18]. *IDH*-mutant gliomas commonly harbor mutations in *PIK3CA*, *TP53*, *CIC*, and 1p/19q co-deletion, Figure 2 [32,56,92]. *IDH*-mutant gliomas have seen promising developments in therapeutics, including the NOA16 phase I clinical trial that employed an IDH1-R132H peptide vaccine that showed strong immunogenicity [25,27]. Although all gliomas are derived from glial cells, these cancers have distinct biomarkers that inform prognosis and therapeutic strategies. Molecular biomarkers for glioma continue to be identified and will be critical in tumor stratification to devise precision therapeutics.

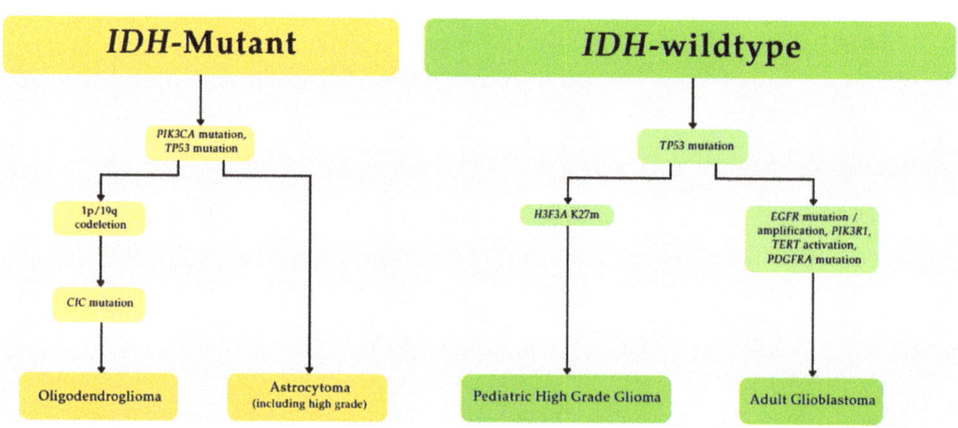

Figure 2. Glioma characteristics associated with *IDH*-mutation status. A flow chart highlights mutations observed in *IDH*-mutant and wildtype gliomas.

Funding: This work was supported by NIH 1R16GM153687-01 (M.K.), UTRGV Presidential Research Fellowship (S.R.) and UTRGV Dean's Scholarship (S.O.).

Acknowledgments: The authors would like to thank Members of the Keniry Laboratory, the UTRGV School of Integrative Biological and Chemical Sciences, the UTRGV School of Mechanical Engineering, the UTRGV College of Engineering, and the UTRGV College of Sciences for their support, reagents, and expertise.

Conflicts of Interest: The authors declare no conflicts of interest.

References

1. Ostrom, Q.T.; Price, M.; Neff, C.; Cioffi, G.; Waite, K.A.; Kruchko, C.; Barnholtz-Sloan, J.S. CBTRUS Statistical Report: Primary Brain and Other Central Nervous System Tumors Diagnosed in the United States in 2016–2020. *Neuro Oncol.* **2023**, *25*, iv1–iv99. [CrossRef] [PubMed]
2. Price, M.; Neff, C.; Nagarajan, N.; Kruchko, C.; Waite, K.A.; Cioffi, G.; Cordeiro, B.B.; Willmarth, N.; Penas-Prado, M.; Gilbert, M.R.; et al. CBTRUS Statistical Report: American Brain Tumor Association & NCI Neuro-Oncology Branch Adolescent and Young Adult Primary Brain and Other Central Nervous System Tumors Diagnosed in the United States in 2016–2020. *Neuro Oncol.* **2024**, *26*, iii1–iii53. [CrossRef] [PubMed]
3. Louis, D.N.; Perry, A.; Wesseling, P.; Brat, D.J.; Cree, I.A.; Figarella-Branger, D.; Hawkins, C.; Ng, H.K.; Pfister, S.M.; Reifenberger, G.; et al. The 2021 WHO Classification of Tumors of the Central Nervous System: A summary. *Neuro Oncol.* **2021**, *23*, 1231–1251. [CrossRef]
4. Parsons, D.W.; Jones, S.; Zhang, X.; Lin, J.C.; Leary, R.J.; Angenendt, P.; Mankoo, P.; Carter, H.; Siu, I.M.; Gallia, G.L.; et al. An integrated genomic analysis of human glioblastoma multiforme. *Science* **2008**, *321*, 1807–1812. [CrossRef] [PubMed]
5. Balss, J.; Meyer, J.; Mueller, W.; Korshunov, A.; Hartmann, C.; von Deimling, A. Analysis of the IDH1 codon 132 mutation in brain tumors. *Acta Neuropathol.* **2008**, *116*, 597–602. [CrossRef]
6. Noushmehr, H.; Weisenberger, D.J.; Diefes, K.; Phillips, H.S.; Pujara, K.; Berman, B.P.; Pan, F.; Pelloski, C.E.; Sulman, E.P.; Bhat, K.P.; et al. Identification of a CpG island methylator phenotype that defines a distinct subgroup of glioma. *Cancer Cell* **2010**, *17*, 510–522. [CrossRef]
7. Han, S.; Liu, Y.; Cai, S.J.; Qian, M.; Ding, J.; Larion, M.; Gilbert, M.R.; Yang, C. IDH mutation in glioma: Molecular mechanisms and potential therapeutic targets. *Br. J. Cancer* **2020**, *122*, 1580–1589. [CrossRef]
8. Sciacovelli, M.; Goncalves, E.; Johnson, T.I.; Zecchini, V.R.; da Costa, A.S.; Gaude, E.; Drubbel, A.V.; Theobald, S.J.; Abbo, S.R.; Tran, M.G.; et al. Fumarate is an epigenetic modifier that elicits epithelial-to-mesenchymal transition. *Nature* **2016**, *537*, 544–547. [CrossRef]
9. Killian, J.K.; Kim, S.Y.; Miettinen, M.; Smith, C.; Merino, M.; Tsokos, M.; Quezado, M.; Smith, W.I., Jr.; Jahromi, M.S.; Xekouki, P.; et al. Succinate dehydrogenase mutation underlies global epigenomic divergence in gastrointestinal stromal tumor. *Cancer Discov.* **2013**, *3*, 648–657. [CrossRef]
10. Cho, U.; Yang, S.H.; Yoo, C. Estimation of the occurrence rates of IDH1 and IDH2 mutations in gliomas and the reconsideration of IDH-wildtype anaplastic astrocytomas: An institutional experience. *J. Int. Med. Res.* **2021**, *49*, 3000605211019258. [CrossRef]
11. Stancheva, G.; Goranova, T.; Laleva, M.; Kamenova, M.; Mitkova, A.; Velinov, N.; Poptodorov, G.; Mitev, V.; Kaneva, R.; Gabrovsky, N. IDH1/IDH2 but not TP53 mutations predict prognosis in Bulgarian glioblastoma patients. *Biomed. Res. Int.* **2014**, *2014*, 654727. [CrossRef] [PubMed]
12. Weller, M.; Wick, W.; Aldape, K.; Brada, M.; Berger, M.; Pfister, S.M.; Nishikawa, R.; Rosenthal, M.; Wen, P.Y.; Stupp, R.; et al. Glioma. *Nat. Rev. Dis. Primers* **2015**, *1*, 15017. [CrossRef]
13. Krell, D.; Assoku, M.; Galloway, M.; Mulholland, P.; Tomlinson, I.; Bardella, C. Screen for IDH1, IDH2, IDH3, D2HGDH and L2HGDH mutations in glioblastoma. *PLoS ONE* **2011**, *6*, e19868. [CrossRef] [PubMed]
14. Verhaak, R.G.; Hoadley, K.A.; Purdom, E.; Wang, V.; Qi, Y.; Wilkerson, M.D.; Miller, C.R.; Ding, L.; Golub, T.; Mesirov, J.P.; et al. Integrated genomic analysis identifies clinically relevant subtypes of glioblastoma characterized by abnormalities in PDGFRA, IDH1, EGFR, and NF1. *Cancer Cell* **2010**, *17*, 98–110. [CrossRef] [PubMed]
15. Venteicher, A.S.; Tirosh, I.; Hebert, C.; Yizhak, K.; Neftel, C.; Filbin, M.G.; Hovestadt, V.; Escalante, L.E.; Shaw, M.L.; Rodman, C.; et al. Decoupling genetics, lineages, and microenvironment in IDH-mutant gliomas by single-cell RNA-seq. *Science* **2017**, *355*, eaai8478. [CrossRef]
16. Glasgow, S.M.; Carlson, J.C.; Zhu, W.; Chaboub, L.S.; Kang, P.; Lee, H.K.; Clovis, Y.M.; Lozzi, B.E.; McEvilly, R.J.; Rosenfeld, M.G.; et al. Glia-specific enhancers and chromatin structure regulate NFIA expression and glioma tumorigenesis. *Nat. Neurosci.* **2017**, *20*, 1520–1528. [CrossRef]

17. Yamauchi, T.; Ohno, M.; Matsushita, Y.; Takahashi, M.; Miyakita, Y.; Kitagawa, Y.; Kondo, E.; Tsushita, N.; Satomi, K.; Yoshida, A.; et al. Radiological characteristics based on isocitrate dehydrogenase mutations and 1p/19q codeletion in grade II and III gliomas. *Brain Tumor Pathol.* **2018**, *35*, 148–158. [CrossRef]
18. Metellus, P.; Coulibaly, B.; Colin, C.; de Paula, A.M.; Vasiljevic, A.; Taieb, D.; Barlier, A.; Boisselier, B.; Mokhtari, K.; Wang, X.W.; et al. Absence of IDH mutation identifies a novel radiologic and molecular subtype of WHO grade II gliomas with dismal prognosis. *Acta Neuropathol.* **2010**, *120*, 719–729. [CrossRef]
19. Cabezas-Camarero, S.; Garcia-Barberan, V.; Perez-Alfayate, R.; Casado-Farinas, I.; Sloane, H.; Jones, F.S.; Perez-Segura, P. Detection of IDH1 Mutations in Plasma Using BEAMing Technology in Patients with Gliomas. *Cancers* **2022**, *14*, 2891. [CrossRef]
20. Gatto, L.; Franceschi, E.; Di Nunno, V.; Tosoni, A.; Lodi, R.; Brandes, A.A. Liquid Biopsy in Glioblastoma Management: From Current Research to Future Perspectives. *Oncologist* **2021**, *26*, 865–878. [CrossRef]
21. Choate, K.A.; Pratt, E.P.S.; Jennings, M.J.; Winn, R.J.; Mann, P.B. IDH Mutations in Glioma: Molecular, Cellular, Diagnostic, and Clinical Implications. *Biology* **2024**, *13*, 885. [CrossRef] [PubMed]
22. Nathan, D.I.; Brander, T.; Gold, J.; Paul, D.; Klein, P.; Cheng, K.; Liu, J.M.; Marcellino, B.K. Diagnostic and Practical Challenges in Applying National Comprehensive Cancer Network Guidelines for Suspected Pathogenic TP53 Mosaicism. *JCO Precis. Oncol.* **2024**, *8*, e2400006. [CrossRef]
23. Yang, Z.; Liu, X.; Xu, H.; Teschendorff, A.E.; Xu, L.; Li, J.; Fu, M.; Liu, J.; Zhou, H.; Wang, Y.; et al. Integrative analysis of genomic and epigenomic regulation reveals miRNA mediated tumor heterogeneity and immune evasion in lower grade glioma. *Commun. Biol.* **2024**, *7*, 824. [CrossRef]
24. Sharma, N.; Mallela, A.N.; Shi, D.D.; Tang, L.W.; Abou-Al-Shaar, H.; Gersey, Z.C.; Zhang, X.; McBrayer, S.K.; Abdullah, K.G. Isocitrate dehydrogenase mutations in gliomas: A review of current understanding and trials. *Neurooncol. Adv.* **2023**, *5*, vdad053. [CrossRef]
25. Sun, X.; Turcan, S. From Laboratory Studies to Clinical Trials: Temozolomide Use in IDH-Mutant Gliomas. *Cells* **2021**, *10*, 1225. [CrossRef]
26. Turkalp, Z.; Karamchandani, J.; Das, S. IDH mutation in glioma: New insights and promises for the future. *JAMA Neurol.* **2014**, *71*, 1319–1325. [CrossRef] [PubMed]
27. Platten, M.; Bunse, L.; Wick, A.; Bunse, T.; Le Cornet, L.; Harting, I.; Sahm, F.; Sanghvi, K.; Tan, C.L.; Poschke, I.; et al. A vaccine targeting mutant IDH1 in newly diagnosed glioma. *Nature* **2021**, *592*, 463–468. [CrossRef]
28. Milella, M.; Falcone, I.; Conciatori, F.; Cesta Incani, U.; Del Curatolo, A.; Inzerilli, N.; Nuzzo, C.M.; Vaccaro, V.; Vari, S.; Cognetti, F.; et al. PTEN: Multiple Functions in Human Malignant Tumors. *Front. Oncol.* **2015**, *5*, 24. [CrossRef] [PubMed]
29. Cetintas, V.B.; Batada, N.N. Is there a causal link between PTEN deficient tumors and immunosuppressive tumor microenvironment? *J. Transl. Med.* **2020**, *18*, 45. [CrossRef]
30. D'Aguanno, S.; Del Bufalo, D. Inhibition of Anti-Apoptotic Bcl-2 Proteins in Preclinical and Clinical Studies: Current Overview in Cancer. *Cells* **2020**, *9*, 1287. [CrossRef]
31. Koul, D.; Takada, Y.; Shen, R.; Aggarwal, B.B.; Yung, W.K. PTEN enhances TNF-induced apoptosis through modulation of nuclear factor-kappaB signaling pathway in human glioma cells. *Biochem. Biophys. Res. Commun.* **2006**, *350*, 463–471. [CrossRef]
32. Brito, C.; Tomas, A.; Azevedo, A.; Esteves, S.; Mafra, M.; Roque, L.; Pojo, M. PIK3CA Mutations in Diffuse Gliomas: An Update on Molecular Stratification, Prognosis, Recurrence, and Aggressiveness. *Clin. Med. Insights Oncol.* **2022**, *16*, 11795549211068804. [CrossRef] [PubMed]
33. Guo, T.; Wu, C.; Zhang, J.; Yu, J.; Li, G.; Jiang, H.; Zhang, X.; Yu, R.; Liu, X. Dual blockade of EGFR and PI3K signaling pathways offers a therapeutic strategy for glioblastoma. *Cell Commun. Signal.* **2023**, *21*, 363. [CrossRef] [PubMed]
34. Zhao, H.-F.; Wang, J.; Shao, W.; Wu, C.-P.; Chen, Z.-P.; To, S.-S.T.; Li, W.-P. Recent advances in the use of PI3K inhibitors for glioblastoma multiforme: Current preclinical and clinical development. *Mol. Cancer* **2017**, *16*, 100. [CrossRef]
35. Choo, E.F.; Ng, C.M.; Berry, L.; Belvin, M.; Lewin-Koh, N.; Merchant, M.; Salphati, L. PK-PD modeling of combination efficacy effect from administration of the MEK inhibitor GDC-0973 and PI3K inhibitor GDC-0941 in A2058 xenografts. *Cancer Chemother. Pharmacol.* **2013**, *71*, 133–143. [CrossRef] [PubMed]
36. El Meskini, R.; Iacovelli, A.J.; Kulaga, A.; Gumprecht, M.; Martin, P.L.; Baran, M.; Householder, D.B.; Van Dyke, T.; Weaver Ohler, Z. A preclinical orthotopic model for glioblastoma recapitulates key features of human tumors and demonstrates sensitivity to a combination of MEK and PI3K pathway inhibitors. *Dis. Model Mech.* **2015**, *8*, 45–56. [CrossRef]
37. Wen, P.Y.; Lee, E.Q.; Reardon, D.A.; Ligon, K.L.; Alfred Yung, W.K. Current clinical development of PI3K pathway inhibitors in glioblastoma. *Neuro Oncol.* **2012**, *14*, 819–829. [CrossRef] [PubMed]
38. Cheung, L.W.; Mills, G.B. Targeting therapeutic liabilities engendered by PIK3R1 mutations for cancer treatment. *Pharmacogenomics* **2016**, *17*, 297–307. [CrossRef]

39. Nonoguchi, N.; Ohta, T.; Oh, J.E.; Kim, Y.H.; Kleihues, P.; Ohgaki, H. TERT promoter mutations in primary and secondary glioblastomas. *Acta Neuropathol.* **2013**, *126*, 931–937. [CrossRef]
40. Cheung, L.W.; Yu, S.; Zhang, D.; Li, J.; Ng, P.K.; Panupinthu, N.; Mitra, S.; Ju, Z.; Yu, Q.; Liang, H.; et al. Naturally occurring neomorphic PIK3R1 mutations activate the MAPK pathway, dictating therapeutic response to MAPK pathway inhibitors. *Cancer Cell* **2014**, *26*, 479–494. [CrossRef]
41. Rodriguez, S.M.B.; Kamel, A.; Ciubotaru, G.V.; Onose, G.; Sevastre, A.S.; Sfredel, V.; Danoiu, S.; Dricu, A.; Tataranu, L.G. An Overview of EGFR Mechanisms and Their Implications in Targeted Therapies for Glioblastoma. *Int. J. Mol. Sci.* **2023**, *24*, 11110. [CrossRef] [PubMed]
42. Eskilsson, E.; Rosland, G.V.; Solecki, G.; Wang, Q.; Harter, P.N.; Graziani, G.; Verhaak, R.G.W.; Winkler, F.; Bjerkvig, R.; Miletic, H. EGFR heterogeneity and implications for therapeutic intervention in glioblastoma. *Neuro Oncol.* **2018**, *20*, 743–752. [CrossRef]
43. Rios, S.A.; Oyervides, S.; Uribe, D.; Reyes, A.M.; Fanniel, V.; Vazquez, J.; Keniry, M. Emerging Therapies for Glioblastoma. *Cancers* **2024**, *16*, 1485. [CrossRef]
44. Zou, Y.; Cao, Y.; Yue, Z.; Liu, J. Gamma-secretase inhibitor DAPT suppresses glioblastoma growth via uncoupling of tumor vessel density from vessel function. *Clin. Exp. Med.* **2013**, *13*, 271–278. [CrossRef]
45. Tanaka, S.; Nakada, M.; Yamada, D.; Nakano, I.; Todo, T.; Ino, Y.; Hoshii, T.; Tadokoro, Y.; Ohta, K.; Ali, M.A.; et al. Strong therapeutic potential of gamma-secretase inhibitor MRK003 for CD44-high and CD133-low glioblastoma initiating cells. *J. Neurooncol.* **2015**, *121*, 239–250. [CrossRef]
46. Fruman, D.A.; Chiu, H.; Hopkins, B.D.; Bagrodia, S.; Cantley, L.C.; Abraham, R.T. The PI3K Pathway in Human Disease. *Cell* **2017**, *170*, 605–635. [CrossRef]
47. Glaviano, A.; Foo, A.S.C.; Lam, H.Y.; Yap, K.C.H.; Jacot, W.; Jones, R.H.; Eng, H.; Nair, M.G.; Makvandi, P.; Geoerger, B.; et al. PI3K/AKT/mTOR signaling transduction pathway and targeted therapies in cancer. *Mol. Cancer* **2023**, *22*, 138. [CrossRef] [PubMed]
48. Cantley, L.C.; Neel, B.G. New insights into tumor suppression: PTEN suppresses tumor formation by restraining the phosphoinositide 3-kinase/AKT pathway. *Proc. Natl. Acad. Sci. USA* **1999**, *96*, 4240–4245. [CrossRef] [PubMed]
49. Tohma, Y.; Gratas, C.; Biernat, W.; Peraud, A.; Fukuda, M.; Yonekawa, Y.; Kleihues, P.; Ohgaki, H. PTEN (MMAC1) mutations are frequent in primary glioblastomas (de novo) but not in secondary glioblastomas. *J. Neuropathol. Exp. Neurol.* **1998**, *57*, 684–689. [CrossRef]
50. Wang, S.I.; Puc, J.; Li, J.; Bruce, J.N.; Cairns, P.; Sidransky, D.; Parsons, R. Somatic mutations of PTEN in glioblastoma multiforme. *Cancer Res.* **1997**, *57*, 4183–4186.
51. Li, Y.; Liang, Y.; Sun, Z.; Xu, K.; Fan, X.; Li, S.; Zhang, Z.; Jiang, T.; Liu, X.; Wang, Y. Radiogenomic analysis of PTEN mutation in glioblastoma using preoperative multi-parametric magnetic resonance imaging. *Neuroradiology* **2019**, *61*, 1229–1237. [CrossRef] [PubMed]
52. Han, F.; Hu, R.; Yang, H.; Liu, J.; Sui, J.; Xiang, X.; Wang, F.; Chu, L.; Song, S. PTEN gene mutations correlate to poor prognosis in glioma patients: A meta-analysis. *Onco Targets Ther.* **2016**, *9*, 3485–3492. [CrossRef] [PubMed]
53. Pan, Y.B.; Wang, S.; Yang, B.; Jiang, Z.; Lenahan, C.; Wang, J.; Zhang, J.; Shao, A. Transcriptome analyses reveal molecular mechanisms underlying phenotypic differences among transcriptional subtypes of glioblastoma. *J. Cell. Mol. Med.* **2020**, *24*, 3901–3916. [CrossRef]
54. Yang, Y.; Shan, N.; Luo, G.; Li, L.; Zheng, L.; Nilsson-Ehle, P.; Xu, N. Mutations of PTEN Gene in Gliomas Correlate to Tumor Differentiation and Short-term Survival Rate. *Anticancer Res.* **2010**, *30*, 981–985.
55. Scheer, M.; Leisz, S.; Sorge, E.; Storozhuk, O.; Prell, J.; Ho, I.; Harder, A. Neurofibromatosis Type 1 Gene Alterations Define Specific Features of a Subset of Glioblastomas. *Int. J. Mol. Sci.* **2021**, *23*, 352. [CrossRef] [PubMed]
56. Yip, S.; Butterfield, Y.S.; Morozova, O.; Chittaranjan, S.; Blough, M.D.; An, J.; Birol, I.; Chesnelong, C.; Chiu, R.; Chuah, E.; et al. Concurrent CIC mutations, IDH mutations, and 1p/19q loss distinguish oligodendrogliomas from other cancers. *J. Pathol.* **2012**, *226*, 7–16. [CrossRef]
57. Chen, H.; Lin, F.; Zhang, J.; Lv, X.; Zhou, J.; Li, Z.C.; Chen, Y. Deep Learning Radiomics to Predict PTEN Mutation Status From Magnetic Resonance Imaging in Patients with Glioma. *Front. Oncol.* **2021**, *11*, 734433. [CrossRef]
58. Palande, V.; Siegal, T.; Detroja, R.; Gorohovski, A.; Glass, R.; Flueh, C.; Kanner, A.A.; Laviv, Y.; Har-Nof, S.; Levy-Barda, A.; et al. Detection of gene mutations and gene-gene fusions in circulating cell-free DNA of glioblastoma patients: An avenue for clinically relevant diagnostic analysis. *Mol. Oncol.* **2022**, *16*, 2098–2114. [CrossRef]
59. Lee, D.Y.; Oh, J.S.; Kim, J.W.; Oh, M.; Oh, S.J.; Lee, S.; Kim, Y.H.; Kim, J.H.; Nam, S.J.; Song, S.W.; et al. Pre-operative dual-time-point [(18)F]FET PET differentiates CDKN2A/B loss and PIK3CA mutation status in adult-type diffuse glioma: A single-center prospective study. *Eur. J. Nucl. Med. Mol. Imaging* **2025**, *52*, 669–682. [CrossRef]

60. Weber, G.L.; Parat, M.O.; Binder, Z.A.; Gallia, G.L.; Riggins, G.J. Abrogation of PIK3CA or PIK3R1 reduces proliferation, migration, and invasion in glioblastoma multiforme cells. *Oncotarget* **2011**, *2*, 833–849. [CrossRef]
61. Quayle, S.N.; Lee, J.Y.; Cheung, L.W.; Ding, L.; Wiedemeyer, R.; Dewan, R.W.; Huang-Hobbs, E.; Zhuang, L.; Wilson, R.K.; Ligon, K.L.; et al. Somatic mutations of PIK3R1 promote gliomagenesis. *PLoS ONE* **2012**, *7*, e49466. [CrossRef] [PubMed]
62. Park, S.W.; Kang, M.R.; Eom, H.S.; Han, J.Y.; Ahn, C.H.; Kim, S.S.; Lee, S.H.; Yoo, N.J. Somatic mutation of PIK3R1 gene is rare in common human cancers. *Acta Oncol.* **2010**, *49*, 125–127. [CrossRef] [PubMed]
63. Thapa, N.; Chen, M.; Cryns, V.L.; Anderson, R. A p85 isoform switch enhances PI3K activation on endosomes by a MAP4- and PI3P-dependent mechanism. *Cell Rep.* **2024**, *43*, 114119. [CrossRef] [PubMed]
64. Park, A.K.; Kim, P.; Ballester, L.Y.; Esquenazi, Y.; Zhao, Z. Subtype-specific signaling pathways and genomic aberrations associated with prognosis of glioblastoma. *Neuro Oncol.* **2019**, *21*, 59–70. [CrossRef]
65. Muench, A.; Teichmann, D.; Spille, D.; Kuzman, P.; Perez, E.; May, S.A.; Mueller, W.C.; Kombos, T.; Nazari-Dehkordi, S.; Onken, J.; et al. A Novel Type of IDH-wildtype Glioma Characterized by Gliomatosis Cerebri-like Growth Pattern, TERT Promoter Mutation, and Distinct Epigenetic Profile. *Am. J. Surg. Pathol.* **2023**, *47*, 1364–1375. [CrossRef]
66. Draaisma, K.; Wijnenga, M.M.; Weenink, B.; Gao, Y.; Smid, M.; Robe, P.; van den Bent, M.J.; French, P.J. PI3 kinase mutations and mutational load as poor prognostic markers in diffuse glioma patients. *Acta Neuropathol. Commun.* **2015**, *3*, 88. [CrossRef]
67. Chen, L.; Yang, L.; Yao, L.; Kuang, X.Y.; Zuo, W.J.; Li, S.; Qiao, F.; Liu, Y.R.; Cao, Z.G.; Zhou, S.L.; et al. Characterization of PIK3CA and PIK3R1 somatic mutations in Chinese breast cancer patients. *Nat. Commun.* **2018**, *9*, 1357. [CrossRef]
68. Punekar, S.R.; Velcheti, V.; Neel, B.G.; Wong, K.K. The current state of the art and future trends in RAS-targeted cancer therapies. *Nat. Rev. Clin. Oncol.* **2022**, *19*, 637–655. [CrossRef]
69. Simanshu, D.K.; Nissley, D.V.; McCormick, F. RAS Proteins and Their Regulators in Human Disease. *Cell* **2017**, *170*, 17–33. [CrossRef]
70. Soriano, O.; Alcon-Perez, M.; Vicente-Manzanares, M.; Castellano, E. The Crossroads between RAS and RHO Signaling Pathways in Cellular Transformation, Motility and Contraction. *Genes* **2021**, *12*, 819. [CrossRef]
71. Knobbe, C.B.; Reifenberger, J.; Reifenberger, G. Mutation analysis of the Ras pathway genes NRAS, HRAS, KRAS and BRAF in glioblastomas. *Acta Neuropathol.* **2004**, *108*, 467–470. [CrossRef] [PubMed]
72. Chang, M.; Sherief, M.; Ioannou, M.; Chinnasamy, V.; Chen, L.; Frost, M.; Mattson-Hoss, M.; Sarnoff, H.; Kamson, D.O.; Holdhoff, M.; et al. NF1 expression profiling in IDH-wildtype glioblastoma: Genomic associations and survival outcomes. *Acta Neuropathol. Commun.* **2024**, *12*, 172. [CrossRef]
73. Gutmann, D.H.; Parada, L.F.; Silva, A.J.; Ratner, N. Neurofibromatosis type 1: Modeling CNS dysfunction. *J. Neurosci.* **2012**, *32*, 14087–14093. [CrossRef]
74. Francis, J.M.; Zhang, C.Z.; Maire, C.L.; Jung, J.; Manzo, V.E.; Adalsteinsson, V.A.; Homer, H.; Haidar, S.; Blumenstiel, B.; Pedamallu, C.S.; et al. EGFR variant heterogeneity in glioblastoma resolved through single-nucleus sequencing. *Cancer Discov.* **2014**, *4*, 956–971. [CrossRef]
75. Heimberger, A.B.; Suki, D.; Yang, D.; Shi, W.; Aldape, K. The natural history of EGFR and EGFRvIII in glioblastoma patients. *J. Transl. Med.* **2005**, *3*, 38. [CrossRef]
76. Ozawa, T.; Brennan, C.W.; Wang, L.; Squatrito, M.; Sasayama, T.; Nakada, M.; Huse, J.T.; Pedraza, A.; Utsuki, S.; Yasui, Y.; et al. PDGFRA gene rearrangements are frequent genetic events in PDGFRA-amplified glioblastomas. *Genes Dev.* **2010**, *24*, 2205–2218. [CrossRef] [PubMed]
77. Yu, R.; Huang, K.; He, X.; Zhang, J.; Ma, Y.; Liu, H. ATRX mutation modifies the DNA damage response in glioblastoma multiforme tumor cells and enhances patient prognosis. *Medicine* **2025**, *104*, e41180. [CrossRef] [PubMed]
78. Vizcaino, M.A.; Shah, S.; Eberhart, C.G.; Rodriguez, F.J. Clinicopathologic implications of NF1 gene alterations in diffuse gliomas. *Hum. Pathol.* **2015**, *46*, 1323–1330. [CrossRef]
79. Martinez-Lage, M.; Lynch, T.M.; Bi, Y.; Cocito, C.; Way, G.P.; Pal, S.; Haller, J.; Yan, R.E.; Ziober, A.; Nguyen, A.; et al. Immune landscapes associated with different glioblastoma molecular subtypes. *Acta Neuropathol. Commun.* **2019**, *7*, 203. [CrossRef]
80. McNulty, S.N.; Schwetye, K.E.; Ferguson, C.; Storer, C.E.; Ansstas, G.; Kim, A.H.; Gutmann, D.H.; Rubin, J.B.; Head, R.D.; Dahiya, S. BRAF mutations may identify a clinically distinct subset of glioblastoma. *Sci. Rep.* **2021**, *11*, 19999. [CrossRef]
81. Prieto, R.; Barrios, L.; Ebrat-Mancilla, E.; Martin, P.; Tejerina, E. The Significance of BRAF Mutation in the Epithelioid Glioblastoma Subtype: A Systematic Literature Review and a Case Report with a Unique Intraventricular Topography. *Int. J. Surg. Pathol.* **2024**, *32*, 649–666. [CrossRef] [PubMed]
82. Sugiura, Y.; Nagaishi, M. Clinical relevance of BRAF status in glial and glioneuronal tumors: A systematic review. *J. Clin. Neurosci.* **2019**, *66*, 196–201. [CrossRef]

83. Lopez-Gines, C.; Gil-Benso, R.; Ferrer-Luna, R.; Benito, R.; Serna, E.; Gonzalez-Darder, J.; Quilis, V.; Monleon, D.; Celda, B.; Cerda-Nicolas, M. New pattern of EGFR amplification in glioblastoma and the relationship of gene copy number with gene expression profile. *Mod. Pathol.* **2010**, *23*, 856–865. [CrossRef] [PubMed]
84. Higa, N.; Akahane, T.; Yokoyama, S.; Yonezawa, H.; Uchida, H.; Takajo, T.; Otsuji, R.; Hamada, T.; Matsuo, K.; Kirishima, M.; et al. Prognostic impact of PDGFRA gain/amplification and MGMT promoter methylation status in patients with IDH wild-type glioblastoma. *Neurooncol. Adv.* **2022**, *4*, vdac097. [CrossRef]
85. Lo, H.W. EGFR-targeted therapy in malignant glioma: Novel aspects and mechanisms of drug resistance. *Curr. Mol. Pharmacol.* **2010**, *3*, 37–52. [CrossRef]
86. Pan, P.C.; Magge, R.S. Mechanisms of EGFR Resistance in Glioblastoma. *Int. J. Mol. Sci.* **2020**, *21*, 8471. [CrossRef]
87. Westphal, M.; Maire, C.L.; Lamszus, K. EGFR as a Target for Glioblastoma Treatment: An Unfulfilled Promise. *CNS Drugs* **2017**, *31*, 723–735. [CrossRef] [PubMed]
88. Peng, G.; Wang, Y.; Ge, P.; Bailey, C.; Zhang, P.; Zhang, D.; Meng, Z.; Qi, C.; Chen, Q.; Chen, J.; et al. The HIF1alpha-PDGFD-PDGFRalpha axis controls glioblastoma growth at normoxia/mild-hypoxia and confers sensitivity to targeted therapy by echinomycin. *J. Exp. Clin. Cancer Res.* **2021**, *40*, 278. [CrossRef]
89. Vuong, H.G.; Altibi, A.M.A.; Duong, U.N.P.; Ngo, H.T.T.; Pham, T.Q.; Fung, K.M.; Hassell, L. BRAF Mutation is Associated with an Improved Survival in Glioma-a Systematic Review and Meta-analysis. *Mol. Neurobiol.* **2018**, *55*, 3718–3724. [CrossRef]
90. Zhu, J.; Ye, J.; Zhang, L.; Xia, L.; Hu, H.; Jiang, H.; Wan, Z.; Sheng, F.; Ma, Y.; Li, W.; et al. Differential Expression of Circular RNAs in Glioblastoma Multiforme and Its Correlation with Prognosis. *Transl. Oncol.* **2017**, *10*, 271–279. [CrossRef]
91. Basindwah, S.; Alkhalidi, H.; Abdelwarith, A.; Elwatidy, S. Ten-year survival in glioblastoma patient with neurofibromatosis type 1: Illustrative case. *J. Neurosurg. Case Lessons* **2022**, *3*, CASE21630. [CrossRef]
92. Gleize, V.; Alentorn, A.; Connen de Kerillis, L.; Labussiere, M.; Nadaradjane, A.A.; Mundwiller, E.; Ottolenghi, C.; Mangesius, S.; Rahimian, A.; Ducray, F.; et al. CIC inactivating mutations identify aggressive subset of 1p19q codeleted gliomas. *Ann. Neurol.* **2015**, *78*, 355–374. [CrossRef]
93. Bunda, S.; Heir, P.; Metcalf, J.; Li, A.S.C.; Agnihotri, S.; Pusch, S.; Yasin, M.; Li, M.; Burrell, K.; Mansouri, S.; et al. CIC protein instability contributes to tumorigenesis in glioblastoma. *Nat. Commun.* **2019**, *10*, 661. [CrossRef]
94. Darabi, S.; Xiu, J.; Samec, T.; Kesari, S.; Carrillo, J.; Aulakh, S.; Walsh, K.M.; Sengupta, S.; Sumrall, A.; Spetzler, D.; et al. Capicua (CIC) mutations in gliomas in association with MAPK activation for exposing a potential therapeutic target. *Med. Oncol.* **2023**, *40*, 197. [CrossRef]
95. Sondka, Z.; Dhir, N.B.; Carvalho-Silva, D.; Jupe, S.; Madhumita, N.; McLaren, K.; Starkey, M.; Ward, S.; Wilding, J.; Ahmed, M.; et al. COSMIC: A curated database of somatic variants and clinical data for cancer. *Nucleic Acids Res.* **2024**, *52*, D1210–D1217. [CrossRef]
96. Zhang, L.; Giuste, F.; Vizcarra, J.C.; Li, X.; Gutman, D. Radiomics Features Predict CIC Mutation Status in Lower Grade Glioma. *Front. Oncol.* **2020**, *10*, 937. [CrossRef]
97. Balana, C.; Castaner, S.; Carrato, C.; Moran, T.; Lopez-Paradis, A.; Domenech, M.; Hernandez, A.; Puig, J. Preoperative Diagnosis and Molecular Characterization of Gliomas with Liquid Biopsy and Radiogenomics. *Front. Neurol.* **2022**, *13*, 865171. [CrossRef]
98. Chen, J. The Cell-Cycle Arrest and Apoptotic Functions of p53 in Tumor Initiation and Progression. *Cold Spring Harb. Perspect. Med.* **2016**, *6*, a026104. [CrossRef]
99. Levine, A.J. Spontaneous and inherited TP53 genetic alterations. *Oncogene* **2021**, *40*, 5975–5983. [CrossRef]
100. Lee, Y.J.; Seo, H.W.; Baek, J.H.; Lim, S.H.; Hwang, S.G.; Kim, E.H. Gene expression profiling of glioblastoma cell lines depending on TP53 status after tumor-treating fields (TTFields) treatment. *Sci. Rep.* **2020**, *10*, 12272. [CrossRef]
101. Jha, P.; Suri, V.; Singh, G.; Jha, P.; Purkait, S.; Pathak, P.; Sharma, V.; Sharma, M.C.; Suri, A.; Gupta, D.; et al. Characterization of molecular genetic alterations in GBMs highlights a distinctive molecular profile in young adults. *Diagn. Mol. Pathol.* **2011**, *20*, 225–232. [CrossRef]
102. Cancer Genome Atlas Research, N. Comprehensive genomic characterization defines human glioblastoma genes and core pathways. *Nature* **2008**, *455*, 1061–1068. [CrossRef]
103. Yang, W.J.; Soares, J.; Greninger, P.; Edelman, E.J.; Lightfoot, H.; Forbes, S.; Bindal, N.; Beare, D.; Smith, J.A.; Thompson, I.R.; et al. Genomics of Drug Sensitivity in Cancer (GDSC): A resource for therapeutic biomarker discovery in cancer cells. *Nucleic Acids Res.* **2013**, *41*, D955–D961. [CrossRef]
104. Wang, X.; Chen, J.X.; Liu, Y.H.; You, C.; Mao, Q. Mutant TP53 enhances the resistance of glioblastoma cells to temozolomide by up-regulating O^6-methylguanine DNA-methyltransferase. *Neurol. Sci.* **2013**, *34*, 1421–1428. [CrossRef]
105. Bieging, K.T.; Mello, S.S.; Attardi, L.D. Unravelling mechanisms of p53-mediated tumour suppression. *Nat. Rev. Cancer* **2014**, *14*, 359–370. [CrossRef]

106. Li, S.; Zhang, W.; Chen, B.; Jiang, T.; Wang, Z. Prognostic and predictive value of p53 in low MGMT expressing glioblastoma treated with surgery, radiation and adjuvant temozolomide chemotherapy. *Neurol. Res.* **2010**, *32*, 690–694. [CrossRef]
107. Garrido-Navas, M.C.; Garcia-Diaz, A.; Molina-Vallejo, M.P.; Gonzalez-Martinez, C.; Alcaide Lucena, M.; Canas-Garcia, I.; Bayarri, C.; Delgado, J.R.; Gonzalez, E.; Lorente, J.A.; et al. The Polemic Diagnostic Role of TP53 Mutations in Liquid Biopsies from Breast, Colon and Lung Cancers. *Cancers* **2020**, *12*, 3343. [CrossRef]
108. Principe, C.; Dionisio de Sousa, I.J.; Prazeres, H.; Soares, P.; Lima, R.T. LRP1B: A Giant Lost in Cancer Translation. *Pharmaceuticals* **2021**, *14*, 836. [CrossRef]
109. Tabouret, E.; Labussiere, M.; Alentorn, A.; Schmitt, Y.; Marie, Y.; Sanson, M. LRP1B deletion is associated with poor outcome for glioblastoma patients. *J. Neurol. Sci.* **2015**, *358*, 440–443. [CrossRef] [PubMed]
110. Yin, D.; Ogawa, S.; Kawamata, N.; Tunici, P.; Finocchiaro, G.; Eoli, M.; Ruckert, C.; Huynh, T.; Liu, G.; Kato, M.; et al. High-resolution genomic copy number profiling of glioblastoma multiforme by single nucleotide polymorphism DNA microarray. *Mol. Cancer Res.* **2009**, *7*, 665–677. [CrossRef] [PubMed]
111. Sergi, C.M. Commentary on: SMARCB1 as a novel diagnostic and prognostic biomarker for osteosarcoma. *Biosci. Rep.* **2022**, *42*, BSR20220040. [CrossRef]
112. Zhang, Z.K.; Davies, K.P.; Allen, J.; Zhu, L.; Pestell, R.G.; Zagzag, D.; Kalpana, G.V. Cell cycle arrest and repression of cyclin D1 transcription by INI1/hSNF5. *Mol. Cell. Biol.* **2002**, *22*, 5975–5988. [CrossRef]
113. Mukherjee, S.; Stroberg, E.; Wang, F.; Morales, L.; Shan, Y.; Rao, A.; Huang, J.H.; Wu, E.; Fonkem, E. SMARCB1 Gene Mutation Predisposes to Earlier Development of Glioblastoma: A Case Report of Familial GBM. *J. Neuropathol. Exp. Neurol.* **2020**, *79*, 562–565. [CrossRef]
114. Cooper, G.W.; Hong, A.L. SMARCB1-Deficient Cancers: Novel Molecular Insights and Therapeutic Vulnerabilities. *Cancers* **2022**, *14*, 3645. [CrossRef]
115. Stockman, D.L.; Curry, J.L.; Torres-Cabala, C.A.; Watson, I.R.; Siroy, A.E.; Bassett, R.L.; Zou, L.; Patel, K.P.; Luthra, R.; Davies, M.A.; et al. Use of clinical next-generation sequencing to identify melanomas harboring SMARCB1 mutations. *J. Cutan. Pathol.* **2015**, *42*, 308–317. [CrossRef]
116. Choi, S.K.; Kim, M.J.; You, J.S. SMARCB1 Acts as a Quiescent Gatekeeper for Cell Cycle and Immune Response in Human Cells. *Int. J. Mol. Sci.* **2020**, *21*, 3969. [CrossRef]
117. Yang, Y.; Chen, Q.; Gou, M.; Wang, X.; Liu, Y.; Liang, R.; Mao, Y.; Luo, J.; Mao, Q. TERT mutation in glioma: Frequency, prognosis and risk. *J. Clin. Neurosci.* **2016**, *26*, 57–62. [CrossRef]
118. Olympios, N.; Gilard, V.; Marguet, F.; Clatot, F.; Di Fiore, F.; Fontanilles, M. TERT Promoter Alterations in Glioblastoma: A Systematic Review. *Cancers* **2021**, *13*, 1147. [CrossRef]
119. Johanns, T.M.; Fu, Y.; Kobayashi, D.K.; Mei, Y.; Dunn, I.F.; Mao, D.D.; Kim, A.H.; Dunn, G.P. High incidence of TERT mutation in brain tumor cell lines. *Brain Tumor Pathol.* **2016**, *33*, 222–227. [CrossRef]
120. El Zarif, T.; Machaalani, M.; Nawfal, R.; Nassar, A.H.; Xie, W.; Choueiri, T.K.; Pomerantz, M. TERT Promoter Mutations Frequency Across Race, Sex, and Cancer Type. *Oncologist* **2024**, *29*, 8–14. [CrossRef] [PubMed]
121. Labussiere, M.; Boisselier, B.; Mokhtari, K.; Di Stefano, A.L.; Rahimian, A.; Rossetto, M.; Ciccarino, P.; Saulnier, O.; Paterra, R.; Marie, Y.; et al. Combined analysis of TERT, EGFR, and IDH status defines distinct prognostic glioblastoma classes. *Neurology* **2014**, *83*, 1200–1206. [CrossRef]
122. Jones, J.J.; Nguyen, H.; Wong, S.Q.; Whittle, J.; Iaria, J.; Stylli, S.; Towner, J.; Pieters, T.; Gaillard, F.; Kaye, A.H.; et al. Plasma ctDNA liquid biopsy of IDH1, TERTp, and EGFRvIII mutations in glioma. *Neurooncol. Adv.* **2024**, *6*, vdae027. [CrossRef]
123. Liu, X.; Wang, J.; Wu, L.J.; Trinh, B.; Tsai, R.Y.L. IMPDH Inhibition Decreases TERT Expression and Synergizes the Cytotoxic Effect of Chemotherapeutic Agents in Glioblastoma Cells. *Int. J. Mol. Sci.* **2024**, *25*, 5992. [CrossRef]
124. Jiao, Y.; Lv, Y.; Liu, M.; Liu, Y.; Han, M.; Xiong, X.; Zhou, H.; Zhong, J.; Kang, X.; Su, W. The modification role and tumor association with a methyltransferase: KMT2C. *Front. Immunol.* **2024**, *15*, 1444923. [CrossRef]
125. Hu, X.; Biswas, A.; De, S. KMT2C-deficient tumors have elevated APOBEC mutagenesis and genomic instability in multiple cancers. *NAR Cancer* **2022**, *4*, zcac023. [CrossRef]
126. Zhang, L.; Liu, Y.; Wang, M.; Wu, Z.; Li, N.; Zhang, J.; Yang, C. EZH2-, CHD4-, and IDH-linked epigenetic perturbation and its association with survival in glioma patients. *J. Mol. Cell Biol.* **2017**, *9*, 477–488. [CrossRef]
127. Lian, J.; Xu, C.; Chen, X.; Huang, S.; Wu, D. Histone methyltransferase KMT2C plays an oncogenic role in prostate cancer. *J. Cancer Res. Clin. Oncol.* **2022**, *148*, 1627–1640. [CrossRef]
128. Liu, X.; Qiu, R.; Xu, M.; Meng, M.; Zhao, S.; Ji, J.; Yang, Y. KMT2C is a potential biomarker of prognosis and chemotherapy sensitivity in breast cancer. *Breast Cancer Res. Treat.* **2021**, *189*, 347–361. [CrossRef]

129. Marei, H.E.; Althani, A.; Afifi, N.; Hasan, A.; Caceci, T.; Felsani, A.; Tringali, G.; Cifola, I.; Pozzoli, G.; Cenciarelli, C. Exome sequencing of glioblastoma-derived cancer stem cells reveals rare clinically relevant frameshift deletion in MLLT1 gene. *Cancer Cell Int.* **2022**, *22*, 9. [CrossRef] [PubMed]
130. Sarker, A.; Uddin, B.; Ahmmed, R.; Mahmud, S.; Ajadee, A.; Pappu, M.A.A.; Aziz, M.A.; Mollah, M.N.H. Discovery of mutated oncodriver genes associated with glioblastoma originated from stem cells of subventricular zone through whole exome sequence profile analysis, and drug repurposing. *Heliyon* **2025**, *11*, e42052. [CrossRef] [PubMed]
131. Rampias, T.; Karagiannis, D.; Avgeris, M.; Polyzos, A.; Kokkalis, A.; Kanaki, Z.; Kousidou, E.; Tzetis, M.; Kanavakis, E.; Stravodimos, K.; et al. The lysine-specific methyltransferase KMT2C/MLL3 regulates DNA repair components in cancer. *EMBO Rep.* **2019**, *20*, e46821. [CrossRef]
132. Wang, N.; Pachai, M.R.; Li, D.; Lee, C.J.; Warda, S.; Khudoynazarova, M.N.; Cho, W.H.; Xie, G.; Shah, S.R.; Yao, L.; et al. Loss of Kmt2c or Kmt2d primes urothelium for tumorigenesis and redistributes KMT2A-menin to bivalent promoters. *Nat. Genet.* **2025**, *57*, 165–179. [CrossRef] [PubMed]
133. Saratsis, A.M.; Knowles, T.; Petrovic, A.; Nazarian, J. H3K27M mutant glioma: Disease definition and biological underpinnings. *Neuro Oncol.* **2024**, *26*, S92–S100. [CrossRef] [PubMed]
134. Sturm, D.; Witt, H.; Hovestadt, V.; Khuong-Quang, D.A.; Jones, D.T.; Konermann, C.; Pfaff, E.; Tonjes, M.; Sill, M.; Bender, S.; et al. Hotspot mutations in H3F3A and IDH1 define distinct epigenetic and biological subgroups of glioblastoma. *Cancer Cell* **2012**, *22*, 425–437. [CrossRef]
135. Harutyunyan, A.S.; Krug, B.; Chen, H.; Papillon-Cavanagh, S.; Zeinieh, M.; De Jay, N.; Deshmukh, S.; Chen, C.C.L.; Belle, J.; Mikael, L.G.; et al. H3K27M induces defective chromatin spread of PRC2-mediated repressive H3K27me2/me3 and is essential for glioma tumorigenesis. *Nat. Commun.* **2019**, *10*, 1262. [CrossRef]
136. Aggarwal, P.; Luo, W.; Pehlivan, K.C.; Hoang, H.; Rajappa, P.; Cripe, T.P.; Cassady, K.A.; Lee, D.A.; Cairo, M.S. Pediatric versus adult high grade glioma: Immunotherapeutic and genomic considerations. *Front. Immunol.* **2022**, *13*, 1038096. [CrossRef] [PubMed]
137. Venneti, S.; Santi, M.; Felicella, M.M.; Yarilin, D.; Phillips, J.J.; Sullivan, L.M.; Martinez, D.; Perry, A.; Lewis, P.W.; Thompson, C.B.; et al. A sensitive and specific histopathologic prognostic marker for H3F3A K27M mutant pediatric glioblastomas. *Acta Neuropathol.* **2014**, *128*, 743–753. [CrossRef]
138. Mohammad, F.; Weissmann, S.; Leblanc, B.; Pandey, D.P.; Hojfeldt, J.W.; Comet, I.; Zheng, C.; Johansen, J.V.; Rapin, N.; Porse, B.T.; et al. EZH2 is a potential therapeutic target for H3K27M-mutant pediatric gliomas. *Nat. Med.* **2017**, *23*, 483–492. [CrossRef]
139. Williams, M.J.; Singleton, W.G.; Lowis, S.P.; Malik, K.; Kurian, K.M. Therapeutic Targeting of Histone Modifications in Adult and Pediatric High-Grade Glioma. *Front. Oncol.* **2017**, *7*, 45. [CrossRef]
140. Chi, A.S.; Tarapore, R.S.; Hall, M.D.; Shonka, N.; Gardner, S.; Umemura, Y.; Sumrall, A.; Khatib, Z.; Mueller, S.; Kline, C.; et al. Pediatric and adult H3 K27M-mutant diffuse midline glioma treated with the selective DRD2 antagonist ONC201. *J. Neurooncol.* **2019**, *145*, 97–105. [CrossRef]
141. MacDonald, B.T.; Tamai, K.; He, X. Wnt/beta-catenin signaling: Components, mechanisms, and diseases. *Dev. Cell* **2009**, *17*, 9–26. [CrossRef] [PubMed]
142. Komiya, Y.; Habas, R. Wnt signal transduction pathways. *Organogenesis* **2008**, *4*, 68–75. [CrossRef] [PubMed]
143. Zhang, Y.; Wang, X. Targeting the Wnt/beta-catenin signaling pathway in cancer. *J. Hematol. Oncol.* **2020**, *13*, 165. [CrossRef] [PubMed]
144. Yu, F.; Yu, C.; Li, F.; Zuo, Y.; Wang, Y.; Yao, L.; Wu, C.; Wang, C.; Ye, L. Wnt/beta-catenin signaling in cancers and targeted therapies. *Signal Transduct. Target. Ther.* **2021**, *6*, 307. [CrossRef] [PubMed]
145. Zhuang, W.; Ye, T.; Wang, W.; Song, W.; Tan, T. CTNNB1 in neurodevelopmental disorders. *Front. Psychiatry* **2023**, *14*, 1143328. [CrossRef]
146. Nager, M.; Sallan, M.C.; Visa, A.; Pushparaj, C.; Santacana, M.; Macia, A.; Yeramian, A.; Canti, C.; Herreros, J. Inhibition of WNT-CTNNB1 signaling upregulates SQSTM1 and sensitizes glioblastoma cells to autophagy blockers. *Autophagy* **2018**, *14*, 619–636. [CrossRef]
147. Denysenko, T.; Annovazzi, L.; Cassoni, P.; Melcarne, A.; Mellai, M.; Schiffer, D. WNT/beta-catenin Signaling Pathway and Downstream Modulators in Low- and High-grade Glioma. *Cancer Genom. Proteom.* **2016**, *13*, 31–45.
148. Moreno, D.A.; Bonatelli, M.; Antoniazzi, A.P.; de Paula, F.E.; Leal, L.F.; Garcia, F.A.O.; de Paula, A.E.; Teixeira, G.R.; Santana, I.V.V.; Saggioro, F.; et al. High frequency of WNT-activated medulloblastomas with CTNNB1 wild type suggests a higher proportion of hereditary cases in a Latin-Iberian population. *Front. Oncol.* **2023**, *13*, 1237170. [CrossRef]
149. Coelho, B.P.; Fernandes, C.F.L.; Boccacino, J.M.; Souza, M.; Melo-Escobar, M.I.; Alves, R.N.; Prado, M.B.; Iglesia, R.P.; Cangiano, G.; Mazzaro, G.R.; et al. Multifaceted WNT Signaling at the Crossroads Between Epithelial-Mesenchymal Transition and Autophagy in Glioblastoma. *Front. Oncol.* **2020**, *10*, 597743. [CrossRef]

150. Kahlert, U.D.; Maciaczyk, D.; Doostkam, S.; Orr, B.A.; Simons, B.; Bogiel, T.; Reithmeier, T.; Prinz, M.; Schubert, J.; Niedermann, G.; et al. Activation of canonical WNT/beta-catenin signaling enhances in vitro motility of glioblastoma cells by activation of ZEB1 and other activators of epithelial-to-mesenchymal transition. *Cancer Lett.* **2012**, *325*, 42–53. [CrossRef]
151. Zechner, D.; Fujita, Y.; Hulsken, J.; Muller, T.; Walther, I.; Taketo, M.M.; Crenshaw, E.B., 3rd; Birchmeier, W.; Birchmeier, C. beta-Catenin signals regulate cell growth and the balance between progenitor cell expansion and differentiation in the nervous system. *Dev. Biol.* **2003**, *258*, 406–418. [CrossRef] [PubMed]
152. Chenn, A.; Walsh, C.A. Regulation of cerebral cortical size by control of cell cycle exit in neural precursors. *Science* **2002**, *297*, 365–369. [CrossRef] [PubMed]
153. Lee, Y.; Lee, J.K.; Ahn, S.H.; Lee, J.; Nam, D.H. WNT signaling in glioblastoma and therapeutic opportunities. *Lab. Investig.* **2016**, *96*, 137–150. [CrossRef]
154. Liu, C.; Tu, Y.; Sun, X.; Jiang, J.; Jin, X.; Bo, X.; Li, Z.; Bian, A.; Wang, X.; Liu, D.; et al. Wnt/beta-Catenin pathway in human glioma: Expression pattern and clinical/prognostic correlations. *Clin. Exp. Med.* **2011**, *11*, 105–112. [CrossRef] [PubMed]
155. Nager, M.; Bhardwaj, D.; Canti, C.; Medina, L.; Nogues, P.; Herreros, J. beta-Catenin Signalling in Glioblastoma Multiforme and Glioma-Initiating Cells. *Chemother. Res. Pract.* **2012**, *2012*, 192362. [CrossRef]
156. Latour, M.; Her, N.G.; Kesari, S.; Nurmemmedov, E. WNT Signaling as a Therapeutic Target for Glioblastoma. *Int. J. Mol. Sci.* **2021**, *22*, 8428. [CrossRef]
157. Yun, E.J.; Kim, S.; Hsieh, J.T.; Baek, S.T. Wnt/beta-catenin signaling pathway induces autophagy-mediated temozolomide-resistance in human glioblastoma. *Cell Death Dis.* **2020**, *11*, 771. [CrossRef]
158. Tyagi, A.; Sharma, A.K.; Damodaran, C. A Review on Notch Signaling and Colorectal Cancer. *Cells* **2020**, *9*, 1549. [CrossRef]
159. Wang, Y.; Sun, Q.; Geng, R.; Liu, H.; Yuan, F.E.; Xu, Y.; Qi, Y.; Jiang, H.; Chen, Q.; Liu, B. Notch intracellular domain regulates glioblastoma proliferation through the Notch1 signaling pathway. *Oncol. Lett.* **2021**, *21*, 303. [CrossRef]
160. Anusewicz, D.; Orzechowska, M.; Bednarek, A.K. Notch Signaling Pathway in Cancer-Review with Bioinformatic Analysis. *Cancers* **2021**, *13*, 768. [CrossRef]
161. Zheng, Z.Q.; Zhang, G.G.; Yuan, G.Q.; Hao, J.H.; Nie, Q.Q.; Zheng, M.C.; Wang, Z. Development and validation of an immune infiltration/tumor proliferation-related Notch3 nomogram for predicting survival in patients with primary glioblastoma. *Front. Genet.* **2023**, *14*, 1148126. [CrossRef] [PubMed]
162. Aoki, K.; Nakamura, H.; Suzuki, H.; Matsuo, K.; Kataoka, K.; Shimamura, T.; Motomura, K.; Ohka, F.; Shiina, S.; Yamamoto, T.; et al. Prognostic relevance of genetic alterations in diffuse lower-grade gliomas. *Neuro Oncol.* **2018**, *20*, 66–77. [CrossRef]
163. Hai, L.; Zhang, C.; Li, T.; Zhou, X.; Liu, B.; Li, S.; Zhu, M.; Lin, Y.; Yu, S.; Zhang, K.; et al. Notch1 is a prognostic factor that is distinctly activated in the classical and proneural subtype of glioblastoma and that promotes glioma cell survival via the NF-kappaB(p65) pathway. *Cell Death Dis.* **2018**, *9*, 158. [CrossRef]
164. Liu, G.; Bu, C.; Guo, G.; Zhang, Z.; Sheng, Z.; Deng, K.; Wu, S.; Xu, S.; Bu, Y.; Gao, Y.; et al. Molecular and clonal evolution in vivo reveal a common pathway of distant relapse gliomas. *iScience* **2023**, *26*, 107528. [CrossRef]
165. Greenwald, A.C.; Darnell, N.G.; Hoefflin, R.; Simkin, D.; Mount, C.W.; Gonzalez Castro, L.N.; Harnik, Y.; Dumont, S.; Hirsch, D.; Nomura, M.; et al. Integrative spatial analysis reveals a multi-layered organization of glioblastoma. *Cell* **2024**, *187*, 2485–2501.E26. [CrossRef]
166. Neftel, C.; Laffy, J.; Filbin, M.G.; Hara, T.; Shore, M.E.; Rahme, G.J.; Richman, A.R.; Silverbush, D.; Shaw, M.L.; Hebert, C.M.; et al. An Integrative Model of Cellular States, Plasticity, and Genetics for Glioblastoma. *Cell* **2019**, *178*, 835–849.e821. [CrossRef]
167. Ren, Y.; Huang, Z.; Zhou, L.; Xiao, P.; Song, J.; He, P.; Xie, C.; Zhou, R.; Li, M.; Dong, X.; et al. Spatial transcriptomics reveals niche-specific enrichment and vulnerabilities of radial glial stem-like cells in malignant gliomas. *Nat. Commun.* **2023**, *14*, 1028. [CrossRef] [PubMed]
168. Park, J.H.; Lee, H.K. Current Understanding of Hypoxia in Glioblastoma Multiforme and Its Response to Immunotherapy. *Cancers* **2022**, *14*, 1176. [CrossRef] [PubMed]
169. Lino, M.M.; Merlo, A.; Boulay, J.L. Notch signaling in glioblastoma: A developmental drug target? *BMC Med.* **2010**, *8*, 72. [CrossRef]
170. Gersey, Z.; Osiason, A.D.; Bloom, L.; Shah, S.; Thompson, J.W.; Bregy, A.; Agarwal, N.; Komotar, R.J. Therapeutic Targeting of the Notch Pathway in Glioblastoma Multiforme. *World Neurosurg.* **2019**, *131*, 252–263.e252. [CrossRef]

biomedicines

MDPI

Review

Microsatellite Instability in Urine: Breakthrough Method for Bladder Cancer Identification

Manuel Alejandro Rico-Méndez [1], María de la Luz Ayala-Madrigal [1], Anahí González-Mercado [1], Melva Gutiérrez-Angulo [2], Jorge Adrián Ramírez de Arellano Sánchez [3], Saul Armando Beltrán-Ontiveros [4], Betsabe Contreras-Haro [5], Itzae Adonai Gutiérrez-Hurtado [6,*] and José Miguel Moreno-Ortiz [1,*]

1 Doctorado en Genética Humana, Instituto de Genética Humana "Dr. Enrique Corona Rivera", Departamento de Biología Molecular y Genómica, Centro Universitario de Ciencias de la Salud, Universidad de Guadalajara, Guadalajara 44340, Jalisco, Mexico; manuel.rico8557@alumnos.udg.mx (M.A.R.-M.); luz.ayala@academicos.udg.mx (M.d.l.L.A.-M.); anahi.gonzalez@academicos.udg.mx (A.G.-M.)

2 Departamento de Ciencias de la Salud, Centro Universitario de los Altos, Universidad de Guadalajara, Tepatitlán de Morelos 47600, Jalisco, Mexico; melva.gutierrez@academicos.udg.mx

3 Instituto de Investigación en Ciencias Biomédicas, Departamento de Biología Molecular y Genómica, Centro Universitario de Ciencias de la Salud, Universidad de Guadalajara, Guadalajara 44340, Jalisco, Mexico; adrian.ramirez@academicos.udg.mx

4 Centrode Investigación y Docencia en Ciencias de la Salud, Universidad Autónoma de Sinaloa, Culiacán Rosales 80030, Sinaloa, Mexico; saul.beltran@uas.edu.mx

5 Unidad de Investigación Biomédica 02, Unidades Médicas de Alta Especialidad, Hospital de Especialidades, Centro Médico Nacional de Occidente, Instituto Mexicano del Seguro Social, Guadalajara 44329, Jalisco, Mexico; betsabecoha@gmail.com

6 Departamento de Biología Molecular y Genómica, Centro Universitario de Ciencias de la Salud, Universidad de Guadalajara, Guadalajara 44340, Jalisco, Mexico

* Correspondence: itzae.gutierrez@academicos.udg.mx (I.A.G.-H.); miguel.moreno@academicos.udg.mx (J.M.M.-O.)

Abstract: Bladder cancer (BC) is the most common neoplasm of the urinary system and ranks tenth in global cancer incidence. Due to its high recurrence rate and the need for continuous monitoring, it is the cancer with the highest cost per patient. Cystoscopy is the traditional method for its detection and surveillance; however, this is an invasive technique, while non-invasive methods, such as cytology, have a limited sensitivity. For this reason, new non-invasive strategies have emerged, analyzing useful markers for BC detection from urine samples. The identification of tumor markers is essential for early cancer detection and treatment. Urine analysis offers a non-invasive method to identify these markers. Microsatellite instability (MSI) has been proposed as a promising marker for tumor cell detection and guided targeted therapies. Therefore, this review aims to explore the evidence supporting the identification of MSI in exfoliated bladder tumor cells (EBTCs) in the urine, emphasizing its potential as a non-invasive and clinically effective alternative for tumor identification. Furthermore, establishing clinical guidelines is crucial for standardizing its application in oncological screening and validating its clinical utility.

Keywords: bladder cancer; microsatellite instability; exfoliated bladder tumor cells; marker; microsatellite instability analysis; urine; pembrolizumab

1. Introduction

Bladder cancer (BC) is the most prevalent neoplasm affecting the urinary system, characterized by a high mutation rate and genomic instability [1]. With a global incidence of 3% and a mortality rate of 2.2%, BC ranks as the tenth most common cancer and the thirteenth leading cause of cancer-related deaths worldwide [2]. In 2020, BC accounted for over half a million cases, with projections indicating that this number could double by 2040 [3].

BC is classified histopathologically into low-grade and high-grade types and based on tumor invasion into non-muscle invasive bladder cancer (NMIBCa) or muscle-invasive bladder cancer (MIBCa). NMIBCa comprises 75% of BC cases and primarily develops in the mucosal layer, exhibiting high recurrence rates. Molecularly, it is identified by deletions in 9q and mutational signatures linked to the APOBEC protein family [4]. In contrast, MIBCa, accounting for 25% of cases, manifests when tumors infiltrate deeper bladder layers, including the muscular and adventitial layers, and has high metastasis rates [5]. Notably, MIBCa has the third-highest mutation rate among all cancers and is characterized by alterations in genes related to DNA damage repair (DDR) pathways [4].

BC is associated with the highest lifetime cost per patient among all cancers, largely due to its high recurrence rate and the need for continuous surveillance [6]. The standard detection and surveillance method involves cystoscopy and cytology. However, these techniques have their limitations [7], leading recent research to identify new urinary biomarkers for BC detection, many of which are Food and Drug Administration (FDA)-approved; however, none have been incorporated into clinical practice guidelines, nor demonstrated clinical utility [6].

Microsatellite instability analysis (MSA) stands out as a promising candidate for inclusion, which is FDA-approved [8] and has been integrated into the clinical practice guidelines for cancers such as colorectal [9], endometrial [10], and gastric cancer [11], but not for BC. The inclusion of this analysis in clinical guidelines is due to the significant benefit that patients with microsatellite instability (MSI)-positive tumors derive from treatment with pembrolizumab. This monoclonal antibody targets and blocks programmed cell death protein 1 (PD-1), an immune checkpoint expressed on T cells, which plays a key role in regulating the immune response. By interrupting the interaction with its ligand, programmed death-ligand 1 (PD-L1), present in tumor cells, the effector capacity of T cells is reactivated, allowing them to recognize and attack tumor cells [12,13]. Therefore, the main goal of this review is to analyze the evidence supporting the detection of MSI in bladder tumor cells present in urine, in order to support the development of clinical guidelines that standardize its use as a genomic alterations test associated with BC and confirm its clinical relevance.

2. Traditional Techniques for Bladder Cancer Detection

The primary symptom of BC is hematuria. Therefore, a urologist must first rule out any potential external causes. If these results are negative, an imaging test is then ordered, along with a cystoscopy to examine the bladder mucosa for any bladder masses. If bladder masses are identified, a tissue sample is obtained through biopsy, or alternatively, a transurethral resection of the bladder tumor is performed for histopathological confirmation and staging. A method that accompanies cystoscopy is cytology, which involves the cytomorphological analysis of a urine sample to detect tumor cells [14]. This loss of cell adhesion is indicative of a high degree of malignancy [15].

Despite cystoscopy and cytology being standard techniques for BC detection, they have limitations. Cystoscopy is an invasive method with a high cost that brings complications for the patient [7]. These include anxiety prior to the procedure, pain during and after the intervention, and temporary alterations in sexual function, such as a reduced libido in both sexes and erectile dysfunction in men. However, these effects are typically short-lived and tend to disappear within a few weeks after the procedure [16]. On the other hand, cytology is a non-invasive method with a limited sensitivity for detecting high-grade tumors (64%). In addition, it has a low sensitivity for detecting low-grade tumors (12%) [17]. Furthermore, inflammatory conditions of the bladder, such as infections or prior procedures, can significantly influence cytology results. Additionally, the reproducibility of this technique is limited, and its reliability heavily depends on the expertise of the technician interpreting the findings [18]. Due to the need to improve the study of BC, there is a search for new non-invasive technologies for the detection of useful genetic markers for the diagnosis, progression, and selection of treatments for cancer. One promising candidate is liquid biopsy, which includes blood, saliva, and urine tests. Urine is an easy resource to obtain, in which compounds such as nucleic acids, proteins, leukocytes, lymphocytes, epithelial cells, kidney cells, and urothelial cells are found [19]. Because the cells of bladder tumors can exfoliate, urine can harbor bladder tumor cells, which can be isolated for analysis. In addition, urine has low amounts of protein and high amounts of free circulating tumor DNA and RNA, which can be used as target markers for the diagnosis of BC [20]. Therefore, several panels have been proposed using urine samples as their subject of study (Table 1), and some of them have been approved by the FDA.

Table 1. Urinary markers for BC management.

Panel	Principle	Detection Unit	Sensitivity	Specificity	References
		Exfoliated bladder tumor cells			
UroVysion *	FISH	Aneuploidies in chromosomes 3, 7, and 17 and deletions in 9p21	73%	83%	[21,22]
Immunocyt *	F-LMab	Carcinoembryonic antigen and sulfated mucin glycoproteins	60–100%	75–84%	[23]
URO17	IHC	Cytokeratin 17	100%	92.6%	[24]
Cell detect	Immunostaining	Malignant cells	82.8%	88.2%	[25]
		Proteins			
BTA-STAT *	ICA	Proteins associated with human complement factor H	76.7%	67.9%	[26,27]
BTA TRAK *	ELISA	Proteins associated with human complement factor H	58%	73%	[21,28]
NMP22 *	ELISA	NMP22 protein	50–70%	60–80%	[21,29]
UBC Rapid test	ELISA	Cytokeratins 8 and 18	72.2%	79.4%	[24,30]
ADXBLADDER	ELISA	MCM5 protein	75.6%	71.1%	[31]
BLCA-4	ELISA	BLCA-4 protein	93%	97%	[32]
Oncuria™	Multiplex Immunoassay	A1AT, APOE, ANG, CA9, IL8, MMP9, MMP10, PAI1, SDC1, and VEGFA proteins	93%	93%	[33]
		mRNA			
Xpert Bladder Cancer Monitor	RT-PCR	mRNA levels of *CRH*, *IGF2*, *UPK1B*, *ANXA10*, and *ABL1* genes.	75%	77%	[34]
CxBladder	RT-PCR	mRNA levels of *MDK*, *HOXA13*, *CDC2*, *IGFBP5*, and *CXCR2* genes	100%	75%	[35]
		DNA alterations			
UroMuTERT	Sequencing	Mutations in *TERT* promoter	87.1%	94.7%	[36]
Uromonitor-V2®	qPCR	Mutations in *TERT*, *FGFR3*, and *KRAS* genes	93.1%	85.4%	[37]
		DNA methylation			
P3 panel	qMSP	Methylation status of *PCDH17*, *POU4F2*, and *PENK* genes	84%	100%	[39]
Bladder Care	qMSP	Methylation status of TRNA-Cys, *SIM2* and *NKX1-1*	93.5%	92.6%	[40]
EpiCheck	qMSP	Methylation status of 15 loci	68.2%	88%	[41]

Table 1. *Cont.*

Panel	Principle	Detection Unit	Sensitivity	Specificity	References
uCAPP-Seq	Sequencing	DNA alterations in regions from 460 genes	83%	97%	[38]
UroMark	Targeted bisulfite sequencing	Methylation status of 150 loci	96%	97%	[42]

FISH: Fluorescence In Situ Hybridization; F-LMab: Fluorescence-labeled monoclonal antibodies; IHC: Immunohistochemistry: BTA: Bladder tumor antigen; ICA: Immunochromatography; ELISA: Enzyme-Linked Immunosorbent Assay; RT-PCR: Reverse Transcription Polymerase Chain Reaction; qMSP: Quantitative Methylation-Specific Polymerase Chain Reaction; *: FDA approval.

The use of urinary markers has been explored as a non-invasive tool for the management of BC. In recent years, various panels of markers have been developed, some of which are FDA-approved, with multiple clinical purposes, including supporting diagnosis, detecting BC, and identifying alterations in nucleic acids and proteins associated with this neoplasm, monitoring the disease, and evaluating recurrence (Table 1).

Although these panels are highly innovative and enhance the accuracy of BC cell detection, none of them have been included in clinical practice guidelines, and their clinical utility has not been fully demonstrated [6]. Taking advantage of these weaknesses is where MSA can come into play.

3. Microsatellite Instability Development

Microsatellites, also known as short tandem repeats, are tandem sequences of a repetitive unit with a size of one to six base pairs. They are distributed throughout the human genome, with a higher frequency in intronic regions. They represent 3% of the human genome, and most of them are polymorphic [43,44]. Due to the repetitive nature of microsatellites, DNA polymerases lead to replication slippage, causing insertions or deletions (indels) in their sequences. The system responsible for correcting these mismatch mistakes is the Mismatch Repair System (MMR), which is mainly composed of the proteins MLH1, MSH2, MSH6, MSH3, and PMS2 [45].

The repair mechanism, using a deletion in a microsatellite as an example, is carried out according to the following steps (Figure 1).

1. Base mismatch: The DNA polymerase (δ or ε, depending on the DNA strand being polymerized) causes a slippage error in the microsatellite sequence, resulting in a deletion.
2. Mismatch recognition: The MutSα heterodimer (MSH2 and MSH6) or MutSβ heterodimer (MSH2 and MSH3) binds to mismatches in the DNA, depending on the size of the mismatch. MutSα recognizes SNVs and indels of 1 to 2 bp, while MutSβ identifies larger indels. This binding induces a conformational change that allows MutSα/β to move along the DNA.
3. Recruitment of MutLα: MutSα/β facilitates the recruitment of MutLα (MLH1 and PMS2), forming a tetrameric complex along with proliferating cell nuclear antigen (PCNA) and replication factor C (RFC), which binds to the DNA strand.
4. Activation of PMS2: PCNA activates MutLα, enabling PMS2 to exert its endonuclease activity specifically on the nascent strand, creating entry sites for exonuclease 1 (EXO1).
5. DNA excision: EXO1 excises the nascent strand from the mismatch to a gap in the single-stranded DNA, with the help of helicase MCM9, forming a protein complex (MutSα/MutLα/EXO1/MCM9).
6. Resynthesis and ligation: Replication protein A (RPA) protects the single-stranded DNA generated, while polymerase correctly resynthesizes the DNA, and finally, DNA ligase 1 seals the gap [46–51].

However, if any of the proteins that compose this system has deficient activity or is not expressed, especially MLH1, the repair process is deficient. This causes the accumulation of indels in microsatellite sequences, altering their allelic size, resulting in a phenotype known as MSI [41].

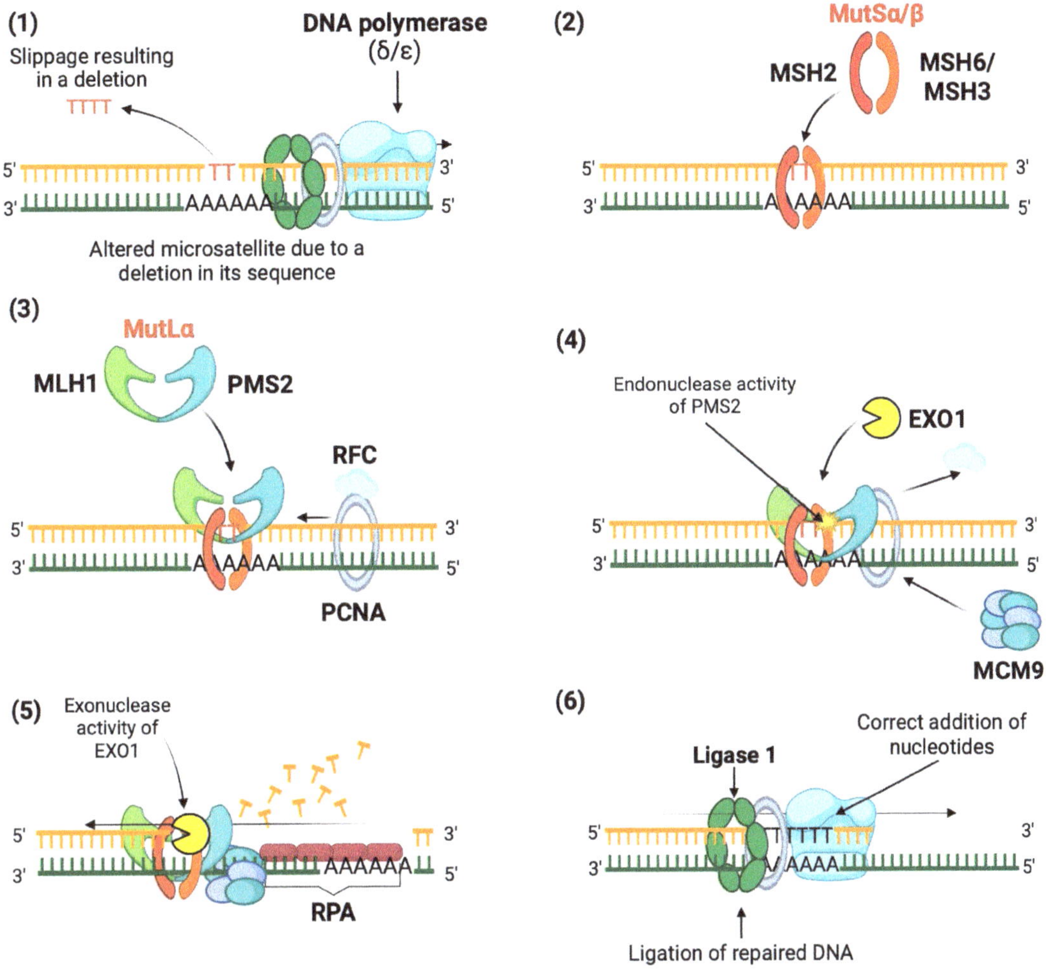

Figure 1. Mechanism of action of the Mismatch Repair System. Mechanism of DNA repair using a microsatellite deletion as an example. (1) A base mismatch occurs due to slippage by DNA polymerase. (2) The mismatch is recognized by MutSα or MutSβ, depending on the size of the indel. (3) MutLα is recruited to form a repair complex with PCNA and RFC. (4) PMS2 is activated to create entry sites for EXO1. (5) EXO1 excises the nascent strand around the mismatch. (6) The gap is resynthesized and sealed by DNA polymerase and DNA ligase 1Created in BioRender.

MSI is classified into the following three categories based on the number of altered loci in the analyzed marker panel: high MSI (MSI-H), when alterations are observed in two or more loci; low MSI (MSI-L), when only one locus shows changes; and microsatellite stability (MSS), when no alterations are detected in any loci [52].

Recent research has demonstrated that patients with MSI-H tumors exhibit a better prognosis in response to immunotherapy compared to those with MSI-L or MSS tumors [53].

This has led to the exploration of specific treatment options for patients with these molecular markers, with pembrolizumab emerging as a leading therapy [8].

A series of trials, collectively known as KEYNOTE studies and sponsored by Merck, the developer of pembrolizumab, have focused on evaluating its efficacy across various cancers characterized by deficiencies in the MMR system (dMMR) and/or MSI-H. Among these, KEYNOTE-016 was one of the first trials to investigate pembrolizumab's impact on MSI-H solid tumors, particularly in colorectal cancer (CRC) [8]. This was followed by a second phase, known as the KEYNOTE-164 trial, which reported an overall survival rate of 33% in MSI-H CRC patients, demonstrating improved outcomes compared to the prior treatments received by the participants [54]. The series culminated in the phase 3 KEYNOTE-177 trial, which compared pembrolizumab to standard chemotherapy in metastatic MSI-H CRC patients, showing a significant improvement in progression-free survival [55]. These trials were instrumental in highlighting the importance of MSI as a marker for predicting response to immunotherapy, which led, in 2017, to FDA approval for the therapeutic use of this monoclonal antibody for oncology patients, both adults and pediatric oncology patients, with solid tumors exhibiting these genetic markers. This was the first time a treatment was approved based on the presence or absence of a single marker [8], and it is now approved in more than 80 countries as a treatment for various types of cancer, including BC [12].

The efficacy of pembrolizumab has also been tested in non-colorectal MSI-H/dMMR-positive cancers. The phase 2 KEYNOTE-158 trial assessed pembrolizumab in 27 different cancer types, with endometrial, gastric, pancreatic, and cholangiocarcinoma cancers being the most frequently studied. The trial reported high response rates and sustained durations of response among patients who benefited from the treatment, further emphasizing pembrolizumab's potential as an effective therapeutic alternative for MSI-H/dMMR cancer patients [56].

4. Role of Microsatellite Instability in Pembrolizumab Response for MSI-H Tumors

The reason why pembrolizumab is effective in patients with MSI-H tumors lies in its inhibition of immune checkpoints (PD-1/PD-L1). MSI-H tumors have a high mutational burden, which leads to the production of tumor-specific neoantigens [8,57]. This triggers a heightened response from antigen-specific cytotoxic T cells. However, prolonged exposure to these antigens causes T cells to enter a state of exhaustion, reducing their cytotoxic capacity and allowing tumor growth. This negative feedback mechanism is driven by inhibitory receptors on T cells that, upon binding to their ligands, limit the effector phase, their clonal expansion, and function, thereby preventing damage to healthy cells [13,58].

PD-1 is an immune checkpoint receptor primarily expressed on activated T cells, B cells, natural killer cells, macrophages, and dendritic cells. It regulates the immune response by preventing the overactivation of T cells, which could otherwise harm healthy tissues. This function is achieved by binding to its ligands, PD-L1, which is expressed in various cell types, including tumor cells, and PD-L2 (programmed death-ligand 2), expressed on immune cells such as dendritic cells and macrophages [13,58].

When PD-1 binds to PD-L1 or PD-L2, it triggers intracellular signaling by phosphorylating its tyrosine inhibitory domain. This phosphorylation recruits the SHP2 phosphatase, which dephosphorylates key proteins involved in T cell activation, primarily the T cell receptor (TCR). This dephosphorylation reduces the activation and effector function of T cells, inhibiting the immune response against tumor cells. Thus, the interaction between PD-1 and its ligands represents a mechanism by which tumors can evade the immune system, allowing them to grow and spread uncontrollably [13,59]. Tumor cells exploit this pathway by overexpressing PD-L1, inhibiting T cell responses, and preventing them from attacking. This phenomenon is accentuated in MSI-H tumors, where T cells are primed to recognize tumor antigens. However, they become inactivated due to PD-1 signaling [13,58].

Pembrolizumab, commercially known as "Keytruda", is a humanized IgG4 Kappa monoclonal antibody targeted against PD-1 on T cells present in tumors, blocking their interaction with PD-L1 on tumor cells. This interrupts the inhibitory signaling pathway and consequently reactivates T cell-mediated immunity, enabling these cells to effectively recognize and attack tumor cells (Figure 2). Therefore, blocking the PD-1/PD-L1 pathway significantly enhances the antitumor response in patients with tumors, promoting tumor regression and improving clinical prognosis. Additionally, the inhibition of the PD-1 pathway can increase cytokine production, further boosting the immune response against tumors [12,13].

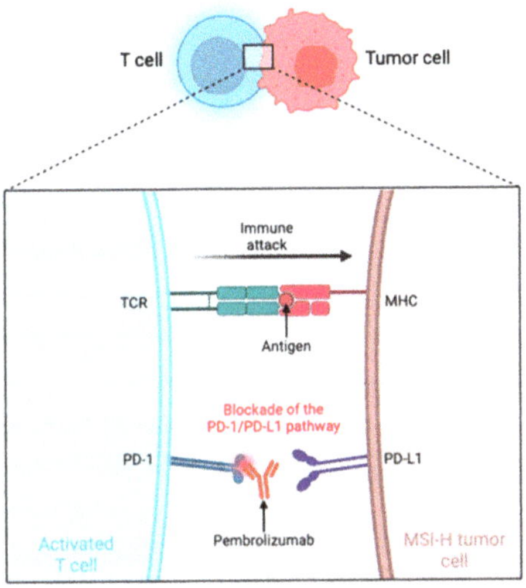

Figure 2. Blockade of PD-1/PD-L1 signaling in tumor immunotherapy. Created in BioRender. TCR: T cell receptor; MHC: Major Histocompatibility Complex; PD-1: Programmed cell death protein 1; PD-L1: Programmed death-ligand 1; MSI-H: High microsatellite instability.

Pembrolizumab has demonstrated a significant efficacy in the treatment of patients with MSI-H CRC, both in early stages [60] and advanced stages [55], offering better overall response and higher progression-free survival rates compared to chemotherapy. Additionally, it reduces the number of severe adverse events [55].

5. Role of Microsatellite Instability in Bladder Cancer Development

MSI is involved in the onset, progression, and prognosis of various types of cancer [53]. It is predominantly represented in CRC, found in 15% of sporadic cases and 90% of hereditary cases [61]. Additionally, it has been evaluated across eighteen types of cancer and detected in fourteen of them, including BC [62].

The finding of MSI in BC is likely to be due to alterations in the DDR pathways, which is a hallmark of BC, especially of the MIBCa subtype [4], involving repair mechanisms such as double-strand breaks (DSBs), homologous recombination, non-homologous end joining, alternative end joining, base excision repair, nucleotide excision repair (NER), and MMR [63]. The pathways with stronger evidence in bladder carcinogenesis are the NER and DSB pathways [64]. While current evidence on the relationship between the MMR pathway and bladder tumorigenesis remains limited, this area presents an opportunity for further research. Recent studies, including those by Fraune et al. (2020) and Mohamedali et al. (2022), highlight that the loss of expression or reduction in the activity of MMR proteins in BC occurs at a very low frequency, underscoring the potential stability of this pathway in the disease [65,66]. On the other hand, research by Catto et al. (2003), Burger et al. (2006), and Vageli et al. (2013) demonstrates higher frequencies of a reduced expression of MMR proteins in bladder tumors [67–69]. Although information about the involvement of the MMR pathway in bladder carcinogenesis is limited, there are additional studies investigating MSI in bladder tumor tissue. These studies report frequencies with a wide range of variation, as shown in Table 2.

Table 2. Reports of MSI frequencies in tumor tissue of patients with BC.

n	MSI Frequency	Analyzed Markers	Reference
44	72.7%	BAT-26, BAT-40, BAX, TGFβ, IGFIIR, MSH3, D2S123, D9S283, D9S1851, and D18S58	[70]
448	1.1%	BAT-25, BAT-26, D2S123, D5S346, D17S250, and MYCL1	[65]
220	39%	ACTBP2, D16S310, D16S476, D18S51, D4S243, D9S162, D9S171, D9S747, FGA, INF-a, MBP, and MJD	[71]
70	65.7%	GSN and D18S51	[72]
84	8%	BAT25, BAT26, D17S250, D2S123, D5S346, BAT40, D10S197, MYC1L, D18S58, D18S69, TGFβR2, BAX, hMSH3, and hMSH6	[67]
117	8.5%	BAT25, BAT26, D2S123, APC, and D17S250	[68]

6. Microsatellite Instability in Urine-Derived Bladder Tumor Cells

Since MSI is a characteristic of tumor cells, and these cells may lose their cell adhesion capacity, it is possible to recover them from the urine sediment of patients with bladder tumors, extract the DNA, and perform MSA (Figure 3) [7,73,74].

The collection, handling, and storage of urine samples are crucial steps in ensuring reliable results for identifying urinary biomarkers, particularly those derived from exfoliated bladder tumor cells (EBTCs) in urine. For optimal collection, samples should come from patients with an active tumor in the bladder. The sample must be placed in a sterile container and should be the first void of the day [73].

As previously noted, urine contains a diverse range of components that can degrade if not processed promptly. Therefore, it is recommended that urine samples be stored at 4 °C and processed within 4 h of collection [73]. To isolate exfoliated urothelial cells, 30 to 50 mL of urine is typically required. The sample should be centrifuged to obtain a pellet, which is then washed with saline solutions. DNA extraction is performed from the cellular pellet following specific protocols, enabling the execution of MSA [73–76].

For better quality control of assays, it has been recommended to filter urine samples using a membrane filter with 8 μm diameter pores. This filter captures urothelial cells, which are typically larger than 20 μm, and removes smaller cells present in the urine [74].

In some cases, urine preservatives may be employed to maintain the composition and integrity of cells and nucleic acids. This is particularly important because microbial growth may occur between sample collection and processing, and preservatives can prevent this. Additionally, preservatives allow the sample to be stored at room temperature [75]. For the long-term storage of urine samples intended for MSA, they can be stored at −80 °C for up to 3 years [76].

Some research groups have performed MSA on EBTCs in urine, reporting variable MSI frequencies (Table 3).

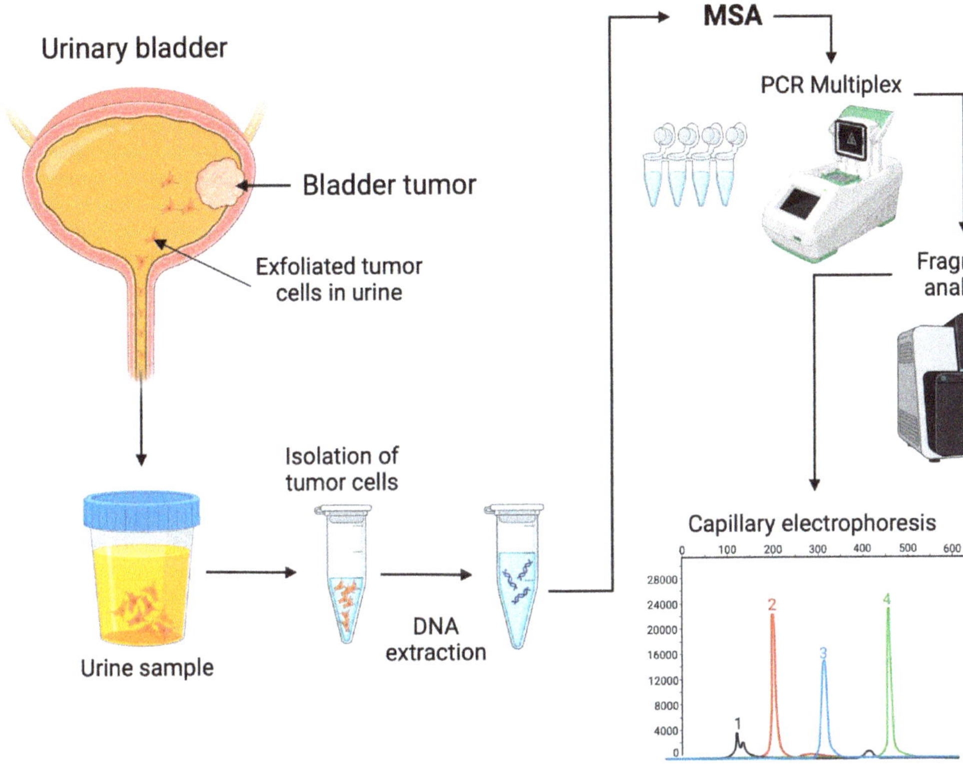

Figure 3. Microsatellite instability analysis in exfoliated bladder tumor cells in urine. In the lower-right corner of the figure is an illustrative image of capillary electrophoresis showing the peaks resulting from the amplification of DNA fragments. The numbered peaks (1, 2, 3, and 4) represent amplified fragments of different sizes detected through capillary analysis. The Y-axis represents relative fluorescence units (RFU), and the X-axis corresponds to base pairs (bp). It should be noted that this figure is purely illustrative and does not represent specific experimental data. Created in BioRender.

Table 3. Reports of MSI frequencies in urine samples of patients with BC.

n	MSI Frequency	Analyzed Markers	Reference
20	95%	ACTBP2, D16S310, FGA, D21S1245, D4S243, D16S476, D9S747, D18S51, MBP, MJD, D9S162, IFNA, and D9S171	[77]
12	83%	D4S243, FGA, ACTBP2, D9S162, D9S171, D9S747, IFNA, MJD52, D16S310, D16S476, D18S51, MBP, and D21S1245	[78]
34	97%	D4S243, FGA, ACTBP2, D8S307, IFNA, D9S162, D9S171, D9S747, D11S488, THO, D13S802, MJD, D16S310, D16S476, D17S695, D17S654, D18S51, MBP, D20S48, and D21S1245	[79]
47	94%	D4S243, FGA, ACTBP2, D9S162, D9S171, D9S747, IFNA, MJD52, D16S310, D16S476, D18S51, MBP, and D21S1245	[80]
150	74%	D9S747, D9S171, D9S162, IFNA, and D4S243	[81]

Table 3. *Cont.*

n	MSI Frequency	Analyzed Markers	Reference
50	76%	D9S63, D9S156, and D9S283	[82]
220	43.5%	ACTBP2, D16S310, D16S476, D18S51, D4S243, D9S162, D9S171, D9S747, FGA, INF-a, MBP, and MJD	[71]

In addition to reporting MSI frequencies in urine samples, some authors mentioned in Table 3 compared MSA with cytology, demonstrating that MSA is more sensitive for detecting BC compared to cytology [77–79,81].

This can be explained by the fact that several patients included in these studies had low-grade tumors and, as previously mentioned, cytology has a low sensitivity for detecting such tumors due to the lower number of tumor cells present in urine [83]. However, this limitation does not apply to MSA, which can detect MSI even when the tumor cell content in the sample is as low as 5–10% [84]. Furthermore, it has been reported that MSA in urine samples has an overall sensitivity ranging from 75% to 96% compared to cytology, whose sensitivity ranges from 13% to 50%. It is important to note that MSA is equally effective in identifying both low- and high-grade tumors [7].

Similarly, comparisons were made between the MSI findings in urine samples and tumor DNA, with concordance reported between the MSI results in both types of samples [72,77]. Moreover, it has been demonstrated that MSA can detect bladder tumor cells in urine sediment and predict recurrence before it is detected by cystoscopy [85].

A wide range of MSI frequencies can be observed in tumor tissue DNA (Table 2), varying from 1.1% to 72.7%, compared to frequencies obtained from urine samples (Table 3), which range from 43.5% and 97%. This disparity may be attributed to the differing sensitivities of the panels used in each study, as each panel is unique. As discussed in the following section, there is a close relationship between the nature of the markers used and their sensitivity for detecting MSI. These variations emphasize the importance of further optimizing MSA in urine samples, which could make them as reliable as tissue samples for MSI detection in BC.

7. Discussion and Conclusions

The detection of MSI in EBTCs from urine samples has emerged as a promising non-invasive method for identifying BC. Traditional diagnostic approaches, such as cystoscopy and cytology, while widely used, present significant limitations. Cystoscopy is an invasive and costly procedure, which can cause discomfort for patients, and cytology, though non-invasive, has a limited sensitivity, particularly in detecting low-grade tumors [7]. These limitations have driven the search for new, more accurate assessment methods.

Urinary markers, including MSI, offer the potential to enhance the detection and monitoring of BC by providing a non-invasive, easily accessible diagnostic tool [7]. MSA has already demonstrated its clinical value in other cancers, such as colorectal, endometrial and gastric cancers, where it has been incorporated into clinical practice guidelines [9–11]. In BC, MSA could serve not only as a disease marker, but also as a guide for personalized treatment.

To ensure accurate MSI detection, it is crucial to use a highly sensitive marker panel. The panels mentioned in Table 3 do not report their sensitivity. However, the markers analyzed vary according to the type of repeat they contain. It is well known that the sensitivity of a marker, as well as its predictive value, decreases as the number of nucleotides in the repeats increases; in other words, they have a polymorphic nature [86,87]. Therefore, an ideal panel for MSA should include non-polymorphic mononucleotide markers, which would ensure more reliable results in the detection of MSI, especially when the goal is to guide specific treatments for cancer patients.

Although several research teams have used multiple markers to analyze MSI in urine samples from patients with BC, to date, there is no validated marker panel due to technical limitations regarding the selection of optimal alleles and the interpretation of results [7]. However, these limitations represent an opportunity for future research to guide the development of an effective marker panel for BC screening, which would benefit patients through these advancements.

There are precedents that may guide the selection of useful markers. MSA panels have been validated in other types of cancer using tumor tissue DNA. However, their results can serve as a foundation to explore their utility in detecting MSI in urine samples.

In 1997, the National Cancer Institute recommended a panel of five markers, which included three dinucleotide markers (D2S123, D5S346, and D17S250) and two mononucleotide markers (BAT-25 and BAT-26). However, this panel had some limitations. The use of dinucleotide markers required comparing the results of MSA in the DNA from tumor tissue and adjacent tissue from each patient to classify MSI [52]. This can be challenging in some types of cancer, where obtaining healthy tissue is difficult. Years later, a new panel for MSA known as the "pentaplex panel" was introduced, consisting of five quasi-monomorphic mononucleotide markers (NR-21, NR-24, NR-27, BAT-26, and BAT-25), proposed by Suraweera et al. (2002) and Buhard et al. (2006). The term "quasi-monomorphic" refers to the fact that the allele sizes of these markers are nearly identical across most populations worldwide. Unlike polymorphic markers, which can introduce biases in analysis due to the variability in the allele sizes among populations, this variation does not indicate MSI, but rather a natural difference in allele size [87,88].

In 2010, Goel et al. evaluated the pentaplex panel and reported a sensitivity of 95.6% for detecting MSI, with a predictive value of 100%. Furthermore, when using this highly sensitive panel, it is not required to compare MSI results with reference DNA. Instead, a range of quasi-monomorphic variation is used to determine the MSI status of each marker. Despite its advantages, the pentaplex panel has not gained widespread acceptance due to a limited understanding of its technical procedure and the lack of reports supporting its validity in laboratories, as well as the fact that its validation has only been tested in CRC. Additionally, it was reported that the markers NR-24 and BAT-25 had a lower predictive power compared to the other three markers. To address this drawback, a triplex panel was proposed with NR-21, NR-27, and BAT-26, which increased the sensitivity of the analysis to 97.4%. However, this panel was unable to detect cases of CRC with deficiencies in MSH6 [52].

To address these limitations, the BAT-52, BAT-59, and BAT-62 markers were added to the pentaplex panel according to Chung et al. (2023), which resulted in an increased sensitivity for detecting MSI in colorectal, endometrial, and gastric cancers [89]. Additionally, Kang et al. (2021) proposed a triplex panel with the CAT-25, BAT-40, and BAT-26 markers, with the advantage that CAT-25 can detect cases of CRC with MSH6 deficiencies, unlike the pentaplex panel. To validate these markers, they used 300 samples from 60 types of cancer, including urothelial cancers such as BC [90]. Therefore, this triplex panel could be a promising option for the detection of MSI in BC.

However, despite the promising data on MSA in urine samples, it is necessary to investigate the identification of highly sensitive and specific markers for effective MSI detection in urine samples, with the aim of establishing a panel for BC screening and, with the necessary validations, integrating it into clinical practice for the management of this neoplasm.

Previously, some KEYNOTE trials were highlighted that validated the efficacy of pembrolizumab across various cancer types. For BC, the phase 2 KEYNOTE-057 clinical trial evaluated the efficacy of pembrolizumab in patients with high-risk NMIBC who were unresponsive to Bacillus Calmette–Guérin (BCG) therapy, as the PD-1 pathway plays a role in BCG resistance. Out of 334 patients screened, 96 met the inclusion criteria and demonstrated a favorable response in terms of antitumor activity. However, 13 patients developed severe treatment-related adverse effects, including arthralgia and hyponatremia [91]. It is important to note that this trial did not include patients with MSI-H, highlighting the need for further investigation of the MSI pathway in BC. Such studies would help validate the use of pembrolizumab not only in tumor tissue DNA, but also in EBTCs in urine, potentially opening up new avenues for more targeted detection, monitoring, and treatment strategies for these patients.

Given this gap in research, there is a clear need for additional large-scale studies to validate the clinical utility of MSI in this context, especially because the use of immunotherapies such as pembrolizumab can bring adverse effects to patients, including impacts in the cutaneous, gastrointestinal, endocrine, neurological, and respiratory systems, among other alterations [13]. Therefore, it is important to select candidate patients based on these genetic markers, as the risks associated with its administration may not justify the benefits in the absence of a significant clinical response.

Such studies would help to determine its effectiveness as a reliable and non-invasive diagnostic tool, as well as its potential role in guiding therapeutic decisions. If successfully validated, the incorporation of MSA as a urine marker in BC detection could improve early diagnosis, reduce the need for invasive procedures, and lead the way for more personalized therapeutic approaches, ultimately improving patient outcomes.

Author Contributions: Conceptualization, J.M.M.-O. and I.A.G.-H.; investigation, M.A.R.-M.; J.A.R.d.A.S. and S.A.B.-O., resources, B.C.-H.; writing—original draft preparation, M.A.R.-M.; writing—review and editing, M.A.R.-M.; M.d.l.L.A.-M. and M.G.-A.; supervision, A.G.-M. All authors have read and agreed to the published version of the manuscript.

Funding: This research received no external funding.

Conflicts of Interest: The authors declare no conflicts of interest.

References

1. Rizzo, A.; Mollica, V.; Cimadamore, A.; Santoni, M.; Scarpelli, M.; Schiavina, R.; Cheng, L.; Lopez-Beltran, A.; Brunocilla, E.; Montironi, R.; et al. TNM staging towards a personalized approach in metastatic urothelial carcinoma: What will the future be like?-a narrative review. *Transl. Androl. Urol.* **2021**, *10*, 1541–1552. [CrossRef] [PubMed]
2. Bray, F.; Laversanne, M.; Sung, H.; Ferlay, J.; Siegel, R.L.; Soerjomataram, I.; Jemal, A. Global cancer statistics 2022: GLOBOCAN estimates of incidence and mortality worldwide for 36 cancers in 185 countries. *CA Cancer J. Clin.* **2024**, *74*, 229–263. [CrossRef] [PubMed]
3. Ferlay, J.; Ervik, M.; Lam, F.; Laversanne, M.; Colombet, M.; Mery, L.; Piñeros, M.; Znaor, A.; Soerjomataram, I.; Bray, F. Global Cancer Observatory: Cancer Today. Lyon, France: International Agency for Research on Cancer. Available online: https://gco.iarc.who.int/today (accessed on 14 September 2024).
4. Fantini, D.; Meeks, J.J. Genomic classification and risk stratification of bladder cancer. *World J. Urol.* **2019**, *37*, 1751–1757. [CrossRef] [PubMed]
5. Dobruch, J.; Oszczudłowski, M. Bladder cancer: Current challenges and future directions. *Medicina* **2021**, *57*, 749. [CrossRef] [PubMed]
6. Soria, F.; Droller, M.J.; Lotan, Y.; Gontero, P.; D'Andrea, D.; Gust, K.M.; Rouprêt, M.; Babjuk, M.; Palou, J.; Shariat, S.F. An up-to-date catalog of available urinary biomarkers for the surveillance of non-muscle invasive bladder cancer. *World J. Urol.* **2018**, *36*, 1981–1995. [CrossRef] [PubMed]
7. Moon, C.; Gordon, M.; Moon, D.; Reynolds, T. Microsatellite instability analysis (MSA) for bladder cancer: Past history and future directions. *Int. J. Mol. Sci.* **2021**, *22*, 12864. [CrossRef]
8. Marcus, L.; Lemery, S.J.; Keegan, P.; Pazdur, R. FDA approval summary: Pembrolizumab for the treatment of microsatellite instability-high solid tumors. *Clin. Cancer Res.* **2019**, *25*, 3753–3758. [CrossRef]
9. Sepulveda, A.R.; Hamilton, S.R.; Allegra, C.J.; Grody, W.; Cushman-Vokoun, A.M.; Funkhouser, W.K.; Kopetz, S.E.; Lieu, C.; Lindor, N.M.; Minsky, B.D.; et al. Molecular biomarkers for the evaluation of colorectal cancer: Guideline from the American Society for Clinical Pathology, College of American Pathologists, Association for Molecular Pathology, and American Society of Clinical Oncology. *J. Mol. Diagn.* **2017**, *19*, 187–225. [CrossRef]
10. Colombo, N.; Creutzberg, C.; Amant, F.; Bosse, T.; González-Martín, A.; Ledermann, J.; Marth, C.; Nout, R.; Querleu, D.; Mirza, M.R.; et al. ESMO-ESGO-ESTRO Endometrial Consensus Conference Working Group. ESMO-ESGO-ESTRO consensus conference on endometrial cancer: Diagnosis, treatment and follow-up. *Ann. Oncol.* **2016**, *27*, 16–41. [CrossRef]
11. Smyth, E.C.; Verheij, M.; Allum, W.; Cunningham, D.; Cervantes, A.; Arnold, D.; ESMO Guidelines Committee. Gastric cancer: ESMO clinical practice guidelines for diagnosis, treatment and follow-up. *Ann. Oncol.* **2016**, *27* (Suppl. S5), v38–v49. [CrossRef] [PubMed]

12. van Vugt, M.J.H.; Stone, J.A.; De Greef, R.H.J.M.M.; Snyder, E.S.; Lipka, L.; Turner, D.C.; Chain, A.; Lala, M.; Li, M.; Robey, S.H.; et al. Immunogenicity of pembrolizumab in patients with advanced tumors. *J. Immunother. Cancer* **2019**, *7*, 212. [CrossRef] [PubMed]
13. Kwok, G.; Yau, T.C.; Chiu, J.W.; Tse, E.; Kwong, Y.L. Pembrolizumab (Keytruda). *Hum. Vaccines Immunother.* **2016**, *12*, 2777–2789. [CrossRef] [PubMed]
14. Busetto, G.M.; Del Giudice, F.; de Cobelli, O.; Carrieri, G.; Porreca, A.; Cimmino, A.; Terracciano, D. Liquid Biopsy Biomarkers in Urine: A Route towards Molecular Diagnosis and Personalized Medicine of Bladder Cancer. *J. Pers. Med.* **2021**, *11*, 237. [CrossRef] [PubMed]
15. Lenis, A.T.; Lec, P.M.; Chamie, K. Bladder cancer: A review. *JAMA* **2020**, *324*, 1980–1991. [CrossRef] [PubMed]
16. Stav, K.; Leibovici, D.; Goren, E.; Livshitz, A.; Siegel, Y.I.; Lindner, A.; Zisman, A. Adverse Effects of Cystoscopy and Its Impact on Patients' Quality of Life and Sexual Performance. *Isr. Med. Assoc. J.* **2004**, *6*, 474–478. [PubMed]
17. Ahmadi, H.; Duddalwar, V.; Daneshmand, S. Diagnosis and Staging of Bladder Cancer. *Hematol. Oncol. Clin. N. Am.* **2021**, *35*, 531–541. [CrossRef]
18. Lee, C.S.; Yoon, C.Y.; Witjes, J.A. The Past, Present and Future of Cystoscopy: The Fusion of Cystoscopy and Novel Imaging Technology. *BJU Int.* **2008**, *102*, 1228–1233. [CrossRef]
19. Chen, D.; Xu, T.; Wang, S.; Chang, H.; Yu, T.; Zhu, Y.; Chen, J. Liquid biopsy applications in the clinic. *Mol. Diagn. Ther.* **2020**, *24*, 125–132. [CrossRef]
20. Crocetto, F.; Barone, B.; Ferro, M.; Busetto, G.M.; La Civita, E.; Buonerba, C.; Di Lorenzo, G.; Terracciano, D.; Schalken, J.A. Liquid biopsy in bladder cancer: State of the art and future perspectives. *Crit. Rev. Oncol. Hematol.* **2022**, *170*, 103577. [CrossRef]
21. Jeong, S.H.; Ku, J.H. Urinary markers for bladder cancer diagnosis and monitoring. *Front. Cell Dev. Biol.* **2022**, *10*, 892067. [CrossRef]
22. Nagai, T.; Naiki, T.; Etani, T.; Iida, K.; Noda, Y.; Shimizu, N.; Isobe, T.; Nozaki, S.; Okamura, T.; Ando, R.; et al. UroVysion fluorescence in situ hybridization in urothelial carcinoma: A narrative review and future perspectives. *Transl. Androl. Urol.* **2021**, *10*, 1908–1917. [CrossRef] [PubMed]
23. Ng, K.; Stenzl, A.; Sharma, A.; Vasdev, N. Urinary biomarkers in bladder cancer: A review of the current landscape and future directions. *Urol. Oncol.* **2021**, *39*, 41–51. [CrossRef] [PubMed]
24. Vasdev, N.; Hampson, A.; Agarwal, S.; Swamy, R.; Chilvers, M.; Hampson, A.; Jahanfard, S.; Kim, N. The role of URO17™ biomarker to enhance diagnosis of urothelial cancer in new hematuria patients—First European data. *BJUI Compass* **2020**, *2*, 46–52. [CrossRef] [PubMed]
25. Shang, D.; Liu, Y.; Xu, X.; Chen, Z.; Wang, D. Diagnostic value comparison of CellDetect, fluorescent in situ hybridization (FISH), and cytology in urothelial carcinoma. *Cancer Cell Int.* **2021**, *21*, 465. [CrossRef]
26. Ecke, T.H.; Meisl, C.J.; Schlomm, T.; Rabien, A.; Labonté, F.; Rong, D.; Hofbauer, S.; Friedersdorff, F.; Sommerfeldt, L.; Gagel, N.; et al. BTA stat®, NMP22® BladderChek®, UBC® Rapid Test, and CancerCheck® UBC® rapid VISUAL as urinary marker for bladder cancer: Final results of a German multicenter study. *Urol. Oncol.* **2023**, *41*, 484.e17–484.e26. [CrossRef]
27. Guo, A.; Wang, X.; Gao, L.; Shi, J.; Sun, C.; Wan, Z. Bladder tumour antigen (BTA stat) test compared to the urine cytology in the diagnosis of bladder cancer: A meta-analysis. *Can. Urol. Assoc. J.* **2014**, *8*, E347–E352. [CrossRef]
28. Malkowicz, S.B. The application of human complement factor H-related protein (BTA TRAK) in monitoring patients with bladder cancer. *Urol. Clin. N. Am.* **2000**, *27*, 63–73. [CrossRef]
29. Wang, J.; Zhao, X.; Jiang, X.L.; Lu, D.; Yuan, Q.; Li, J. Diagnostic performance of nuclear matrix protein 22 and urine cytology for bladder cancer: A meta-analysis. *Diagn. Cytopathol.* **2022**, *50*, 300–312. [CrossRef]
30. Ecke, T.H.; Weiß, S.; Stephan, C.; Hallmann, S.; Barski, D.; Otto, T.; Gerullis, H. UBC® Rapid Test for detection of carcinoma in situ for bladder cancer. *Tumour Biol.* **2017**, *39*, 1010428317701624. [CrossRef]
31. Roupret, M.; Gontero, P.; McCracken, S.R.C.; Dudderidge, T.; Stockley, J.; Kennedy, A.; Rodriguez, O.; Sieverink, C.; Vanié, F.; Allasia, M.; et al. Diagnostic accuracy of MCM5 for the detection of recurrence in nonmuscle invasive bladder cancer follow-up: A blinded, prospective cohort, multicenter European study. *J. Urol.* **2020**, *204*, 685–690. [CrossRef]
32. Cai, Q.; Wu, Y.; Guo, Z.; Gong, R.; Tang, Y.; Yang, K.; Li, X.; Guo, X.; Niu, Y.; Zhao, Y. Urine BLCA-4 exerts potential role in detecting patients with bladder cancers: A pooled analysis of individual studies. *Oncotarget* **2015**, *6*, 37500–37510. [CrossRef] [PubMed]
33. Hirasawa, Y.; Pagano, I.; Chen, R.; Sun, Y.; Dai, Y.; Gupta, A.; Tikhonenkov, S.; Goodison, S.; Rosser, C.J.; Furuya, H. Diagnostic performance of Oncuria™, a urinalysis test for bladder cancer. *J. Transl. Med.* **2021**, *19*, 141. [CrossRef] [PubMed]
34. Sharma, G.; Sharma, A.; Krishna, M.; Devana, S.K.; Singh, S.K. Xpert bladder cancer monitor in surveillance of bladder cancer: Systematic review and meta-analysis. *Urol. Oncol.* **2022**, *40*, 163.e1–163.e9. [CrossRef] [PubMed]
35. Chai, C.A.; Yeoh, W.S.; Rajandram, R.; Aung, K.P.; Ong, T.A.; Kuppusamy, S.; Nazran, A.; Kumaran, K.; Razack, A.H.A.; Teoh, J.Y. Comparing CxBladder to urine cytology as adjunct to cystoscopy in surveillance of non-muscle invasive bladder cancer—A pilot study. *Front. Surg.* **2021**, *8*, 659292. [CrossRef]
36. Avogbe, P.H.; Manel, A.; Vian, E.; Durand, G.; Forey, N.; Voegele, C.; Zvereva, M.; Hosen, M.I.; Meziani, S.; De Tilly, B.; et al. Urinary TERT promoter mutations as non-invasive biomarkers for the comprehensive detection of urothelial cancer. *EBioMedicine* **2019**, *44*, 431–438. [CrossRef]

37. Sieverink, C.A.; Batista, R.P.M.; Prazeres, H.J.M.; Vinagre, J.; Sampaio, C.; Leão, R.R.; Máximo, V.; Witjes, J.A.; Soares, P. Clinical validation of a urine test (Uromonitor-V2®) for the surveillance of non-muscle-invasive bladder cancer patients. *Diagnostics* **2020**, *10*, 745. [CrossRef] [PubMed]
38. Dudley, J.C.; Schroers-Martin, J.; Lazzareschi, D.V.; Shi, W.Y.; Chen, S.B.; Esfahani, M.S.; Trivedi, D.; Chabon, J.J.; Chaudhuri, A.A.; Stehr, H.; et al. Detection and surveillance of bladder cancer using urine tumor DNA. *Cancer Discov.* **2019**, *9*, 500–509. [CrossRef]
39. Fang, Q.; Zhang, X.; Nie, Q.; Hu, J.; Zhou, S.; Wang, C. Improved urine DNA methylation panel for early bladder cancer detection. *BMC Cancer* **2022**, *22*, 237. [CrossRef]
40. Piatti, P.; Chew, Y.C.; Suwoto, M.; Yamada, T.; Jara, B.; Jia, X.Y.; Guo, W.; Ghodoussipour, S.; Daneshmand, S.; Ahmadi, H.; et al. Clinical evaluation of Bladder CARE, a new epigenetic test for bladder cancer detection in urine samples. *Clin. Epigenetics* **2021**, *13*, 84. [CrossRef]
41. Witjes, J.A.; Morote, J.; Cornel, E.B.; Gakis, G.; van Valenberg, F.J.P.; Lozano, F.; Sternberg, I.A.; Willemsen, E.; Hegemann, M.L.; Paitan, Y.; et al. Performance of the Bladder EpiCheck™ methylation test for patients under surveillance for non-muscle-invasive bladder cancer: Results of a multicenter, prospective, blinded clinical trial. *Eur. Urol. Oncol.* **2018**, *1*, 307–313. [CrossRef] [PubMed]
42. Feber, A.; Dhami, P.; Dong, L.; de Winter, P.; Tan, W.S.; Martínez-Fernández, M.; Paul, D.S.; Hynes-Allen, A.; Rezaee, S.; Gurung, P.; et al. UroMark—A urinary biomarker assay for the detection of bladder cancer. *Clin. Epigenetics* **2017**, *9*, 8. [CrossRef]
43. Bagshaw, A.T.M. Functional mechanisms of microsatellite DNA in eukaryotic genomes. *Genome Biol. Evol.* **2017**, *9*, 2428–2443. [CrossRef] [PubMed]
44. Kristmundsdottir, S.; Jonsson, H.; Hardarson, M.T.; Palsson, G.; Beyter, D.; Eggertsson, H.P.; Gylfason, A.; Sveinbjornsson, G.; Holley, G.; Stefansson, O.A.; et al. Sequence variants affecting the genome-wide rate of germline microsatellite mutations. *Nat. Commun.* **2023**, *14*, 3855. [CrossRef] [PubMed]
45. Söreide, K.; Janssen, E.A.M.; Söiland, H.; Körner, H.; Baak, J.P.A. Microsatellite instability in colorectal cancer. *Br. J. Surg.* **2006**, *93*, 395–406. [CrossRef] [PubMed]
46. Tamura, K.; Kaneda, M.; Futagawa, M.; Takeshita, M.; Kim, S.; Nakama, M.; Kawashita, N.; Tatsumi-Miyajima, J. Genetic and genomic basis of the mismatch repair system involved in Lynch syndrome. *Int. J. Clin. Oncol.* **2019**, *24*, 999–1011. [CrossRef] [PubMed]
47. Gupta, D.; Heinen, C.D. The mismatch repair-dependent DNA damage response: Mechanisms and implications. *DNA Repair* **2019**, *78*, 60–69. [CrossRef] [PubMed]
48. Kadyrova, L.Y.; Kadyrov, F.A. Endonuclease activities of MutLα and its homologs in DNA mismatch repair. *DNA Repair* **2016**, *38*, 42–49. [CrossRef] [PubMed]
49. Li, S.; Martin, A. Mismatch repair and colon cancer: Mechanisms and therapies explored. *Trends Mol. Med.* **2016**, *22*, 274–289. [CrossRef]
50. Kunkel, T.A.; Erie, D.A. Eukaryotic mismatch repair in relation to DNA replication. *Annu. Rev. Genet.* **2015**, *49*, 291–313. [CrossRef]
51. Traver, S.; Coulombe, P.; Peiffer, I.; Hutchins, J.R.; Kitzmann, M.; Latreille, D.; Méchali, M. MCM9 is required for mammalian DNA mismatch repair. *Mol. Cell* **2015**, *59*, 831–839. [CrossRef]
52. Goel, A.; Nagasaka, T.; Hamelin, R.; Boland, C.R. An optimized pentaplex PCR for detecting DNA mismatch repair-deficient colorectal cancers. *PLoS ONE* **2010**, *5*, e9393. [CrossRef]
53. Yang, G.; Zheng, R.Y.; Jin, Z.S. Correlations between microsatellite instability and the biological behaviour of tumours. *J. Cancer Res. Clin. Oncol.* **2019**, *145*, 2891–2899. [CrossRef] [PubMed]
54. Le, D.T.; Kim, T.W.; Van Cutsem, E.; Geva, R.; Jäger, D.; Hara, H.; Burge, M.; O'Neil, B.; Kavan, P.; Yoshino, T.; et al. Phase II Open-Label Study of Pembrolizumab in Treatment-Refractory, Microsatellite Instability-High/Mismatch Repair-Deficient Metastatic Colorectal Cancer: KEYNOTE-164. *J. Clin. Oncol.* **2020**, *38*, 11–19. [CrossRef] [PubMed]
55. Diaz, L.A.; Shiu, K.K.; Kim, T.W.; Jensen, B.V.; Jensen, L.H.; Punt, C.; Smith, D.; Garcia-Carbonero, R.; Benavides, M.; Gibbs, P.; et al. KEYNOTE-177 Investigators. Pembrolizumab versus chemotherap for microsatellite instability-high or mismatch repair-deficient metastatic colorectal cancer (KEYNOTE-177): Final analysis of a randomised, open-label, phase 3 study. *Lancet Oncol.* **2022**, *23*, 659–670. [CrossRef] [PubMed]
56. Marabelle, A.; Le, D.T.; Ascierto, P.A.; Di Giacomo, A.M.; De Jesus-Acosta, A.; Delord, J.P.; Geva, R.; Gottfried, M.; Penel, N.; Hansen, A.R.; et al. Efficacy of Pembrolizumab in Patients With Noncolorectal High Microsatellite Instability/Mismatch Repair-Deficient Cancer: Results From the Phase II KEYNOTE-158 Study. *J. Clin. Oncol.* **2020**, *38*, 1–10. [CrossRef] [PubMed]
57. Luchini, C.; Bibeau, F.; Ligtenberg, M.J.L. ESMO recommendations on microsatellite instability testing for immunotherapy in cancer, and its relationship with PD-1/PD-L1 expression and tumour mutational burden: A systematic review-based approach. *Ann. Oncol.* **2019**, *30*, 1232–1243. [CrossRef]
58. Liu, J.; Chen, Z.; Li, Y.; Zhao, W.; Wu, J.; Zhang, Z. PD-1/PD-L1 checkpoint inhibitors in tumor immunotherapy. *Front. Pharmacol.* **2021**, *12*, 731798. [CrossRef]
59. Selvajaran, G. Pembrolizumab: The Nut Cracker. *Indian J. Med. Paediatr. Oncol.* **2020**, *41*, 393–396.
60. André, T.; Cohen, R.; Salem, M.E. Immune checkpoint blockade therapy in patients with colorectal cancer harboring microsatellite instability/mismatch repair deficiency in 2022. *Am. Soc. Clin. Oncol. Educ. Book* **2022**, *42*, 233–241. [CrossRef]
61. De' Angelis, G.L.; Bottarelli, L.; Azzoni, C.; De' Angelis, N.; Leandro, G.; Di Mario, F.; Gaiani, F.; Negri, F. Microsatellite instability in colorectal cancer. *Acta Biomed.* **2018**, *89*, 97–101.

62. Hause, R.J.; Pritchard, C.C.; Shendure, J.; Salipante, S.J. Classification and characterization of microsatellite instability across 18 cancer types. *Nat. Med.* **2016**, *22*, 1342–1350. [CrossRef] [PubMed]
63. Huang, R.; Zhou, P.K. DNA damage repair: Historical perspectives, mechanistic pathways, and clinical translation for targeted cancer therapy. *Signal Transduct. Target. Ther.* **2021**, *6*, 254. [CrossRef] [PubMed]
64. Mouw, K.W. DNA repair pathway alterations in bladder cancer. *Cancers* **2017**, *9*, 28. [CrossRef]
65. Fraune, C.; Simon, R.; Hube-Magg, C.; Makrypidi-Fraune, G.; Kähler, C.; Kluth, M.; Höflmayer, D.; Büscheck, F.; Dum, D.; Luebke, A.M.; et al. MMR deficiency in urothelial carcinoma of the bladder presents with temporal and spatial homogeneity throughout the tumor mass. *Urol. Oncol. Semin. Orig. Investig.* **2020**, *38*, 488–495. [CrossRef] [PubMed]
66. Mohamedali, R.; Adhya, A.K.; Mandal, S.; Mitra, S. Expression of mismatch repair proteins in urothelial carcinoma of the urinary bladder. *Indian J. Cancer* **2022**, *59*, 279–281. [CrossRef]
67. Catto, J.W.F.; Xinarianos, G.; Burton, J.L.; Meuth, M.; Hamdy, F.C. Differential expression of hMLH1 and hMSH2 is related to bladder cancer grade, stage and prognosis but not microsatellite instability. *Int. J. Cancer* **2003**, *105*, 484–490. [CrossRef]
68. Burger, M.; Burger, S.J.; Denzinger, S.; Wild, P.J.; Wieland, W.F.; Blaszyk, H.; Obermann, E.C.; Stoehr, R.; Hartmann, A. Elevated microsatellite instability at selected tetranucleotide repeats does not correlate with clinicopathologic features of bladder cancer. *Eur. Urol.* **2006**, *50*, 770–776. [CrossRef] [PubMed]
69. Vageli, D.P.; Giannopoulos, S.; Doukas, S.G.; Kalaitzis, C.; Giannakopoulos, S.; Giatromanolaki, A.; Koukouli, G.K.; Touloupidis, S. Mismatch repair hMSH2, hMLH1, hMSH6 and hPMS2 mRNA expression profiles in precancerous and cancerous urothelium. *Oncol. Lett.* **2013**, *5*, 283–294. [CrossRef]
70. Vaish, M.; Mandhani, A.; Mittal, R.; Mittal, B. Microsatellite instability as a prognostic marker in bladder tumors: Clinical significance. *BMC Urol.* **2005**, *5*, 2. [CrossRef]
71. Awadalla, A.; Harraz, A.M.; Abol-Enein, H.; Laymon, M.; Ahmed, A.E.; Abdel-Rahim, M.; Zekri, A.-R.N.; Shokeir, A.A. Prognostic influence of microsatellite alterations of muscle-invasive bladder cancer treated with radical cystectomy. *Urol. Oncol. Semin. Orig. Investig.* **2022**, *40*, e9–e64. [CrossRef]
72. Saidi, S.; Popov, Z.; Stavridis, S.; Panov, S. Alterations of microsatellite loci GSN and D18S51 in urinary bladder cancer. *Hippokratia* **2015**, *19*, 200–204. [PubMed]
73. Walz, S.; Pollehne, P.; Geng, R.; Schneider, J.; Maas, M.; Aicher, W.K.; Stenzl, A.; Amend, B.; Harland, N. A protocol for organoids from the urine of bladder cancer patients. *Cells* **2023**, *12*, 2188. [CrossRef] [PubMed]
74. Andersson, E.; Dahmcke, C.M.; Steven, K.; Larsen, L.K.; Guldberg, P. Filtration Device for On-Site Collection, Storage and Shipment of Cells from Urine and Its Application to DNA-Based Detection of Bladder Cancer. *PLoS ONE* **2015**, *10*, e0131889. [CrossRef] [PubMed]
75. Jordaens, S.; Arora, A.; MacDonald, K.W.; Wood, C.; Hendrickx, J.O.; Zwaenepoel, K.; Deben, C.; Tjalma, W.; Pauwels, P.; Beyers, K.; et al. UAS™-A Urine Preservative for Oncology Applications. *Cancers* **2023**, *15*, 3119. [CrossRef]
76. Linn, J.F.; Lango, M.; Halachmi, S.; Schoenberg, M.P.; Sidransky, D. Microsatellite Analysis and Telomerase Activity in Archived Tissue and Urine Samples of Bladder Cancer Patients. *Int. J. Cancer* **1997**, *74*, 625–629. [CrossRef]
77. Mao, L.; Schoenberg, M.P.; Scicchitano, M.; Erozan, Y.S.; Merlo, A.; Schwab, D.; Sidransky, D. Molecular detection of primary bladder cancer by microsatellite analysis. *Science* **1996**, *271*, 659–662. [CrossRef]
78. Mourah, S.; Cussenot, O.; Vimont, V.; Desgrandchamps, F.; Teillac, P.; Cochant-Priollet, B.; Le Duc, A.; Fiet, J.; Soliman, H. Assessment of microsatellite instability in urine in the detection of transitional-cell carcinoma of the bladder. *Int. J. Cancer* **1998**, *79*, 629–633. [CrossRef]
79. Seripa, D.; Parrella, P.; Gallucci, M.; Gravina, C.; Papa, S.; Fortunato, P.; Alcini, A.; Flammia, G.; Lazzari, M.; Fazio, V.M. Sensitive detection of transitional cell carcinoma of the bladder by microsatellite analysis of cells exfoliated in urine. *Int. J. Cancer* **2001**, *95*, 364–369.
80. Amira, N.; Mourah, S.; Rozet, F.; Teillac, P.; Fiet, J.; Aubin, P.; Cortesse, A.; Desgrandchamps, F.; Le Duc, A.; Cussenot, O.; et al. Non-invasive molecular detection of bladder cancer recurrence. *Int. J. Cancer* **2002**, *101*, 293–297. [CrossRef]
81. Molina Burgos, R.; Millán Salvador, J.M.; Oltra Soler, J.S.; Jiménez Cruz, J.F. Microsatellite analysis in exfoliated cells from urine sediment. Utility for bladder cancer detection. Comparative study with urinary cytology. *Actas Urol. Esp.* **2003**, *27*, 618–628. [CrossRef] [PubMed]
82. Wadhwa, N.; Mathew, B.B.; Tandon, S.; Biju, V.G.; Tiwari, A. Assessment of microsatellite instability for screening bladder cancer in a high-risk population. *J. Cancer Res. Ther.* **2018**, *14*, 916–920. [CrossRef] [PubMed]
83. Andersson, E.; Steven, K.; Guldberg, P. Size-based enrichment of exfoliated tumor cells in urine increases the sensitivity for DNA-based detection of bladder cancer. *PLoS ONE* **2014**, *9*, e94023. [CrossRef]
84. Brennetot, C.; Buhard, O.; Jourdan, F.; Flejou, J.F.; Duval, A.; Hamelin, R. Mononucleotide repeats BAT-26 and BAT-25 accurately detect MSI-H tumors and predict tumor content: Implications for population screening. *Int. J. Cancer* **2005**, *113*, 446–450. [CrossRef] [PubMed]
85. Reynolds, T.; Bertsche, K.; Moon, D.; Moon, C. Qualification of the microsatellite instability analysis (MSA) for bladder cancer detection: The technical challenges of concordance analysis. *Int. J. Mol. Sci.* **2023**, *25*, 209. [CrossRef] [PubMed]
86. Haghighi, M.M.; Javadi, G.R.; Parivar, K. Frequent MSI mononucleotide markers for diagnosis of hereditary nonpolyposis colorectal cancer. *Asian Pac. J. Cancer Prev.* **2010**, *11*, 1033–1035. [PubMed]

87. Suraweera, N.; Duval, A.; Reperant, M.; Vaury, C.; Furlan, D.; Leroy, K.; Seruca, R.; Iacopetta, B.; Hamelin, R. Evaluation of tumor microsatellite instability using five quasimonomorphic mononucleotide repeats and pentaplex PCR. *Gastroenterology* **2002**, *123*, 1804–1811. [CrossRef]
88. Buhard, O.; Cattaneo, F.; Wong, Y.F.; Yim, S.F.; Friedman, E.; Flejou, J.F.; Duval, A.; Hamelin, R. Multipopulation analysis of polymorphisms in five mononucleotide repeats used to determine the microsatellite instability status of human tumors. *J. Clin. Oncol.* **2006**, *24*, 241–251. [CrossRef]
89. Chung, Y.; Nam, S.K.; Chang, H.E.; Lee, C.; Kang, G.H.; Lee, H.S.; Park, K.U. Evaluation of an eight marker-panel including long mononucleotide repeat markers to detect microsatellite instability in colorectal, gastric, and endometrial cancers. *BMC Cancer* **2023**, *23*, 1100. [CrossRef]
90. Kang, S.Y.; Kim, K.M. Highly sensitive duplex MSI test and BAT40 germline polymorphism. *APMIS* **2021**, *129*, 607–615. [CrossRef]
91. Balar, A.V.; Kamat, A.M.; Kulkarni, G.S.; Uchio, E.M.; Boormans, J.L.; Roumiguié, M.; Krieger, L.E.M.; Singer, E.A.; Bajorin, D.F.; Grivas, P.; et al. Pembrolizumab monotherapy for the treatment of high-risk non-muscle-invasive bladder cancer unresponsive to BCG (KEYNOTE-057): An open-label, single-arm, multicentre, phase 2 study. *Lancet Oncol.* **2021**, *22*, 919–930. [CrossRef]

biomedicines

MDPI

Case Report

NSD3::NUTM1 Fusion Sarcoma Mimicking Malignant Peripheral Nerve Sheath Tumor with Prolonged Survival

Jing Di [1,*], Ali M. Alhaidary [1], Chi Wang [2,3], Jinge Liu [3], Sainan Wei [1], Joseph Valentino [4] and Therese J. Bocklage [1,*]

1 Department of Pathology & Laboratory Medicine, University of Kentucky, Lexington, KY 40536, USA; ali.alhaidary@uky.edu (A.M.A.); sainan.wei@uky.edu (S.W.)

2 Division of Cancer Biostatistics, Department of Internal Medicine, College of Medicine, University of Kentucky, Lexington, KY 40536, USA; chi.wang@uky.edu

3 Biostatistics and Bioinformatics Shared Resource Facility, Markey Cancer Center, University of Kentucky, Lexington, KY 40536, USA; jinge.liu@uky.edu

4 Head, Neck & Respiratory Clinic, Markey Cancer Center, University of Kentucky, Lexington, KY 40536, USA; joseph.valentino@uky.edu

* Correspondence: jingdi2015@gmail.com (J.D.); therese.bocklage@uky.edu (T.J.B.); Tel.: +1-(505)-506-3351 (T.J.B.)

Abstract: Nuclear Protein in Testis (NUT)-rearranged tumors comprise predominantly NUT carcinoma but also include certain lymphomas, leukemias, skin appendage tumors, and sarcomas. Although histologically diverse, all are genetically identified by oncogenic rearrangement in the NUTM1 gene. Many fusion partners occur, and NSD3 is NUT carcinoma's third most common partner. Herein, we present a case of a 26-year-old man with an *NSD3::NUTM1* fusion sarcoma. The patient presented at the age of 13 months with a scalp nodule. Over the next 24 years, he experienced five local recurrences and ultimately expired of a rapidly progressive recurrence. His treatment included surgical resections, radiation, and various chemotherapies. Deceptively, the clinical presentation and histopathology aligned with a malignant peripheral nerve sheath tumor, a diagnosis rendered at initial resection with concurrence by a national soft tissue tumor expert. The patient's exceptionally long survival could be due to *NSD3* as the fusion partner, aided by the initial small tumor size and young patient age. Thus, this case expands NUT fusion sarcomas' histologic and immunohistochemical profile to include mimicking a malignant peripheral nerve sheath tumor (MPNST). Additionally, it indicates that the *NSD3::NUTM1* fusion can drive sarcoma genesis.

Keywords: malignant peripheral nerve sheath tumor; *NSD3::NUTM1* fusion; RNA sequencing; neurofibroma; NUT sarcoma

1. Introduction

Here, we present a case of a 26-year-old man with a history of a multiply recurrent malignant peripheral nerve sheath tumor (MPNST) whose tumor was found to harbor an oncogenic *NSD3::NUTM1* fusion. NUT fusion tumors comprise a diversity of tumor types that include NUT carcinoma and specific types of lymphomas/leukemias, skin appendage tumors, and sarcomas [1]. Uniting these tumors is an oncogenic *NUTM1* rearrangement with various fusion partners. NUT carcinoma is the most well characterized of the NUT fusion tumors, a poorly differentiated carcinoma considered a subtype of highly aggressive squamous cell carcinoma, previously known as NUT midline carcinoma [2,3]. NUT carcinomas exhibit histologic features of a malignant epithelial tumor, including the expression of epithelial antigens. The most common fusion gene partners in NUT carcinoma are *BRD4*, *BRD3*, and *NSD3*. The *NSD3::NUTM1* fusion has not been previously reported in a sarcoma. Moreover, an *NUTM1* fusion has not been previously reported in a tumor diagnostically consistent with MPNST. *NSD3::NUTM1* fusions in sarcomas and their poorly understood biological implications necessitate a deeper examination of their oncogenic activity and clinical significance [1–4]. Different fusion partners in NUT carcinomas can significantly influence tumor behavior and patient prognoses, underscoring the need for identifying specific fusion types to inform clinical practice and potential therapeutic targets [5].

Our patient's tumor, based on its morphology and immunohistochemistry expression profiling, aligned with a diagnosis of MPNST initially. MPNST is a rare and aggressive soft tissue sarcoma that may arise sporadically, associated with neurofibromatosis type 1, or secondary to radiation [6]. Genetically, MPNSTs are characterized by frequent inactivating mutations in *NF1*, *CDKN2A/2B*, and *PRC2* core components' (*EED* or *SUZ12*) three pathways, resulting in complete loss of function [7,8]. Traditional sarcoma classification, dominated by aggregating clinical findings, histologic features, and the immunohistochemical expression profile, generally enables an accurate diagnosis. However, our patient's case, which fit the traditional classification profile for MPNST but instead harbored an unexpected *NSD3::NUTM1* fusion, provides an example of discordance between histology and genetics. Thus, our case underscores the value of comprehensive genomic profiling in managing sarcomas to identify potential therapeutic targets and appropriately classify tumors.

2. Case Presentation

2.1. Clinical History

A 26-year-old male with a history of MPNST presented with two recurrent scalp and neck masses measuring 4 × 3 cm located in the right occipital scalp and 7 × 5 cm located in the right neck, respectively. The patient's disease course was exceptionally extended (see Table 1 for timeline). He was first diagnosed at age 13 months, presenting with a posterior scalp mass. Over the next 25 years, he experienced five local recurrences. His first recurrence occurred at age six and was managed with surgical resection followed by external beam radiation therapy (EBRT). Subsequent recurrences at ages 12 and 20 were treated similarly with resections and additional EBRT. His participation in the COG D9902 clinical trial offered a period of remission. However, at age 22, imaging revealed a fourth recurrence, leading to wide local re-excision, and included the finding of a plexiform neurofibroma, with the absence of other classic neurofibromatosis signs. At 23, a dull ache in his scalp and a hypermetabolic scalp nodule hinted at yet another recurrence, which was confirmed via fine needle aspiration. Subsequent wide local re-excision revealed a recurrent sarcoma. At 26, during his sixth recurrence, rapid and deep local tumor progression was evident through serial imaging. Complications escalated with the confirmation of leptomeningeal carcinomatosis and skull base metastases via MRI, which corresponded with clinical symptoms of hydrocephalus, hyponatremia, and respiratory challenges. His condition deteriorated, marked by pain, numbness, neck swelling, diplopia, and weakness in his lower extremities. After personal reflection and consultation with family and caregivers, the patient declined additional aggressive therapy and entered hospice care. He died of tumor complications 25 years after his initial presentation at age 13 months.

Table 1. Histologic, immunohistochemical, and genetic findings and treatments.

Tumors	H&E Morphology	Mitosis (Count/mm^2)	Necrosis	Immunohistochemistry	Genetic Tests	Treatment
Initial tumor at 13 months	Not recorded	Not recorded	None	Not recorded	Not performed	Resection
Recurrence #1 at age 6	Not recorded	Not recorded	None	Positive for neurofilament, collagen IV, Leu 7, and vimentin; negative for S-100, EMA CD99, desmin, and keratin	Not performed	Resection and EBRT

Table 1. *Cont.*

Tumors	H&E Morphology	Mitosis (Count/mm^2)	Necrosis	Immunohistochemistry	Genetic Tests	Treatment
Recurrence #2 at age 12	Mix of plump spindled and epithelioid tumor cells in sheets	5	None	Negative for NUT; H3K27me3 weakly patchy positive	Not performed	Resection and EBRT; enrolled in COG D9903
Recurrence #3 at age 20	Mix of plump epithelioid and spindled cells in sheets	4	None	Not performed	Not performed	Resection and XRT 6100 cGy
Recurrence #4 at age 22	Large cells with vesicular nuclei	15	None	Not performed	Not performed	Resection
Recurrence #5 at age 23	Small round cells with patchy rhabdoid cells	12	None	Negative for S-100, SOX10, HMB45, and Melan-A	Negative for *NF1* alterations by Invitae; Whole Genome NGS by CARIS Life Sciences	Resection and expectant management
Recurrence #6 at age 26	Mix of small round blue cells and rhabdoid cells in a myxoid background	13	<50% geographic necrosis	Positive for vimentin; patchy positive for NUT, S-100, and SOX10; INI1 retained; focal positive for neurofilament; patchy positive for H3K27me3	Whole Genome NGS by ORIEN AVATAR	Incomplete resection

2.2. Morphologic and Immunohistochemical Overview of Tumor Recurrences

The initial surgical pathology report describing the patient's tumor at age 13 months was not available. At his first recurrence at age 6, the immunohistochemical analysis showed neurofilament, collagen IV, Leu 7, and vimentin expression, with negative results for S-100, EMA, CD99, desmin, and keratin. At the second recurrence at age 12, the tumor comprised a mixture of plump and spindle epithelial cells, with a mitotic count of 5 per mm^2 (Figure 1A,B). The third recurrence at age 20 revealed a similar mix of predominantly plump epithelial and spindle cells, with a mitotic count of 4 per mm^2.

The patient's fourth recurrence at age 22 featured large cells with vesicular nuclei and an increased mitotic count of 15 per mm^2 (Figure 2A). Additionally, adjacent plexiform neurofibroma-like nerve bundles were observed with intermingled atypical cells (Figure 2B,C). The fifth recurrence at age 23 involved small round cells and patchy rhabdoid cells (Figure 2D), a mitotic count of 12 per mm^2, and a negative expression of S-100, SOX10, HMB45, and Melan-A. Adjacent neurofibroma-like nerve bundles were noted, exhibiting patchy S-100 expression (Figure 2E,F). The sixth recurrence at age 26 revealed a heterogeneous mixture of small round blue cells and rhabdoid cells set in a myxoid background (Figure 2G), with a mitotic count of 13 per mm^2 and less than 50% geographic necrosis. The immunohistochemical analysis was positive for vimentin, focally positive for the neurofilament (Figure 2H), and variably positive for S-100 and SOX10 (Figure 2I,J), with INI1 retained.

2.3. Advanced Immunohistochemical Analysis

Immunohistochemistry for NUT protein and H3K27me3 was performed on formalin-fixed paraffin-embedded tissues from recurrences #2 to #6 at Mayo Clinic Laboratories with interpretation in the UK. The nuclear expression of NUT protein and loss of H3K27me3 were assessed relative to internal controls. The recurrence #2 tumor showed the patchy expression of NUT and patchy loss of H3K27me3 expression (Figure 1C,D). The recurrence #6 tumor showed the expression of H3K27me3 and NUT (Figure 2K,L), demonstrating a complex and evolving immunophenotypic profile.

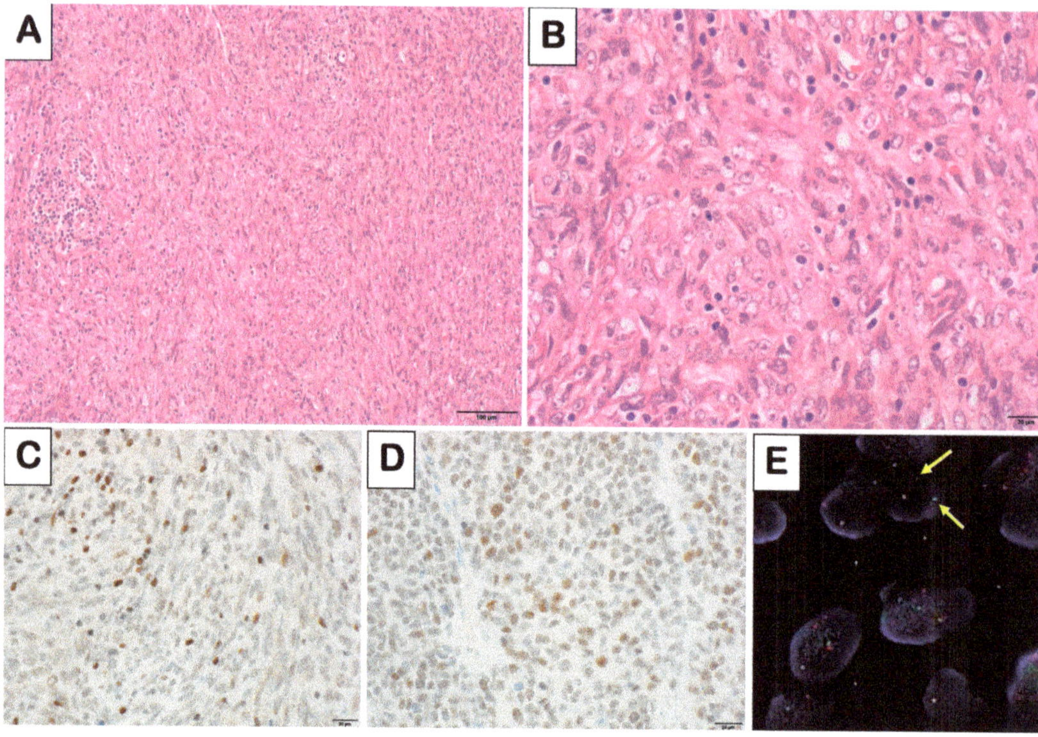

Figure 1. Histological, immunohistochemical, and genetic analyses of the recurrence #2 tumor sample. (**A**,**B**): Hematoxylin and eosin-stained sections displaying epithelioid tumor cells at two magnifications: 200× in panel A and 600× in panel B, highlighting cellular morphology. (**C**): Immunohistochemical staining for H3K27me3 at 600× magnification, showing weak to absent expression in most tumor cells. (**D**): Immunohistochemical staining for NUT protein at 600× magnification, illustrating NUT protein expression in tumor nuclei. (**E**): Fluorescence in situ hybridization (FISH) results at 600× magnification demonstrating the separation of 5′ and 3′ NUTM1 gene probes, with yellow arrows indicative of NUTM1 gene rearrangement in tumor cells.

2.4. Genetic Testing

2.4.1. Karyotype (Performed on Recurrence #6)

In total, 75% of metaphase cells examined showed chromosomal abnormalities with two translocations, t(7;12)(q22; q24.3) and t(8;15)(p11.2; q11.2).

2.4.2. Fluorescence In Situ Hybridization (FISH) (Performed on Recurrences #2, #5, and #6)

To detect the presence of *NUTM1* rearrangement, a break-apart probe set (NUTM1 Break Apart DNA probes; NUTM1BA-20-GROR, Empire Genomics) was used, which targets sequences flanking the NUM1 gene (CHR15: 34343314-34357736). Formalin-fixed paraffin-embedded tissue sections were prepared, and the probes were applied and allowed to hybridize overnight. Post-hybridization washes removed unbound probes, and DAPI was used for counterstaining. Under a fluorescence microscope, the separation of 5′ and 3′ probes indicated a break within the NUTM1 gene. This study scored 40 cells per sample, revealing that approximately 70% of the cells exhibited NUTM1 rearrangement (Figure 1E).

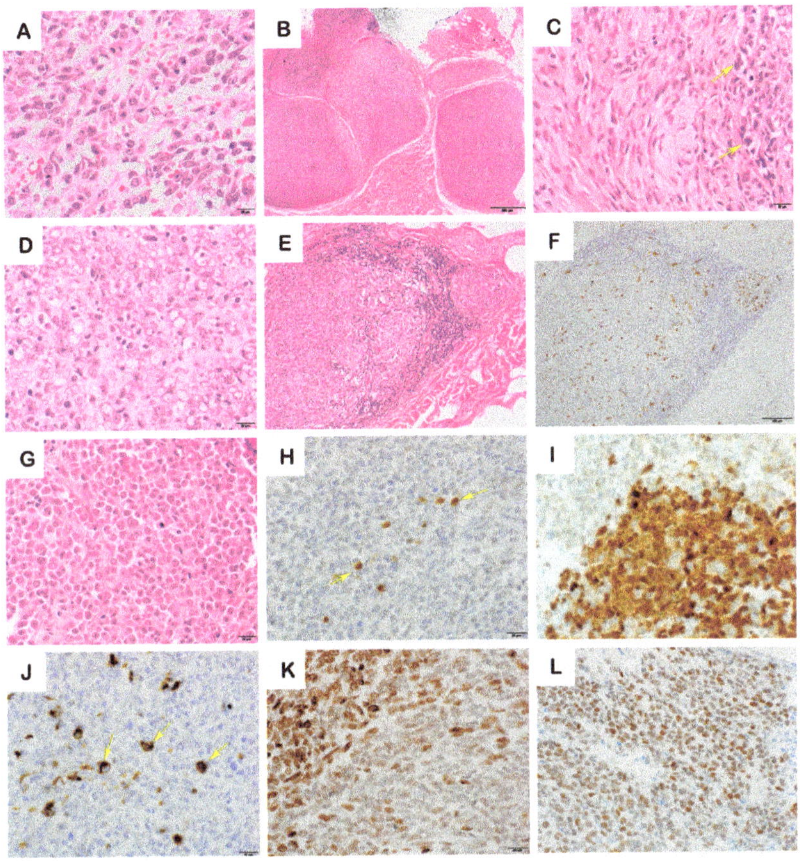

Figure 2. Morphological and immunohistochemical characterization features of the recurrence #4, #5, and #6 tumors with adjacent plexiform neurofibroma-like nerve bundles. (**A–C**): Hematoxylin and eosin-stained sections of the recurrence #4 tumor: (**A**): Display of plump epithelial tumor cells at 600× magnification, emphasizing their dense, eosinophilic cytoplasm. (**B**): The visualization of adjacent nerve bundles, highlighting their structural alignment and density at 100× magnification. (**C**): The depiction of atypical cells within the nerve bundles, noted for their irregular morphology and nuclear features (yellow arrows), at 600× magnification. (**D–F**): Hematoxylin and eosin-stained sections of the recurrence #5 tumor: (**D**): Presentation of plump tumor cells at 600× magnification, similar in appearance to those in recurrence #4. (**E**): Illustration of adjacent neurofibroma-like tumor cells, showing their integration with the nerve bundles at 200× magnification. (**F**): Immunohistochemical staining showing the patchy positive expression of S-100, indicating variable antigen expression across the tumor cells at 200× magnification. (**G–L**): Hematoxylin and eosin- and immunohistochemical-stained sections of the recurrence #6 tumor at 600× magnification—(**G**): Hematoxylin and eosin-stained section, showing the heterogeneous cellular architecture of the tumor. (**H**): Immunohistochemical staining for the neurofilament, focally positive, highlighting the presence of nerve cell markers in tumor cells (yellow arrows). (**I**): Immunohistochemical staining for S-100, partially positive, demonstrating the expression of this neural crest marker in a subset of tumor cells. (**J**): Immunohistochemical staining for SOX-10, focally positive, with yellow arrows indicating the presence of this transcription factor involved in neural crest development. (**K**): Immunohistochemical staining for H3K27me3, showing weak to moderate expression and providing insights into the epigenetic landscape of the tumor. (**L**): Immunohistochemical staining for NUT protein, showing expression consistent with the *NSD3::NUTM1* fusion in the tumor.

2.4.3. Germline Assessment (Performed on Recurrence #5)

Germline assessment was conducted using Invitae genetic testing (Invitae, San Francisco, CA, USA) and was negative for NF1 alterations.

2.4.4. Next-Generation Sequencing (NGS)

RNA-seq analyses were conducted on recurrence #5 and #6 tumor tissues using two NGS platforms (CARIS Life Sciences, Phoenix, AZ, USA, and AVATAR, ORIEN Oncology Research Information Exchange Network, Hudson, FL, USA). An *NSD3::NUTM1* fusion was found at two distinct breakpoints. In the recurrence #5 sample, the fusion occurred at the exon 7 (breakpoint at chromosome 8 position 38318895) and exon 3 (at chromosome 15 position 38318895) splice site. In the recurrence #6 sample, the fusion was identified at the exon 9 (chromosome 8 position 38176413) and exon 3 (chromosome 15 position 34640170) splice site. The transcript IDs corresponding to these findings are NM_017778.2 and NM_175741.2. Unclassified translocations *NT5C2::SNRPD2* and *SOX11::ZKSCAN1* in recurrence #5 and ARHGAP42::CNTN5 in recurrence #6 were identified.

Gene expression was examined with Gene Set Enrichment Analysis (GSEA 4.3.2) software to assess over 2000 differentially expressed genes (DEGs), which were then ranked and visualized (Figure 3). The top 40 DEGs were analyzed, revealing a spectrum of gene upregulation and downregulation differences between the recurrence #5 and #6 tumors (Supplementary Figure S1 and Supplementary Table S1).

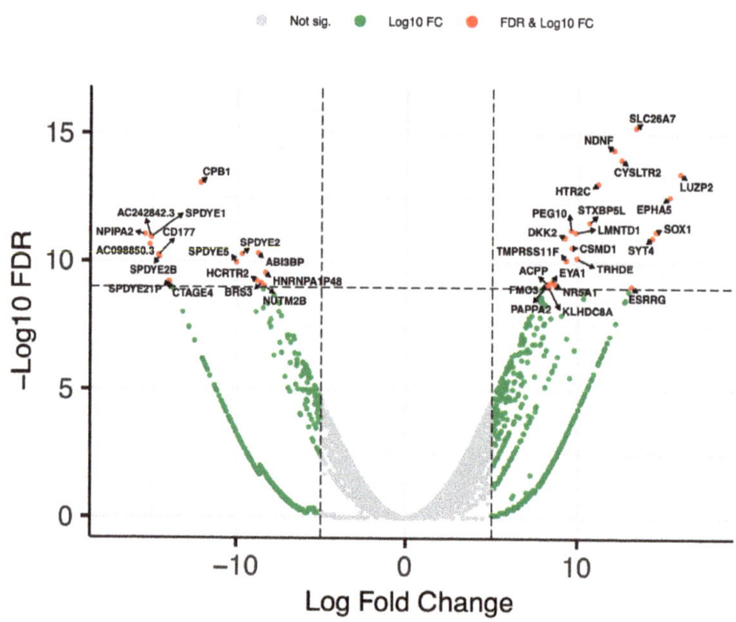

Figure 3. A volcano plot displaying the differential gene expression recurrence #5 and #6 tumor samples, where the x-axis represents log2 fold change and the y-axis indicates −log10 (FDR), highlighting genes significantly upregulated (to the right) and downregulated (to the left) with the top 20 genes marked with the red color and labeled. Total = 18,901 variables.

2.4.5. Methylation Profiling Testing

Genomic DNA was extracted from the recurrence #6 formalin-fixed paraffin-embedded (FFPE) tissue sections. Macro-dissection was performed to enrich tumor content, and DNA was bisulfite-converted and analyzed using the Infinium Methylation EPIC kit on an iScan reader. Tumor classification and molecular profiling were conducted using established classifiers and an in-house pipeline. The integrative diagnosis was determined by combining methylation profiling, next-generation sequencing (NGS) results, histopathology, clinical history, and the relevant literature. The Laboratory of Pathology at NCI developed and performed the tests according to CLIA requirements. The material available was deemed adequate for molecular evaluation, with an estimated 70% fraction of viable lesional cells. Despite using versions 11b6 and 12b6 of the Heidelberg and the NCI/Bethesda classifier, no matching methylation class was identified.

3. Discussion

This novel case of a 26-year-old man with a long-standing diagnosis of MPNST but who exhibited an *NSD3::NUTM1* fusion as early as his second recurrence at age 12 years presents a complex diagnostic and therapeutic challenge. Diagnosing sporadic MPNSTs is challenging due to genetic and immunohistochemical heterogeneity, often necessitating a diagnosis by exclusion [6]. Histologically, the tumors can consist of spindle, mixed spindle and epithelioid, or entirely epithelioid cells, and cellular pleomorphism varies [7]. Some tumors exhibit biphasic differentiation with epithelial components, including well-formed glands [7]. Immunohistochemical antibodies to S-100 and SOX-10 are variably expressed [8]. The patient's first recurrence expressed the neurofilament, Leu 7, and vimentin but lacked S-100 protein, EMA, and keratin. This supported an interpretation of neuronal differentiation and, given the tumor's histologic features and location in soft tissue, was consistent with a diagnosis of MPNST. Moreover, in recurrence # 4 and #5, the tumor displayed features of involvement of a plexiform neurofibroma, a cancer found almost exclusively in patients with neurofibromatosis type 1 [9]. However, there was no clinical evidence of NF1 nor a germline or tumor mutation in the *NF1* gene.

Notably, patchy loss of H3K27me3 expression in #2 and #6 recurrences suggests a perturbance of regular H3K27me3 expression but not to the point of complete loss as is notable in ~80% of MPNSTs [6,7]. Morphologically, the tumors showed consistent features over two decades, comprising sheets and lobules of monotonous, plump, epithelioid cells ± plump spindle cells with abundant eosinophilic cytoplasm. The final recurrences, however, also featured rhabdoid cell morphology, small round epithelioid cells, and a significantly elevated mitotic rate.

The *NSD3::NUTM1* fusion is reported exclusively in NUT carcinoma, an aggressive cancer typically characterized by epithelial differentiation and considered a subtype of squamous cell carcinoma [6,7]. The presence of this specific *NUTM1* fusion in what otherwise met histologic and IHC diagnostic criteria for an MPNST required a re-examination of the MPNST diagnosis and consideration of a diagnosis of either NUT carcinoma (albeit in an unusual location) or a NUT sarcoma with phenotypic peripheral nerve sheath cell differentiation. It is unlikely that the patient had a pre-existing typical MPNST that then underwent random molecular alterations that included a NUT fusion because somatic genetic evidence for MPNST in the patient's tumor is lacking. *NF1* was neither mutated nor lost in cancer, germline sequencing was negative for an *NF1* mutation, and the patient's karyotype lacked complex aneuploidy typical of MPNST. On the sequencing analysis, the patient's recurrence #6 showed a low tumor mutation burden of 2 mut/Mb and a low level of loss of heterozygosity at 1% of tested genomic segments, also atypical for MPNST [6]. Furthermore, the NUT fusion was established by age 12 years (recurrence #2), suggesting that the NUT fusion was present probably at tumor initiation and that additional molecular alterations accruing at recurrence #6 accelerated tumor aggressiveness.

NSD3, a histone lysine methyltransferase from the NSD family, modulates gene expression via histone marks and interacts with BRD4's ET domain in the NSD3::NUTM1 fusion process, critical for the function of the BRD4-NUTM1 oncoprotein and potentially influencing gene transcription in neuroectodermal (NC) cells by regulating H3K36 methylation or macroH2A1 interaction [4,10–12]. The *NSD3::NUTM1* fusion protein is necessary and sufficient for maintaining the undifferentiated state in NC cells [12]. Notably, patients with NUT carcinoma in the head and neck region and who exhibit the *NSD3::NUTM1* fusion tend to have a notably improved prognosis compared to the typical NUT carcinoma median survival of 6.5 months, with a median overall survival of 36.5 months [13]. In an extraordinary case from a recent series, the patient survived for an impressive duration of 14 years post-positive identification of the NUTM1 break-apart in the tumor [14]. Thus, there is precedence for prolonged survival in patients whose NUT fusion tumors harbor *NSD3::NUTM1* fusions.

The gene set enrichment analysis performed on recurrence #5 and #6 showed over 2000 differentially expressed genes (DEGs). Repeated bouts of radiation therapy and chemotherapy could have affected the gene expression and selection of subclones. Notably, four genes involved in neural development or function (*SOX1, NDNF, HTR2C, SYT4*) were significantly overexpressed in recurrence #6 in keeping with persistent aberrant differentiation toward a neural-like phenotype [15]. This patient was not treated with Bromodomain and extra-terminal (BET) inhibitors, which may potentially target NSD3-driven tumorigenesis [16,17]. The number of NSD3 inhibitors available for cancer therapy is currently limited, and no drugs targeting NSD3 are available on the market [4]. Future research should focus on the development of specific inhibitors to target NSD3 fusion proteins in order to improve therapeutic outcomes for patients with such rare sarcomas [16].

The limitations of this study are rooted in its nature as a case report. Whether our findings can be applied to other MPNST cases remains unknown. Possibly, sarcomas that appear compatible with a diagnosis of MPNST but show NUT fusions could be analogous to *CIC::NUTM1* fusion tumors, in which the CIC fusion protein drives the phenotypic and methylation profile of the cancer to align with classic *CIC*-fused sarcomas [18].

In summary, our patient's tumor is the first "MPNST" to show an *NSD3::NUTM1* fusion, expanding the phenotypic profile of NUT fusion sarcomas. The facility of *NUTM1* fusion tumors to develop into multiple different tumor types, with corresponding corroborating histologic features and immunohistochemical profiles, suggests that it is prudent to include a molecular genetic analysis in cases where a sarcoma such as an MPNST exhibits unusual features. Our case also indicates that the *NSD3* fusion partner can drive carcinogenesis and sarcoma genesis, with the resulting tumor phenotype most likely dependent on the originating cell type.

Supplementary Materials: The following supporting information can be downloaded at: https://www.mdpi.com/article/10.3390/biomedicines12081709/s1, Figure S1: The top 40 ranked genes show a range of upregulated and downregulated gene expressions between Recurrence #5 and #6 tumor samples, as indicated by their log FC; Table S1: The top 40 ranked genes' expression changes (listed in the order according to the degree of up- or downregulation) and potential roles in sarcoma pathogenesis.

Author Contributions: J.D. conceptualized and designed the study, conducted pathological analysis, interpreted data, and drafted the manuscript. A.M.A. contributed to data collection, performed clinical assessments, and assisted in manuscript revision. C.W. conducted statistical analysis and biostatistical interpretation, providing critical insights into data interpretation. J.L. assisted with genetic and molecular analysis and contributed to the interpretation of RNA sequencing data. S.W. performed cytogenetics and FISH evaluations and manuscript preparation. J.V. provided clinical insights, supervised the patient's clinical management, and reviewed the manuscript for clinical relevance. T.J.B. supervised the entire project, provided critical revisions of the manuscript, and approved the final version for publication. All authors have read and agreed to the published version of the manuscript.

Funding: This research was supported by the Biospecimen Procurement & Translational Pathology Shared Resource Facility, the Cancer Research Informatics Shared Resource Facility, and the Biostatistics and Bioinformatics Shared Resource Facility of the University of Kentucky Markey Cancer Center, funded by grant P30CA177558 from the National Cancer Institute.

Institutional Review Board Statement: This study was conducted according to the ethical standards of the institutional and national re-search committee, along with the 1964 Helsinki Declaration and its later amendments or compa-rable ethical standards. Approval was waived due to the fact that the patient was deceased prior to the conduct of the research.

Informed Consent Statement: Informed consent was obtained from the participant involved in the study. All patient data were anonymized, and confidentiality was maintained throughout the research.

Data Availability Statement: The datasets generated and analyzed during the current study are available from the corresponding author upon reasonable request. Additional data supporting the findings of this study are included within the article and its Supplementary Materials. All relevant data are contained within the manuscript, and high-resolution data are stored securely by the corresponding research institution and are available under specific conditions to researchers who meet the criteria for confidential data access.

Acknowledgments: The authors thank the ORIEN Network, Connie Haney, for her assistance in pulling blocks and coordinating send-out tests, and Janna Neltner and Kimberly Roberts for their assistance with ob-taining methylation profiling.

Conflicts of Interest: The authors declare that they have no conflicts of interest relevant to the content of this article. No funding was received for conducting this study, and there are no financial or personal relationships with other people or organizations that could inappropriately influence our work.

References

1. Agaimy, A.; Tögel, L.; Stoehr, R.; Meidenbauer, N.; Semrau, S.; Hartmann, A.; Mantsopoulos, K. NSD3-NUTM1-rearranged carcinoma of the median neck/thyroid bed developing after recent thyroidectomy for sclerosing mucoepidermoid carcinoma with eosinophilia: Report of an extraordinary case. *Virchows Arch.* **2021**, *479*, 1095–1099. [CrossRef] [PubMed]
2. Agaimy, A.; Haller, F.; Renner, A.; Niedermeyer, J.; Hartmann, A.; French, C.A. Misleading Germ Cell Phenotype in Pulmonary NUT Carcinoma Harboring the ZNF532-NUTM1 Fusion. *Am. J. Surg. Pathol.* **2022**, *46*, 281–288. [CrossRef] [PubMed]
3. Allison, D.B.; Rueckert, J.; Cornea, V.; Lee, C.Y.; Dueber, J.; Bocklage, T. Thyroid Carcinoma with NSD3::NUTM1 Fusion: A Case with Thyrocyte Differentiation and Colloid Production. *Endocr. Pathol.* **2022**, *33*, 315–326. [CrossRef] [PubMed]
4. French, C.A.; Rahman, S.; Walsh, E.M.; Kühnle, S.; Grayson, A.R.; Lemieux, M.E.; Grunfeld, N.; Rubin, B.P.; Antonescu, C.R.; Zhang, S.; et al. NSD3-NUT fusion oncoprotein in NUT midline carcinoma: Implications for a novel oncogenic mechanism. *Cancer Discov.* **2014**, *4*, 928–941. [CrossRef] [PubMed]
5. French, C. NUT midline carcinoma. *Nat. Rev. Cancer* **2014**, *14*, 149–150. [CrossRef] [PubMed]
6. Somatilaka, B.N.; Sadek, A.; McKay, R.M.; Le, L.Q. Malignant peripheral nerve sheath tumor: Models, biology, and translation. *Oncogene* **2022**, *41*, 2405–2421. [CrossRef] [PubMed]
7. Nielsen, P.; Chi, P. *WHO Classification of Tumours of Soft Tissue and Bone*, 5th ed.; International Agency for Research on Cancer: Lyon, France, 2022.
8. Yao, C.; Zhou, H.; Dong, Y.; Alhaskawi, A.; Hasan Abdullah Ezzi, S.; Wang, Z.; Lai, J.; Goutham Kota, V.; Hasan Abdulla Hasan Abdulla, M.; Lu, H. Malignant Peripheral Nerve Sheath Tumors: Latest Concepts in Disease Pathogenesis and Clinical Management. *Cancers* **2023**, *15*, 1077. [CrossRef] [PubMed]
9. Chen, Z.; Liu, C.; Patel, A.J.; Liao, C.P.; Wang, Y.; Le, L.Q. Cells of origin in the embryonic nerve roots for NF1-associated plexiform neurofibroma. *Cancer Cell* **2014**, *26*, 695–706. [CrossRef] [PubMed]
10. Charlab, R.; Racz, R. The expanding universe of NUTM1 fusions in pediatric cancer. *Clin. Transl. Sci.* **2023**, *16*, 1331–1339. [CrossRef] [PubMed]
11. McEvoy, C.R.; Fox, S.B.; Prall, O.W.J. Emerging entities in NUTM1-rearranged neoplasms. *Genes Chromosomes Cancer* **2020**, *59*, 375–385. [CrossRef] [PubMed]
12. Moreno, V.; Saluja, K.; Pina-Oviedo, S. NUT Carcinoma: Clinicopathologic Features, Molecular Genetics and Epigenetics. *Front. Oncol.* **2022**, *12*, 860830. [CrossRef] [PubMed]
13. Chau, N.G.; Ma, C.; Danga, K.; Al-Sayegh, H.; Nardi, V.; Barrette, R.; Lathan, C.S.; DuBois, S.G.; Haddad, R.I.; Shapiro, G.I.; et al. An Anatomical Site and Genetic-Based Prognostic Model for Patients with Nuclear Protein in Testis (NUT) Midline Carcinoma: Analysis of 124 Patients. *JNCI Cancer Spectr.* **2020**, *4*, pkz094. [CrossRef] [PubMed]
14. Wang, H.; Weiss, V.L.; Hoffman, R.D.; Abel, T.; Ho, R.H.; Borinstein, S.C.; Mannion, K.; Bridge, J.A.; Black, J.; Liang, J. Salivary Gland NUT Carcinoma with Prolonged Survival in Children: Case Illustration and Systematic Review of Literature. *Head Neck Pathol.* **2021**, *15*, 236–243. [CrossRef] [PubMed]
15. Lei, X.X.; Wang, S.L.; Xia, Y.; Yan, M.; He, B.; Wang, B.; Long, Z.J.; Liu, Q. SOX1 acts as a tumor hypnotist rendering nasopharyngeal carcinoma cells refractory to chemotherapy. *Cell Death Discov.* **2023**, *9*, 194. [CrossRef] [PubMed]

16. Liu, Z.; Piao, L.; Zhuang, M.; Qiu, X.; Xu, X.; Zhang, D.; Liu, M.; Ren, D. Silencing of histone methyltransferase NSD3 reduces cell viability in osteosarcoma with induction of apoptosis. *Oncol. Rep.* **2017**, *38*, 2796–2802. [CrossRef] [PubMed]
17. Xiu, S.; Chi, X.; Jia, Z.; Shi, C.; Zhang, X.; Li, Q.; Gao, T.; Zhang, L.; Liu, Z. NSD3: Advances in cancer therapeutic potential and inhibitors research. *Eur. J. Med. Chem.* **2023**, *256*, 115440. [CrossRef] [PubMed]
18. Le Loarer, F.; Laffont, S.; Lesluyes, T.; Tirode, F.; Antonescu, C.; Baglin, A.C.; Delespaul, L.; Soubeyran, I.; Hostein, I.; Pérot, G.; et al. Clinicopathologic and Molecular Features of a Series of 41 Biphenotypic Sinonasal Sarcomas Expanding Their Molecular Spectrum. *Am. J. Surg. Pathol.* **2019**, *43*, 747–754. [CrossRef] [PubMed]

MDPI AG
Grosspeteranlage 5
4052 Basel
Switzerland
Tel.: +41 61 683 77 34

Biomedicines Editorial Office
E-mail: biomedicines@mdpi.com
www.mdpi.com/journal/biomedicines

www.ingramcontent.com/pod-product-compliance
Lightning Source LLC
Chambersburg PA
CBHW061445210926
51850CB00008B/1623